Techniques in Interventional R

Series Editors

Michael J. Lee

Anthony F. Watkinson

For further volumes:
http://www.springer.com/series/8281

Other titles in this Series:

Robert A. Morgan · Eric Walser
Editors

Handbook of Angioplasty and Stenting Procedures

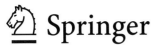 Springer

Series Editors

Michael J. Lee, MD
Professor of Interventional Radiology
Beaumont Hospital and Royal College
  of Surgeons in Ireland
Dublin
Ireland

Anthony F. Watkinson, BSc MSc(Oxon)
  MBBS FRCS FRCR
Professor of Interventional Radiology
The Royal Devon and Exeter Hospital
  and Peninsula Medical School
Exeter
UK

Editors

Robert A. Morgan MB ChB, MRCP, FRCR
St George's Hospital NHS Trust
London
UK

Eric Walser, MD
Mayo Clinic
Jacksonville
Florida
USA

ISBN 978-1-84800-398-9   e-ISBN 978-1-84800-399-6
DOI 10.1007/978-1-84800-399-6
Springer London Dordrecht Heidelberg New York

British Library Cataloguing in Publication Data
A catalogue record for this book is available from the British Library

Library of Congress Control Number: 2009940403

Printed on acid-free paper

Springer is part of Springer Science+Business Media (www.springer.com)

Foreword

Despite the fact that Interventional Radiology is steadily moving toward a clinical specialty with the need for broad medical training, daily craftsmanship will always remain fundamental to what an interventional radiologist does. Without basic catheter and wire skills IR would not be what it is today. When I watch experienced colleagues work I am always surprised to see that, concerning the technique and the materials, we all make the same choices. There is apparently a common IR skill, which is universal and can be learned with experience. I always see this with new IR fellows, that it takes time to step away from improvising and letting the procedure take the lead to logic and standardized control over a procedure. Choosing the right materials for the right job and building a level of confidence with these materials is a very important part of any IR fellowship. Why can a supervisor get a stable catheter position with a new wire in no time, whereas the fellow almost gives up? The difference is knowing your materials for this specific indication and combining routine and standardized operational procedures. Hands-on workshops are always very popular at every IR meeting because one can really learn about basic skills. Lectures with the title "How I do it," can always count on a full audience.

A handbook that describes the technique of performing the various interventional radiology procedures is not available and would be very useful as the amount of IR procedures increases almost everyday. This book will bridge the gap between books on pathology and more organ-specific IR books. This new series of technique-specific books will be primarily of benefit to those in training in general radiology and more specifically for residents and fellows who are training in interventional radiology. Experienced interventional radiologists can also use a book like this. This is a book that should be available in every IR cath lab.

Jim A. Reekers
The Netherlands

Preface from the Series Editors

Interventional radiology treatments now play a major role in many disease processes and continue to mushroom with novel procedures appearing almost on a yearly basis. Indeed, it is becoming more and more difficult to be an expert in all facets of interventional radiology. The interventional trainee and practising interventional radiologist will have to attend meetings and read extensively to keep up to date. There are many IR textbooks which are disease specific, but incorporate interventional radiology techniques. These books are important to understand the natural history, epidemiology, pathophysiology, and diagnosis of disease processes. However, a detailed handbook that is technique based is a useful addition to have in the Cath Lab, the office, or at home where information can be accessed quickly, before or even during a case. With this in mind we have embarked on a series of books which will provide technique-specific information on IR procedures. Initially, technique handbooks on angioplasty and stenting, transcatheter embolization, biopsy, and drainage and ablative techniques will comprise the series. In the future we hope to add books on pediatric and neurointervention.

We have chosen two editors, who are experts in their fields, for each book. One editor is an European and the other is an American so that the knowledge of detailed IR techniques is balanced and representative. We have tried to make the information easy to access using a consistent bullet point format with sections on clinical features, anatomy, tools, patient preparation, technique, aftercare, complications, and key points at the end of each chapter.

These technique-specific books will be of benefit to those residents and fellows who are training in interventional radiology and who may be taking subspeciality certificate examinations in interventional radiology. In addition, these books will be of help to most practicing interventional radiologists in academic or private practice. We hope that these books will be left in the interventional lab where they should also be of benefit to ancillary staff, such as radiology technicians, radiographers, or nurses who are specializing in the care of patients referred to interventional radiology.

We hope that you will use these books extensively and that they will be of help during your working IR career.

Michael J. Lee
Dublin, Ireland
Anthony F. Watkinson
Exeter, UK

Preface from the Editors

In creating this handbook, the first in a new series *Techniques in Interventional Radiology*, we compiled a list of relevant topics and distributed them to world-renowned surgeons and interventional radiologists in Europe and the United States. Their task was simple – rely on your wealth of experience and the best available research and create a document outlining the optimal treatment for vascular disorders. Give us everything you know about, say, venous angioplasty, and then condense it into a list of what *really* matters. We fielded authors' queries as to the length of the text, the number of pictures, and the reference list with the answers *short, few, and fewer* with the objective of providing you with an easily readable, yet powerful handbook of angioplasty and vascular intervention – a presentation of topics that can function as a textbook in the hands of a novice or as a reference in the hands of a seasoned interventionalist.

This work begins with a series of introductory chapters describing the basics of vascular intervention, such as tools, drugs, hemodynamics, vascular access, and closure and then proceeds to treat specific topics using a consistent framework. After reviewing the clinical features and diagnostic evaluation of a particular disorder, the authors describe the indications, contraindications, and preparations for the procedure; the performance of the procedure itself; and finally the expected outcomes and complications.

The editors shared a brief, yet intense storm of interventional experiences on a small island in the ocean many years ago, from which they emerged as lasting friends and frequent collaborators on medical (and not so medical) projects. While we remain separated by continents, we hope that we have used this disadvantage to your benefit by accumulating expert contributors for this handbook from both sides of the Atlantic.

We wish to thank Professors Michael Lee and Anthony Watkinson for their clear purpose and valuable guidance. We also deeply appreciate the assistance of the staff at Springer-Verlag publishing, including Gavin Finney, Melissa Morton, Denise Roland, and Lauren Stoney. Finally, we thank our wives (Jeannie and Caroline)

for their patience and support for the time we spent in discussion and in the editing
process, much of it late at night, in the creation of this handbook.

Robert Morgan
London, UK
Eric Walser
Jacksonville, FL, USA

Contents

Contributors

Efthymia Alexopoulou Second Department of Radiology, Attikon University Hospital, University of Athens, Medical School, Chaidari, Athens, Greece

George Behrens Department of Radiology, Rush University Medical Center, Chicago, IL, USA

Anna-Maria Belli Department of Radiology, St George's Hospital, London, UK

Laurent Bellmann Cardiovascular Radiology, Hospital Européen Georges, Pompidou, Paris, France

Clare L. Bent Department of Interventional Radiology, University Health Network – Toronto General Hospital, Toronto, ON, Canada

Jean-Paul Beregi Department of Cardiovascular Imaging and Intervention, Hôpital Cardiologique – University Hospital of Lille, Lille, France

Haraldur Bjarnason Division of Vascular and Interventional Radiology, Mayo Clinic, Rochester, MN, USA

Elias N. Brountzos Second Department of Radiology, Attikon University Hospital, University of Athens, Medical School, Chaidari, Athens, Greece

Trevor John Cleveland Sheffield Vascular Institute, Sheffield Teaching Hospitals NHSFT, Sheffield, UK

Stephen P. D'Souza Department of Interventional Radiology, Lancashire Teaching Hospitals NHS Foundation Trust, Preston, UK

Hector Ferral Department of Radiology, Rush University Medical Center, Chicago, IL, USA

Guy Fishwick X-Ray Department, University Hospitals Leicester, Leicester Royal Infirmary, Leicester, UK

Robert A. Hieb Department of Vascular and Interventional Radiology, Medical College of Wisconsin, Froedtert Memorial Lutheran Hospital, Milwaukee, WI, USA

Basic Tools Required to Perform Angioplasty and Stenting Procedures

David O. Kessel

Introduction

This chapter deals with selection of basic tools needed to perform angioplasty and stenting procedures. The key to success in angioplasty and stenting as in most interventional procedures is preparation.

Before starting you should ensure that you have

- A clear understanding of the indications and contraindications for the procedure.
- Reviewed the preprocedure imaging to assess lesion location, morphology, and length.
- A plan of campaign, a backup plan, and an exit strategy.
- Considered the likely approach to be used.

Other chapters will detail the requirements in specific cases. Here, we will reflect on the basic principles, which in conjunction with your knowledge and experience, will allow you to select the correct catheters, guidewires, sheaths, guide catheters, balloons, and stents to treat the patient and to manage any emergent problems.

The equipment below (Table 1) can be considered as essential tools for the following steps:

Each type of equipment will be considered in turn. Procedural techniques, contrast, and injection pumps will not be discussed.

Table 1 Essentials tools	
Stage	Equipment
Vascular access	Sheaths and guide catheters
Crossing the lesion	Catheters and guidewires
Angiography	Catheters, contrast, and injector
Treating the lesion	Angioplasty balloons and stents
Managing complications	Mainly stents and stent grafts
Puncture site	Closure device; not routinely indicated

R.A. Morgan, E. Walser (eds.), *Handbook of Angioplasty and Stenting Procedures*, Techniques in Interventional Radiology, DOI 10.1007/978-1-84800-399-6_1, © Springer-Verlag London Limited 2010

Sheaths and Guide Catheters

A vascular sheath is advisable for all but the simplest angiographic procedure, especially if there will be catheter and wire exchanges.

A guide catheter is simply a catheter with a large lumen. This allows other catheters and devices to be deployed through it and "guided" to their target.

There are three principal differences between a long sheath and a guide catheter:

- Sizing: Remember that for a vascular sheath, the French size refers to the circumference of the inner lumen as opposed to a catheter, where the French size is the outer circumference. In other words, a 6F sheath will accommodate a 6F catheter but not vice versa.
- A long sheath comes with an introducer, allowing direct placement into a vessel. A guide catheter does not have an introducer and so is inserted through an appropriately sized sheath.
- A sheath has a hemostatic valve, which will accommodate devices up to the French size of the sheath. To prevent bleeding around the guidewire, a guide catheter needs to be fitted either with a removable hemostatic valve or a Tuohy-Borst adapter. In either case make sure that any device you plan to insert will pass through the catheter and valve!

The most important factors when deciding what to use are

- What is the largest device that will be needed during the procedure?
This determines the size of the sheath.

  - The simplest strategy is to start with a sheath that will accommodate the largest device that you are likely to require. This means that you will not need to spend time making sheath exchanges while you are in a precarious position. The disadvantage of this strategy is that you will be left with the biggest puncture site hole, even if you are unsuccessful.
  - Alternatively, if there is a significant chance that the procedure will not be technically possible, consider starting with a smaller sheath until you have traversed the lesion. At this point a larger sheath can be inserted which can accommodate the device to be used, taking care not to lose access across the lesion.

- Will additional stability be helpful?

  - If so, consider using a long sheath or guide catheter, which can be positioned close to the target lesion.
  - This effectively shortens the working distance from the operator, e.g., when working with monorail systems over 0.014" guidewires.

- How far is it to the target lesion?

  - This determines the length of the sheath/guide catheter.

- o If the sheath is purely to allow vascular access and catheter exchange, a conventional short sheath will suffice.
- o When the sheath is also used to provide support to the working catheter and guidewire, it must be long enough to reach from the point of access to the target lesion.
- o It is self-evident that your catheters and guidewires must be long enough to pass through the sheath/guide catheter. While it is obvious that a 65 cm catheter will be too short in a 90 cm sheath, it is less evident that the lengths on the packaging can be misleading. For example, some 100 cm catheters will barely reach the tip of a 90 cm guide catheter.
- o The time to experiment with this is before starting the case! If there is any doubt, check the lengths before starting the case.

- What shape to use?

  - o Guide catheters can be obtained in a variety of shapes.
  - o Some long sheaths have an angled tip like a multipurpose catheter. The shape allows a combination of steering as well as support.
  - o Choose the optimal shape as you would any catheter by assessing the angle of the target vessel from its parent artery.
  - o In general, simple shapes are easier to use and are usually just as effective.

Angiographic Catheters

Catheters are needed for two tasks:

- Diagnostic angiography:

  - o In many cases, the anatomy will have been defined by the preprocedural imaging. If there are unanswered questions, formal angiography will be required. This is best performed with a catheter with multiple side holes.
  - o When choosing the catheter consider the flow rate necessary and bear in mind that the catheter lumen diameter and length will affect this so that a 4F pigtail catheter suitable for a distal aortic run might not give sufficient flow for an arch aortogram.

- Traversing the lesion:
  A catheter and a guidewire combination is used to traverse a lesion. The techniques for doing this are discussed in subsequent chapters. Simple principles and personal preferences should influence selection. Follow these basic rules:

  1. Select a catheter that points in the general direction you wish to travel. For example, if you want to cross the aortic bifurcation, you need at least the curvature of a cobra catheter but may find it easier with a renal double curve

       catheter or even a true reverse facing catheter such as a shepherd's hook shape (Sidewinder/Simmons/Sos).

2.   Select a catheter that affords enough torque and trackability. The catheter performance will be affected by its size and construction. Stiffer catheters have greater torque control, but tend to be more reluctant to track around curves. In general, a mid-range catheter is the best option. Hydrophilic catheters offer little support. Highly braided catheters, while having excellent torque control, tend to be rather "all or nothing" in their response.

3.   Select the smallest suitable catheter that will do the job effectively. In practice, there is little that cannot be managed with the appropriate modern 4F catheter.

4.   Select a long enough catheter to reach your target, taking into account any sheath or guide catheter.

5.   Use a catheter that fits snugly on the guidewire. Trying to advance a catheter with a 0.038" lumen over a 0.035" or 0.018" wire may lead to frustration, as the catheter will tend to snag on any stenosis it encounters.

6.   Keep it simple. Choose the access point and the catheter, which maximizes the chance of succeeding. This is usually the most obvious straightforward route.

Guidewires

Think of wires in terms of steerability, tip length, support, and coating.

- Steerability: Just about any wire can be pointed in the correct direction using a catheter, but not all wires allow additional steering. For example, neither J-wires nor straight-tip wires are steerable. To be steered, a wire must have an angled tip and sufficient torquability to allow rotation of the shaft to transmit to the wire tip.
- Tip length: All guidewires have a variable length flexible tip. This is usually 2–4 cm long. Wires designed for use where there is limited access will have 1 cm flexible tips. Other wires have very long flexible tips and are intended to be very atraumatic; the corollary of this is that the wire will only be stable when it is deeply engaged in the target vessel.
- Support: The support afforded by a guidewire varies considerably and depends on the wire diameter and its construction. The commonest guidewire sizes are 0.035", 0.018", and 0.014", but other sizes such as 0.038" and 0.021" wires also exist. In general, thinner wires are less supportive than their thicker counterparts. It is essential to use a wire, which will pass through your catheter (see the Table 2 below).

Table 2 Catheter and wire compatibility

Device	Typical guidewire	Comments
Conventional 4F catheter	0.035"	Some take 0.038" wire or microcatheter
3F catheter, low profile over the wire angioplasty balloon	0.018"	Some 0.018" wires are surprisingly supportive
Microcatheter or low-profile monorail balloon/stent	0.014"	Will need guiding catheter or long sheath

The construction of the wire will markedly affect how supportive it is. You can gauge this by seeing what length of wire can be held out horizontally. Very stiff wires are intended to be used for support and not for negotiating through a vessel. To advance a stiff wire into place, a catheter must first be guided to the site using a conventional wire. The wire is subsequently exchanged for the stiff wire. Take care while doing this, as the stiff wire will have a propensity to dislodge the catheter.

- Coating: Hydrophilic wires have a coating, which is designed to be slippery when it is wet. Never pass a hydrophilic wire through a puncture needle as the coating may be stripped off and may embolize into the distal circulation. A pin vice is indispensable for gripping and turning a hydrophilic wire. As hydrophilic wires dry, they tend to become sticky and can readily stick to the operator's gloves or a gauze swab. This is a common cause for losing position.

Selecting the right wire: Once again it is a case of each to his own, but these simple considerations may help you choose:

1. Several different wires may be needed during the course of a procedure.
2. Steerable hydrophilic wires are excellent for manipulating across stenoses and into branch vessels. They are mandatory for subintimal angioplasty.
3. Straight-tipped wires in conjunction with a steerable catheter are helpful for gently probing occlusions to try to identify the true lumen.
4. Supportive wires are extremely useful once a position has been obtained.
5. Regarding guidewire length, make sure that the guidewire is long enough to reach the target and to enable catheter exchanges. This sounds trivial and obvious, but is a guaranteed source of frustration and is a potential complication if it is not taken into account. Remember the following formula to allow catheter exchange:

Guidewire length $\geq$ total length in the body + length outside the body in the sheath or guide catheter + length of any over the wire catheter to be used.

As a rule of thumb, 180-cm long wires will enable the exchange of most standard angiographic catheters within the abdomen. Longer wires should be considered when working in the aortic arch vessels or with long guide catheters/sheaths.

6. Regarding wire diameter, as previously stated, it may be necessary to use several wires during a procedure. Use the right wire for each stage, but plan ahead and keep the number of wire exchanges to a minimum, as these will predispose to losing access.

Treating the Lesion

The aim of angioplasty is to increase the vessel lumen by stretching the wall and tearing the lining, the mechanism for this is discussed in Chapter "General Principles of Angioplasty and Stenting".

Angioplasty Balloons

There are hundreds of different angioplasty balloons available. They all have three things in common:

- A balloon near the end
- A channel for inflating and deflating the balloon
- A channel for the guidewire

Most of the time, a simple workhorse balloon will suffice, but in some circumstances a thoroughbred with special features is necessary.

Balloons can be made of different materials. This can affect the profile, but otherwise is of little practical interest. In most cases, the factors that influence choice are listed in Table 3.

Special Purpose Balloons

- *High-pressure balloons:* Some stenoses particularly associated with dialysis fistulae can be very resistant to balloon dilatation. There are special balloons with very high-rated burst pressures to use in these circumstances. Unfortunately, these normally have higher profiles.
- *Cutting balloons:* These provide an alternative to high-pressure balloons. There are "atherotomes" (tiny blades measuring 0.127 mm in depth) attached to the balloon. When the balloon is inflated the blades make tiny incisions in the vessel lining allowing the vessel to be dilated. Cutting balloons have a low burst pressure, which should not be exceeded.
- *Rapid exchange balloons (monorail):* Conventional angioplasty balloons are constructed with guidewire channels running the length of the catheter and supporting the entire catheter. Rapid exchange balloons typically use 0.014"

Table 3 Properties of angioplasty balloons

Characteristic	Comment
Balloon diameter	This should correspond to the diameter + approximately 10% of the artery adjacent to the site to be treated
Balloon length	The length of vessel that can be dilated with single balloon inflation. Typically the balloon is 2–10 cm long. It is normally recommended to use the shortest balloon, which will cover the lesion. This is because angioplasty of normal artery has the potential to cause neointimal hyperplasia. In practice, this is unlikely unless the vessel is markedly over-dilated. In practice, short balloons have a tendency to migrate out of position as they are inflated. This can also damage the adjacent vessel, so there is a trade-off between length and positional stability
Catheter shaft length	Make sure that the working length of the catheter is sufficient to reach the target
French size	Note that this relates to the sheath size required to insert/remove the balloon. It is not the shaft size of the balloon catheter, which is often much less!
Wire diameter	Varies from 0.014 to 0.038 inch
Speed of inflate deflate	This is determined by the strength/viscosity of contrast used to inflate the balloon and the diameter of the inflation/deflation channel of the balloon
Nominal pressure	The pressure at which the balloon reaches its rated diameter
Burst pressures	The *rated burst pressure** is the highest pressure to which a balloon can be inflated with almost no chance of bursting. The *burst pressure* is the average pressure required to rupture a balloon and is usually several atmospheres higher than the rated burst pressure
Balloon compliance	The degree by which the balloon stretches between the nominal and rated burst pressure. Most angioplasty balloons are of low compliance and the diameter will increase by about 10% over this pressure range

*Maximum pressure to which balloons may be inflated without bursting with 99.9% confidence 95% of the time.

guidewires. The wire only runs in the distal portion of the catheter leaving most of the shaft unsupported. The result is a low-profile system, which allows a much shorter guidewire to be used. This in turn makes control of the catheter and wire much easier. The term rapid exchange refers to the fact that when the balloon is removed the wire is held at the sheath hub, the catheter can be rapidly pulled back until the exit point of the wire channel is reached. The balloon is then handled exactly like a conventional catheter. The disadvantage of monorail systems is that they must be used with a guiding catheter, as there is minimal support from the guidewire. Rapid exchange balloons are typically used in interventional cardiology and also during carotid stenting procedures.

Modified Balloons

Several variations on the theme of angioplasty balloons have been developed to try to improve the outcomes of angioplasty and also to increase the range of possible therapies. These are largely experimental:

Drug delivery: This can be achieved in several ways:

- Drugs can be coated onto the surface of balloons. Drug transfer to the vessel wall is facilitated by pressure, heat, or laser light.
- Balloons can be manufactured with multiple tiny pores. This enables topical drug delivery.

Energy delivery:

- Laser: Balloon catheters can be used to transmit laser light to a focal area. This can either be used to cause heating of the tissues or in conjunction with enhancers in photodynamic therapy.
- Heat transfer: Balloons can be used to conduct heat into or out of tissue, for example, cooling in cryoplasty.

Vascular Stents and Stent Grafts

Stents

Bare metal stents are simply mechanical scaffolds, which can be placed within blood vessels (and other tubular structures). They are used as an adjunct to angioplasty to

- Manage vascular recoil following angioplasty.
- Manage arterial dissection.
- Prevent distal embolization when treating iliac occlusions.

Additional uses of stents include

- Managing emboli.
- Drug delivery.
- Radiation delivery.

Vascular stents have certain desirable properties:

- High expansion ratios: so that they can be introduced through small holes and expanded to relatively large diameters.
- Visibility: so that they can be seen during deployment. Visibility is either related to the intrinsic radio-opacity of the stent material or the presence of additional markers.
- Radial strength: once expanded, the stent must resist compression to an appropriate degree. There is a considerable variation in radial strengths between different stents.
- Flexibility: to ensure that the stent conforms to any vessel tortuosity
- Ease of deployment: allowing simple precise placement.
- Long-term patency.

Vascular stents are available in two main variants:

- *Balloon expandable*: These stents are mounted onto an angioplasty balloon. They are deployed by balloon dilatation. The same stent can usually safely be expanded to a range of final diameters depending on the balloon on which it is mounted:
  - Balloon-expandable stents tend to have high radial strength, but relatively limited flexibility. That is to say they tend to maintain their expanded diameter but cannot readily be deployed over bifurcations or in tortuous vessels.
  - Balloon-mounted stents can be crushed and should not be used in locations where they may be compressed by external forces, such as over joints and the carotid artery.
  - The majority of balloon-expandable stents purchased are already mounted. Some stents are not premounted at the factory and have to be fixed or crimped to the balloon by hand. These stents are less stable compared with the premounted variety, and there is a risk of dislodgement during the insertion procedure.

- *Self-expanding*: These stents have a spring-like tendency to expand to reach their nominal diameter. There are many different types of stent construction, each with particular advantages and disadvantages.
  - In general, self-expanding stents have the advantage of flexibility but less radial force. It is invariably necessary either to pre- or postdilate the lesion to allow the stent to expand.
  - Self-expanding stents can be delivered over the aortic bifurcation and will conform to tortuous vessels.
  - Self-expanding stents will tend to re-expand if they are crushed. However, they are generally avoided at sites where they will be subject to repeated flexion due to the risk of stent fracture.

Table 4 Stent properties

Parameter	Balloon Expandable	Self Expanding
Radial strength	+++	Highly variable
	Remember that the mechanism of expansion is not the sole determinant here. There are some very strong self expanding stents but this is usually at the expense of flexibility.	
Flexibility	Limited	+++
	Remember that a flexible stent is only as good as the delivery catheter on which it is mounted.	
Delivery catheter	Relatively rigid	Variable – many are very flexible but very tight curves will challenge any device.
Ability to conform to different diameters	Limited	+++
	Most operators will choose a self expanding stent when there is a significant discrepancy in the target vessel sizes e.g. common/external iliacartery, SVC stenting. Balloon expandable stents can be tailored by modelling with different diameter balloons.	
Precision of deployment	Tends to be accurate but has the same tendency to migrate as a short balloon.	Variable – most are very accurate. Some stents (e.g. Wallstents). shorten during deployment making length difficult to predict
	Remember that the real limitations to precise stent deployment are: positioning angiogram, patient co-operation and operator skill rather than the device.	
Delivery catheter	Relatively rigid	Variable – many are very flexible
	Remember very tight curves will challenge any device. Even if the delivery catheter will reach the target it may not function properly if kinked.	
Range of diameters	Excellent	Smallest usually 5 mm
	With large stents the choice is more likely to be influenced by other factors such as radial strength and size of delivery catheter.	
Range of lengths	Limited	Excellent some up to 20 cm
	When you need to overlap stents make sure that you have at least a centimetre of coverage	

Almost all self-expanding stents conform to one of the following designs:

- Nitinol cells — the vast majority of stents are made of nitinol alloy, a metal with "thermal memory". Various open- and closed-cell configurations exist, which affect radial strength, flexibility, and the ability to "trap" material against the vessel wall.
- Braided steel fibres, e.g., Wallstent — one of the earliest stents with a braided structure akin to the braiding in a hosepipe. Strength and shortening relate to the number of braids and the braiding angle.
- Stainless steel Z type, e.g., Gianturco stent — this design is now confined to stent grafts.

The vast majority of self-expanding stents or stent grafts are held compressed and constrained by a sheath. They are deployed by retracting the outer sheath. A few stent grafts are constrained by a thin fabric covering, which is opened by pulling a "rip cord". It is impossible to detail all the variations on the theme of deployment as each manufacturer has their own theme. The best approach is to ask the sales representative to show you how their device works.

Choosing between self-expanding and balloon-expanding stents.

Table 4 will give you some suggestions. Suffice it to say that there is no perfect device in the market, and not a great deal to choose between most of the products. Importantly, there is almost complete absence of patency data on the various stents available.

Stent Grafts

These are simply stents covered with a graft material. They are used to manage emergencies such as arterial rupture and also the exclusion of aneurysms.

Covered stents are also available in balloon-expandable and self-expanding varieties. The fabric covering means that they have a significantly higher profile than a bare stent, so they must be used with correspondingly larger sheaths.

Summary

There is a vast and potential bewildering array of equipment available for angioplasty and stenting. Understanding the basic principles of your intended procedure and following some simple algorithms will help you select the optimal equipment and approach.

Arterial Pressure Measurements

Thomas B. Kinney

Angiographic Assessment of Peripheral Vascular Disease

1. Detection of peripheral vascular disease (PVD)

   - History
   - Physical examination
   - Non-invasive vascular laboratory findings.

2. Angiography is relegated for patients with diagnostic uncertainty and when candidates are considered for surgical or transcatheter revascularization.
3. Angiography provides a highly detailed view of the location and morphology of peripheral vascular disease. Both the distribution of disease along with assessment of severity is included.
4. Angiography also provides an excellent assessment of the visceral arteries and the inflow and outflow arteries surrounding vascular stenoses or occlusions.
5. Despite the detailed depiction of vascular disease, catheter angiography has several inherent limitations, primarily because angiography may underestimate the functional or hemodynamic significance of individual lesion(s).

   - Significant stenoses of the iliac arteries are often missed on angiography but may be associated with up to a 60% systolic pressure gradient. Iliac occlusions, however, are readily apparent on contrast angiography and typically are associated with a marked reduction in the systolic pressure downstream from the obstruction.
   - Single-plane angiography provides a 2D representation of a 3D structure; the degree of narrowing may depend upon the imaging plane used to measure this quantity. The degree of stenosis is typically measured as the percentage of narrowing of the "normal" luminal diameter. Experimental studies have shown that no method exists to accurately determine the area of narrowing, which is the best indicator of flow obstruction by the lesion. The errors are compounded in eccentric lesions more than concentric lesions. In order to reduce errors, it is recommended that several views be obtained (AP, lateral, bilateral obliques).

R.A. Morgan, E. Walser (eds.), *Handbook of Angioplasty and Stenting Procedures*,
Techniques in Interventional Radiology, DOI 10.1007/978-1-84800-399-6_2,
© Springer-Verlag London Limited 2010

6. Four situations cause particular problems for contrast angiographic assessment of the hemodynamic significance:

- Lesions of moderate severity
- Arteries with diffuse disease
- Arteries with tandem lesions
- Lesions with abrupt transitions

Particular arterial trees where pressure measurements are used extensively include the aorto-iliac system, renal arteries, and mesenteric arteries. In particular, pressure measurements in the iliac arteries are important before and after angioplasty/stenting if a femoral bypass procedure is being contemplated.

Intra-arterial Pressure Measurements

1. Intra-arterial pressures were first used in assessment of aorto-iliac disease by simultaneous measurement of femoral and brachial pressures (1956). Normal controls were found to have average femoral systolic pressures *higher* than the corresponding brachial pressures (range 1.03–1.27; mean 1.14).

   - This occurs because the increased peripheral resistance while approaching more distal circulations has the effect of differentiating the pulse wave (acting as a high-pass filter) so that the systolic pressure wave peaks higher the more distally one moves in the circulation.

2. Peak systolic pressure gradients are the most sensitive indicators of arterial disease, while measurements of mean arterial pressure may not show any change at all.
3. The use of pressure measurements to document significant disease predicts a good response from surgical and hence endovascular therapies.
4. While the resting systolic pressure gradients are diagnostically adequate when evaluating patients with critical ischemia – including rest pain or ischemic ulcers – patients with claudication may only show significant pressure gradients across suspected lesions with augmented flow (either based upon exercise, induced ischemia by reactive hyperemia (blood pressure cuffs), or pharmacological augmentation with vasodilators).

   - These maneuvers may increase the flow rates from 2 to 4 times resting, basal flow rates. Papaverine is one such vasodilator that can be used at a dose of 20 mg given intra-arterially.
   - In many studies, the use of pressure measurements has proven more accurate in assessment of hemodynamic significance than single-plane angiography, and in many instances, multi-plane angiography.

5. Most angiographers rate very well in determining the hemodynamic significance of high-grade lesions (i.e., nearly occlusive) and alternatively lesions with minimal luminal narrowing.

   - The largest variability in assessing hemodynamic significance is in those lesions judged to be moderately narrow by angiography.
   - Intra-arterial pressure measurements add to the objectivity in quantifying the hemodynamic significance of such lesions.

Intra-arterial Pressure Measurements and Therapeutic End Points

1. The functional impact of an endovascular procedure can be assessed in the same way that the initial hemodynamic assessment was determined. The elimination of a previously detected systolic gradient either at rest or preferably with augmented flow is a desired end point of successful endovascular treatment of obstructing arterial lesions.
2. Hemodynamic pressure measurements are more accurate than angiography for determining satisfactory end points for angioplasty or stenting.

   - The Society of Cardiovascular and Interventional Radiology guidelines define successful aorto-iliac artery angioplasty/stenting as alleviation of systolic pressure gradients.

Technical Considerations During Intra-arterial Pressure Measurements

1. Factors influencing the accuracy of intra-arterial pressure measurements include the frequency response of the detector system and optimized damping coefficient. The components of this measurement system consist of an end-hole catheter of sufficient size to transmit pressure waves, properly flushed connector tubing, and a pressure transducer.

   - The minimum frequency response of the system has to be at least 20 Hz based upon experimental and theoretical considerations.
   - The presence of air within the pressure-measuring conduit may adversely affect the damping − compromising the fidelity of the pressure waveform measurements.

2. The most accurate method of aorto-iliac artery pressure measurements uses a two-transducer system with one catheter in the aorta and a second in the femoral or external iliac artery. The use of simultaneous measurements eliminates variability related to changes in systemic pressure, which becomes more problematic when pharmacologic flow augmentation is done.

- An alternative to the two-catheter method is the unilateral pullback technique. At resting conditions this is relatively reproducible unless the patient has cardiac rhythm disturbances such as atrial fibrillation.
- In situations where flow augmentation is done, changes in systemic pressure may result in false-positive findings.

3. Antegrade measurement of pressure gradients is complicated by the flow disturbance contributed by the flow restriction of the cross-section occupied by the catheter in relation to the luminal narrowing.

   - Examples include pressure measurements for renal and infra-inguinal arterial lesions. As the catheter lumen subtends more of the luminal area, the exaggeration of the pressure gradient increases. This can be mitigated by using smaller catheter or even pressure guidewires.

4. The actual threshold values of significant pressure gradients vary depending upon the fidelity of pressure measurements in each catheterization laboratory.

   - Our thresholds have included resting systolic gradients greater than 5–10 mmHg and augmented flow systolic gradients of 10 mmHg or greater.
     - *Keypoints*: The measurement of intra-arterial pressure gradients is a direct estimation of the arterial energy loss associated with a particular arterial lesion.
     - Estimation of the hemodynamic significance of lesions solely based upon angiographic data is fraught with errors, particularly in situations of moderately severe or diffuse lesions.
     - The use of pressure gradients is highly correlated with successful clinical outcomes from endoluminal or surgical interventions.

Patients with IC may not show any change in pressure measurements at rest across a particular lesion. Vasodilators can be used to augment flow to determine if there is a significant gradient across the lesion.

Suggested Reading

1. Kinney TB, Rose SC. Intraarterial pressure measurements during angiographic evaluation of peripheral vascular disease: Techniques, interpretation, applications, and limitations. AJR 1996; 166:277–284

Drugs — Pre-, Peri- and Post-intervention

Raman Uberoi

Medications Preintervention

Managing Risk Factors Before Intervention

Smoking

- The most important etiological risk factor for PAD.
- Smoking increases the risk for PAD by 4.23 times.
- Smoking increases the risk of amputation in persons with intermittent claudication.
- Patency in lower extremity bypass grafts is worse in smokers than in non-smokers.
- Smoking cessation decreases the progression of PAD to critical leg ischemia and decreases the risk of myocardial infarction (MI) and death from vascular causes.
- Smoking cessation is the most clinically efficacious and cost-effective intervention for the treatment of PAD.
- Management includes

  - Use of nicotine patches or nicotine polacrilex gum.
  - If this is unsuccessful, nicotine nasal spray and/or treatment with the antidepressant bupropion should be considered.
  - A nicotine inhaler is also available.

Hypertension (Systolic >130 mmHg and diastolic >80 mmHg)

- Established risk factor for PAD
- Increases the risk of PAD by 1.75 times
- Management includes

  - Lifestyle modifications
  - Drug therapy

- Indications for therapy:

  - Very high blood pressure values (>180/110 mmHg)

R.A. Morgan, E. Walser (eds.), *Handbook of Angioplasty and Stenting Procedures*,
Techniques in Interventional Radiology, DOI 10.1007/978-1-84800-399-6_3,
© Springer-Verlag London Limited 2010

- ○ Cardiovascular disease
- ○ Three or more cardiovascular risk factors (age: men >55 years, women >65 years, smoking, dyslipidemia, positive family history, obesity, CRP >1 mg/dL)
- ○ End-organ disease (LVH, microalbuminuria, elevated serum creatinine)
- ○ Diabetes mellitus

- There are many different regimes, which are equally effective, i.e., diuretics, beta-blockers, and newer agents such as calcium channel blockers and ACE inhibitors.

  - ○ There is no evidence that beta-blockers adversely affect claudication.
  - ○ An ACE inhibitor should be the first-line medication in the presence of congestive heart failure, diabetes mellitus with proteinuria, and a previous MI with systolic left ventricular dysfunction. For example, ramipril — commence at 1.25 mg/day increasing to a maximum dose of 10 mg/day.
  - ○ A beta-blocker should be prescribed following an acute MI, e.g., bisopropolol — 10 mg/day.
  - ○ A diuretic (Bendroflumethiazide 2.5 mg/day) or a long-acting calcium channel blocker (e.g., Amlodipine 5 mg/day to a maximum of 10 mg/day) may be more effective in elderly patients with isolated hypertension.

Diabetes

- Diabetes is a risk factor for PAD.
- Increases risk of PAD 2.08 times.
- Diabetes should be treated so that the hemoglobin A_{1c} level decreases to <7%.
- In addition to diet control, oral hypoglycemic drugs, e.g., Metformin (500 mg/day initially, increasing to a maximum dose of 2 g/day), glitazones (rosiglitazone 4 mg –8 mg), and sulfonylureas (gliclazide 40–80 mg to max of 160 mg/day) may be required for type 2 or non-insulin-dependent diabetes.
- Insulin therapy is indicated if the HgA1C remains >7% and for type 1 diabetes.

Dyslipidemia

- Hypercholesterolemia increases the risk of PAD by 1.67 times.
- Treatment with statin medication reduces the incidence of mortality, cardiovascular events, and stroke in PAD with and without coronary artery disease (CAD).
- Simvastatin reduces significantly the incidence of intermittent claudication by 38% compared with placebo.
- Statins also reduce atherosclerotic aneurysm formation.
- Therefore, all patients with PAD and hypercholesterolemia should be treated with statins to reduce cardiovascular mortality and morbidity, and reduce the progression of PAD.

- The aim of therapy is to maintain the serum LDL level less than 100 mg/dL. In patients over 40 years of age with overt cardiovascular disease, the serum LDL level should be reduced by 30–40%, regardless of the baseline LDL level before treatment. A typical regime is simvastatin 10–80 mg given as a single dose at night.

Medical Treatment of Claudication

- Five oral drugs have been licensed for the treatment of claudication. Two of these drugs, inositol nicotinate and cinnarizine, have not been established as effective when compared with placebo. The evidence is limited for efficacy of the drugs mentioned below.
- Pentoxifylline (400 mg three times per day) improves the walking distance by 50% compared with placebo.
- Pentoxigylline has been shown to provide an additional 30% improvement in the walking distance compared with pentoxifylline.
- Naftidrofuryl has shown an increased walking distance by up to 30% compared with placebo at 6 months.
- Cilostazol (100 mg orally twice a day), a phosphodiesterase inhibitor, shows a 40% increase in the walking distance at 3 months and is the drug of choice in the medical management of claudication.

Medical Treatment of Ulcers

- Ticlopidine has been shown to be effective in ulcer healing.
- The use of low molecular weight heparin (LMWH) has shown beneficial results in the healing of ischemic ulcers. Oral anticoagulant medication confers no additional benefit.
- Prostaglandin analogues, e.g., intravenous PGI2 and PGE or oral beraprost have antiplatelet and vasodilator actions. Iloprost has been shown to heal arterial ulcers.

Management of Pre-existing Medications Before Intervention

Warfarin

- If possible, this drug should be discontinued at least 3 days before the procedure and the INR should be checked the day before. An INR of 1.5 or less is desirable.

- If warfarin cannot be discontinued, e.g., if there is a mechanical heart valve, the patient requires admission a few days before the procedure and should be converted to heparin medication.
- If the procedure is very urgent, the situation can be managed by fresh frozen plasma and the use of vascular closure devices.

Heparin

- Stopping heparin 3 h before the procedure is usually adequate without the need to check the APTT.

Aspirin

- All patients should be commenced on lifelong aspirin therapy (75–325 mg/day) as soon as the diagnosis of peripheral vascular disease is made.
- Although platelet function is impaired in patients taking aspirin, there is no agreement on whether or not aspirin requires cessation before the procedure.

Clopidogrel

- It is usually not possible to discontinue clopidogrel in patients with coronary stents.
- Closure devices should be used in all procedures.

Diabetic Medication

- Metformin
  - Stop for 48 h after the procedure.
  - Check renal function before restarting.
- Other oral hypoglycemic drugs:
  - Withhold medication the morning of the procedure.
  - Medication should be restarted when food is taken after the procedure.
- Insulin:
  - Reduce the morning dose by 50%.
  - 5% dextrose infusion.
  - Monitor the blood glucose regularly.
  - A sliding scale is not generally necessary.

Prescription of Medications Before Intervention

Prevention of Contrast-Induced Nephropathy (CIN)

- Defined as elevation of the serum creatinine >25% or 44 mmol/L within 3 days of contrast administration.
- Risk factors for CIN are pre-existing renal failure, age, dehydration, heart failure, and the ongoing usage of NSAIDs.
- If possible, NSAIDS, diuretics, and Metformin should be held 48 h prior to the procedure in patients susceptible to CIN.
- Patients at risk of CIN should be well hydrated before the procedure.

  ○ This is usually achieved by an intravenous infusion of saline (100 mL/h).
  ○ The infusion should be commenced 4 h prior to the procedure and should be continued for 24 h.
  ○ Use a contrast medium suited to patients at risk of CIN, e.g., Visipaque.
  ○ *N*-Acetyl cysteine (150 mg/kg i.v. pre- and 50 mg/kg i.v. post-procedure) and ascorbic acid may be valuable in very high-risk patients although the evidence is limited.
  ○ Alternatively, an oral dose (600 mg BID) of *N*-acetyl cysteine can be given the day before and day of the procedure.

Antiplatelet Medication

- Platelet aggregation is 30% higher in patients with peripheral vascular disease.
- A number of antiplatelet agents are available.
- Aspirin (COX inhibitor) is the commonest.

  ○ Patients treated by peripheral angioplasty benefit from receiving aspirin at a dose of 50–300 mg daily, commenced before PTA and continued indefinitely.

- Clopidogrel (Plavix) and Ticlopidine (Ticlid) (ADP receptor blockers) are powerful antiplatelet agents. Clopidogrel is the most common of these agents used in IR.

  ○ Clopidogrel (loading dose 300 mg PO then 75 mg/day) is a useful alternative if aspirin is not tolerated because of GI side effects or if there is aspirin resistance.
  ○ Clopidogrel may be used in combination therapy with aspirin if there is an increased risk of re-occlusion post-procedure.
  ○ Clopidogrel shows a greater cardiovascular risk reduction compared with aspirin.
  ○ Ticlopidine-loading dose is 500 mg PO than 250 mg BD.
  ○ Clopidogrel and Ticlopidine are more expensive.

- Abciximab, eptifibatide, and tirofiban (glycoprotein IIb/IIIa receptor blockers)

  ○ Abciximab (ReoPro) is used in coronary interventions and has been advocated for extended infrainguinal interventions in patients with a high risk of peri-procedural re-occlusion.
  ○ Typical regime – 250 mcg i.v. over 1 min than 125 ng/kg/min to a maximum dose of 10 mcg/min.

Medications During Intervention

Local Anesthetic Agents

- Lidocaine/lignocaine:

  ○ Rapid onset (2–5 min).
  ○ Median duration of action (60 min).
  ○ Commonly used at needle puncture sites prior to interventional procedures.

- Co-administration with epinephrine can increase the duration of action up to 3 h. Avoid epinephrine in areas of limited blood supply (ears, noses) or in distal appendages (fingers, toes, penis) to reduce the risk of local necrosis.
- Bupivacaine:

  ○ Slow onset (5–10 min) with a long duration (4 h) of action.
  ○ Action can also be prolonged with epinephrine.

- A combination of lidocaine, bupivacaine, and epinephrine can be used to produce a rapid onset with prolonged analgesic effect.
- EMLA:

  ○ A mixture of lidocaine and prilocaine
  ○ Provides local anesthesia on application to the skin
  ○ Useful for minor procedures in children

Anticoagulation

- Heparin:

  ○ It is standard practice to give 3–5,000 units during the procedure in divided doses. This may be increased for longer procedure, i.e., longer than 2 h.
  ○ Ideally, the dose of heparin should be titrated with the activated clotting time (desired range: 250–300 sec).
  ○ Heparin effects can be reversed by Protamine sulfate. The latter binds to heparin to negate its anticoagulant effects. Dose is 1 mg protamine sulfate for every 100 IU of active heparin. Give by slow i.v. injection. Dose should not exceed 50 mg in any 10-min period.

- ○ Low molecular weight heparins (e.g., Dalteparin sodium 2,500 units) might be superior to unfractionated heparin in the prevention of early and mid-term re-occlusion/restenosis. Bivalirudin may be used as an alternative (750 mcg/kg i.v. pre-procedure than 1.75 mg/kg/h for upto 4 h).

- • Thrombolytics

  - ○ Fibrinolysis occurs by the degradation of fibrin by plasmin. The latter is generated form plasminogen in response to tissue activators like t-PA, urokinase, and streptokinase.
  - ○ These agents are used for thrombolysis.
  - ○ t-PA

    - ■ t-PA has a half-life of 5–10 min and is available as the recombinant varieties of alteplase and reteplase
    - ■ t-PA is widely used in Europe as a thrombolytic agent

  - ○ Streptokinase

    - ■ Obtained from b-hemolytic streptococci with a half-life of 40–80 min
    - ■ Large doses are needed because antibodies develop and allergic reactions can also occur. Nowdays it is seldom used.

  - ○ Urokinase

    - ■ Made from cultured human kidney cells with a half-life of 15–20 min
    - ■ With t-PA widely used for thrombolysis.

Vasodilators

- • Calcium channel blockers

  - ○ Verapamil, dialtiazem, nifedipine, and nicardipine

    - ■ Inhibit the influx of calcium into the cell via calcium channels.
    - ■ Mycocardial and arterial smooth muscle cells relax causing dilatation of the peripheral vasculature.
    - ■ Verapamil and dialtiazem suppress atrioventricular conduction and have negative inotropic and chronotropic effect. They should be used with caution in patients with heart failure or AV block. Nicardipine is not associated with AV node suppression.
    - ■ Verapamil is used for cerebral vasospasm in subarachnoid hemorrhage (SAH) at a dose of 3–8 mg intra-arterially per vessel. It can also be used for hand angiography at 100 μg in 10 mL normal saline, 30 sec before CM injection.
    - ■ Nicardipine is also used for cerebral vasospasm in SAH at a dose of 1-5 mg intra-arterially per vessel.

- Nifedipine is available in a sublingual form for immediate release and extended release oral preparations.
- Its effect on blood pressure is unpredictable and it can exacerbate myocardial ischemia.
- There is now controversy regarding its use for emergency lowering of blood pressure. Use with caution.

- Nitrates
  - Glyceryl trinitrate (GTN)

    - GTN is converted to nitric oxide, which causes dilatation of arterial and venous beds.
    - Widely used in IR when encountering spasm to deliberately vasodilate a vascular bed (GI bleeding study) or to prophylactically reduce spasm.
    - Given intra-arterially in 100–150-μg doses
    - May be combined with a GTN patch (5 mg over 24 h)

  - Molsidomine (Corvasol)

    - Orally active long-acting nitric oxide releasing vasodilator
    - Can be used for infrapopliteal intervention
    - Dose 1 mg orally before procedure

- Other vasodilators
  - Papaverine

    - Nonspecific smooth muscle relaxant causing arterial and arteriolar vasodilatation
    - Can be used for cerebral vasospasm in SAH (300 mg papaverine in 0.9% saline) given to affected artery over 20–30 min
    - Widely used for pressure study measurements. Dose is 20 mg intra-arterially

  - Tolazoline

    - Direct effect on peripheral vascular smooth muscle with moderate alpha-adrenergic blocking activity and histamine agonist activity
    - 5-mg doses intra-arterially up to 10–15 mg
    - Withdrawn in the US in 2002
    - Safer agents such as GTN and papaverine are available

Medications Post-intervention

- Aspirin (50–330 mg), with or without dipyridamole, reduces arterial restenosis and re-occlusion at 6 to 12 months compared to placebo or vitamin K antagonists. Ideally aspirin should be continued lifelong.

- Clopidogrel (75 mg/day) is indicated for lesions considered to be at very high risk for re-occlusion. Most experience has involved coronary artery interventions. Long-term Clopidogrel therapy is being used by many interventionalists for a variety of lesions in various locations. However, evidence for its efficacy or cost effectiveness is scanty.
- Long-term combination therapy with aspirin and Clopidogrel can be used for selected indications. The most common group of patients in this category are patients who have undergone carotid stenting.
- All risk factors should continue to be managed with continuation of appropriate drug therapy as described previously.

Key Points

- Managing risk factors before interventions can optimize outcomes.
- It may be necessary to change specific medications in patients about to undergo interventions.
- Antiplatelet medication is indicated for patients with peripheral vascular disease.
- Antiplatelet medication should be continued indefinitely after angioplasty and stenting.

Arterial Access

Dimitrios K. Tsetis

Preparation of Access Site

- Identify the arterial pulse.
- Shave the skin over the vessel, clean the puncture site with povidone iodine and cover with sterile towels.
- Gently tension the skin over the palpated pulse.
- Infiltrate the skin each side of the artery with lignocaine 1%, and leave the needle in situ to mark the skin incision point.
- Make a small skin incision and use a curved mosquito forceps to spread subcutaneous tissues.

Selection of Needle Type

Seldinger Needle

- Two-part needle.
- 18-gauge hollow needle with a sharp stylet.
- Used for "double-wall" puncture of the common femoral artery (CFA).
- During puncture, the needle is supported with the right middle and index fingers on each flange and with the thumb placed over the stylet.
- Not as frequently used as single-part needles (see below).

Needle Without a Stylet

- Standard arterial puncture needle used for most procedures.
- Sharp hollow needle lacking a stylet, appropriate for single-wall puncture of the artery.
- The entry of the needle tip into the artery is recognized immediately by the passage of blood through the needle lumen.
- Indications for single-wall puncture technique:

  ○ Generally the first choice needle for femoral, popliteal, pedal, radial, brachial, and axillary artery access.

R.A. Morgan, E. Walser (eds.), *Handbook of Angioplasty and Stenting Procedures*, Techniques in Interventional Radiology, DOI 10.1007/978-1-84800-399-6_4, © Springer-Verlag London Limited 2010

- ○ Femoral artery access when the patient has abnormal clotting parameters or when thrombolysis is contemplated.
- ○ The direct puncture of synthetic grafts.

- The main drawback of single-part needles is that small pieces of tissue or clot may occlude the needle and prevent the return of blood even though the needle tip has entered the arterial lumen. For this reason, the needle must be flushed before each repeated puncture attempt.

General Principles of Arterial Puncture

- The needle should be inserted at an angle of approximately 45° to the skin.
- The direction of the needle should match the palpated or expected course of the vessel.
- Advance the needle until the arterial pulsations are felt or are transmitted through the needle.
- Enter the artery with a steady forward thrust.
- If the needle is a single-part needle, entry of the needle tip into the vessel will be accompanied by the exit of pulsating blood through the needle.
- If using a Seldinger needle, advance the needle until it encounters the femoral head.
- Remove the stylet and slowly withdraw the needle until a jet of blood emerges through the needle.
- With the needle tip within the arterial lumen, a standard guidewire with a J tip should be gently advanced through the needle into the arterial lumen.
- If there is resistance to the passage of the guidewire, do not use force to push the wire harder as this may cause dissection of the vessel wall. Use fluoroscopy to exclude buckling or deformation of the wire.

Troubleshooting

- If the blood return through the needle is not pulsatile, the following are possible causes:

- ○ Venous puncture (repeat the puncture more laterally or medially).
- ○ There may be severe occlusive disease of the access artery (check with small injections of contrast).
- ○ The needle may be partially within the vessel wall (reposition the needle).

- If the guidewire cannot be advanced beyond the needle tip, the following possibilities exist:

- ○ The bevel of the needle is partially embedded in the wall of the artery. To rectify this, remove the wire and check if pulsatile blood continues to return.

If not, slowly withdraw the needle until pulsatile backflow is established and reinsert the wire.

- ○ The needle tip is abutting plaque (typically in the far CFA wall). Flatten the needle against the skin and reinsert the wire.
- ○ The needle tip is in a small branch artery. Remove the needle, obtain hemostasis and try another puncture.

- If there is good backflow of blood but difficulties with wire insertion remain, perform the following steps:

  - ○ Using tight collimation, inject a small amount of contrast through the needle to reveal the direction of the vessel (a roadmap can be helpful).
  - ○ A very floppy-tipped guidewire (e.g., Bentson wire) will usually negotiate plaque with a minimal risk of dissection. In this situation, a hydrophilic wire (e.g., Terumo, Tokyo, Japan) should be avoided, because the hydrophilic coating may be sheared off by the cutting bevel of the needle
  - ○ If the above measures fail, remove the needle, compress the artery for 5–10 min, and try again or consider another access.

- If the wire stops after a short distance:

  - ○ Exclude fluoroscopically that the wire has entered a branch vessel. If this occurs, the wire needs redirecting under fluoroscopic or roadmap guidance.
  - ○ Introduce a 4–5F dilator and inject contrast medium to detect the obstacle. This may be a severe atherosclerotic lesion or a tortuous vascular segment.
  - ○ Try to negotiate the obstacle with an angled hydrophilic wire passed through the dilator, preferably under roadmap guidance.

Access Sites

Femoral Artery Access

Retrograde Common Femoral Artery (CFA)

- By far the most commonly used vascular access route.
- The ideal location for arterial puncture is the middle third of the CFA. Here, the artery lies in front of the femoral head. As a result, the femoral pulse is most prominent here and the artery can be securely compressed against the underlying bone to ensure optimal hemostasis after the procedure.
- The course of the artery is palpated by three fingers in a straight line with the distal phalanges flattened rather than with the finger tips end on. The three fingers are placed just cephalad to the skin entry site and over the intended arterial entry point.
- If the femoral pulse is weak or absent, due to severe obesity or a high-grade iliac stenosis, fluoroscopy of the femoral region may help:

- To direct blind puncture over the medial aspect of the femoral head.
- To detect the CFA route by identifying calcification in the arterial wall.

- Alternatively, ultrasound (US) may be used in difficult cases to assist in femoral puncture.

Contralateral Retrograde CFA (Cross-Over)

Enables percutaneous intervention of the contralateral CFA, the profunda femoris artery, and the proximal superficial femoral artery (SFA):

- Some operators also use the cross-over technique to treat more distal contralateral lesions, although this technique can be problematic because of the necessity to use much longer catheters, balloons, and guidewires to reach the lesions.
- To access the opposite iliac artery across the aortic bifurcation, a suitably shaped diagnostic 4–5F catheter (e.g., cobra, Simmons 1, Sos-Omni) is positioned at the aortic bifurcation and manipulated so that the tip of the catheter "engages" the ostium of the contralateral common iliac artery (CIA).
- An angled 0.035-inch hydrophilic wire is advanced down the contralateral iliac artery into the common, superficial, or deep femoral artery. The diagnostic catheter is advanced over the guidewire and is positioned in the contralateral femoral artery.
- For most interventional procedures, a cross-over sheath should be placed to enable check angiography and to provide support for multiple catheter and guidewire exchanges across the aortic bifurcation.
- The hydrophilic wire is exchanged for a stiff guidewire (e.g., Amplatz superstiff guidewire (Boston Scientific Corp.), which is advanced into the distal femoral artery.
- A 6 or 7Fr cross-over sheath is advanced over the stiff guidewire and is positioned with the tip in the contralateral external iliac artery (EIA). Thus angiograms can be obtained before, during, and after lesion dilation.
- In patients with excessive calcification at the aortic bifurcation or an extremely acute angle between the origins of both CIAs, this type of access may be very difficult or impossible because of difficulties in manipulating catheters and sheaths across the aortic bifurcation.

Ipsilateral Antegrade CFA

The standard vascular access for infrainguinal interventions:

- Antegrade femoral access is preferable to the cross-over technique unless the lesion is close to the origin of the SFA.
- Complex distal interventions such as suction thrombectomy can only be performed from an ipsilateral antegrade access.

- Single-wall puncture is recommended to avoid bleeding complications, especially if thrombolysis is contemplated.
- Similar to retrograde puncture, the entry point into the CFA should be over the femoral head.
- The angle of entry should be 45–60° with respect to the femoral artery.
- Vertical punctures may result in buckling of introducer sheaths and catheters.
- In obese patients, the skin entry site may appear to be several centimeters above the inguinal ligament because of the excess soft tissue. In such circumstances the redundant soft tissues should be pulled cephalad and taped and/or flattened by an assistant. Alternatively, a pillow can be placed under the patient's buttocks. After this maneuver the pulse is generally easier to palpate, is nearer to the skin, and is more obviously below the inguinal ligament.
- During antegrade puncture, it is important to avoid suprainguinal puncture of the external iliac artery because this may result in intraperitoneal hemorrhage because of difficulties in achieving hemostasis after puncture of the external iliac artery.

Important Technical Points

- If the arterial entry point is in the proximal or the mid-CFA and the guidewire persists in passing down the profunda, the following maneuvers can help to guide the wire into the SFA:

  ○ Simple external rotation of the ipsilateral limb.
  ○ Flattening the needle against the patient's abdomen elevates the tip of the needle, which may facilitate selection of the SFA by the guidewire
  ○ Redirection of the needle tip with the assistance of a roadmap (without losing the puncture site access) may make it easier to guide the wire into the SFA. During this deflection maneuver, the guidewire should not be completely withdrawn into the needle.

- If the arterial entry point is very close to the CFA bifurcation and the guidewire enters the profunda, there is a risk of dislodging the needle during the deflection maneuver described above:

  ○ In this situation, a cobra, a multipurpose or vertebral catheter, can be passed into the profunda and slowly withdrawn, while injecting contrast medium slowly, until the origin of the SFA is identified.
  ○ At this point, the catheter is rotated so that the catheter tip points down the SFA and the guidewire can then be passed down the SFA.

- If the needle enters the proximal SFA (over or just below the femoral head) and the guidewire advances freely, the procedure is continued.
- If the needle enters directly into the profunda, the needle must be removed, the artery compressed, and a repeat puncture performed at a higher level.

- ○ However, before the needle is removed, it is advisable to gradually withdraw the needle to see whether a second jet of arterial blood is obtained because occasionally the needle will have passed through the SFA before it reaches the profunda.

Ipsilateral Retrograde CFA Access with Reversal of the Catheter (i.e., Conversion to an Antegrade Access)

This is an option favored by some interventionalists. There are few firm indications for this technique although it is useful to be familiar with it for some specific situations. (Fig. 1)

- Indications – It may be performed for infrainguinal recanalization in the following situations:
  - ○ Obese patients with a large overhanging "apron"
  - ○ Patients who fail ipsilateral antegrade catheterization and have an acute aortic bifurcation, or tortuous and severely diseased iliac arteries, which prevents the cross-over technique.
  - ○ When iliac angiography is required and the operator wishes to avoid a second puncture or the cross-over technique.

Technique

- It is important that the angle of entry into the artery is near vertical, in order to facilitate reversal of the direction of the catheter.
- After retrograde catheterization of the femoral artery, a reverse curved catheter such as a Sos-Omni or Simmons 1 catheter is advanced over a standard guidewire, and is formed in the lower aorta.
- The standard guidewire is exchanged for an angled-tip 0.035″ hydrophilic wire, which is advanced back down the ipsilateral iliac artery and both the wire and catheter are withdrawn into the CFA.
- At this point, the wire is further advanced into the proximal SFA (it is usually helpful to access the SFA using a roadmap).
- The catheter is withdrawn further until the apex of its curve is located at the puncture site.
- When it is at this location, it should be possible to advance the catheter antegradely over the guidewire into the SFA.
- After the catheter has been advanced into the SFA, the hydrophilic wire is exchanged for a stiff wire and a sheath is inserted antegradely, enabling intervention to be performed on the SFA or a more distal lesion.
- The main drawback of this technique is the increased screening time and radiation dose to the operator's hand because it is difficult to keep the hands out of the main fluoroscopy beam.

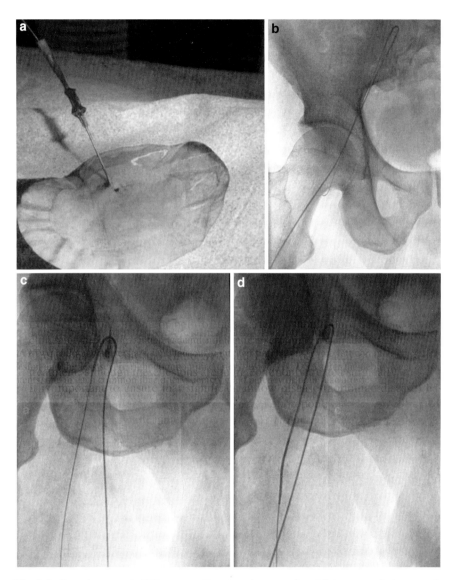

Fig. 1 Ipsilateral retrograde CFA access with antegrade conversion. (**a**) A near vertical retrograde puncture 1–2 cm above the inguinal crease is performed. (**b**) A 5F Sos-Omni catheter and an angled 0.035-inch glidewire, which has been advanced down the ipsilateral SFA, are pulled back together. (**c**) The catheter is gently "right sided" rotated and further pulled back until it is just traversing the puncture site. (**d**) The glidewire and catheter are advanced well deep into SFA in order to achieve sufficient support for placement of a sheath

Popliteal Artery Access

This access route is usually only performed in patients with critical limb ischemia:

- The popliteal artery should be relatively free of disease.
- Indications:

  ○ Failure of antegrade recanalization of SFA occlusions.
  ○ SFA occlusions without a visible stump of SFA at the CFA bifurcation, i.e., a flush occlusion of the SFA.

Technique

- The patient is turned to the prone position and the popliteal artery is punctured just above the knee joint under ultrasound guidance:

  ○ The popliteal artery is imaged with the probe directed from the medial side of the popliteal vessels so that the artery is visualized side by side to the vein.
  ○ Anatomically, the vein lies posterior to the artery.
  ○ If the probe is placed directly posterior to the artery, puncture of the artery from this position may result in the needle passing though the vein on the way to the artery, which may cause an arteriovenous fistula.

- The needle is directed toward the popliteal artery from medial to lateral avoiding the popliteal vein.
- It is sensible to use a small caliber access system such as a micropuncture kit (W. Cook) with a 21-gauge needle to minimize arterial trauma in case arterial cannulation is difficult.
- If a catheter or sheath is already placed in the ipsilateral external iliac or femoral artery, the popliteal artery puncture can be performed with the assistance of roadmap fluoroscopy after injection of contrast medium through the proximal access.
- After insertion of a sheath (up to 6Fr), intra-arterial heparin (5000 Iu) and GTN (100-150 mcg) are administered to prevent pericatheter thrombosis and spasm.

Pedal Artery Access

A possible access route if recanalization of a tibial artery occlusion cannot be achieved from above.

- Has been described as a component of the SAFARI technique (subintimal arterial flossing with antegrade−retrograde intervention).
- Should only be used in patients with critical limb ischemia (CLI).

- Clearly, the technique can only be performed if the pedal vessel supplied by the occluded tibial vessel is patent.
- Either the anterior or posterior tibial artery can be used as the access vessel.
- The selected vessel is punctured under US or fluoroscopic guidance with a micropuncture system.
- After puncture, the 0.018-inch straight-tip guidewire is advanced retrogradely into the artery, followed by insertion of a 4Fr short sheath.

Brachial Artery Access

This is an alternative approach for aortic, visceral artery, and lower extremity diagnostic and interventional angiographic procedures. It is a useful access for diagnostic angiography if there is an aortoiliac occlusion.

Upper extremity access also provides an alternative approach for interventional procedures on visceral arteries, e.g., renal, superior mesenteric, celiac artery, if these vessels arise at an acute angle to the aorta, i.e., have an inferior angulation, which causes problems in their cannulation from a femoral access.

The left brachial artery approach is preferred as it is usually the nondominant arm and this route avoids crossing the aortic arch, with the attendant risk of vertebral artery embolization.

Technique

- The artery is punctured in its distal portion in the cubital fossa just above the elbow joint with the joint extended and the arm supinated. At this level, the artery is relatively superficial and can be compressed against the humerus to obtain hemostasis.
- The vessel can be punctured with a standard 18 gauge, single-wall puncture needle, although a micropuncture system is preferable to minimize trauma, particularly arterial dissection, and its risk.
- After insertion of a sheath, intra-arterial GTN to prevent spasm and heparin to prevent pericatheter thrombosis should be administered.
- Sheath size should generally not exceed 6Fr; however, percutaneous introduction of a 7F sheath is possible. For larger sheath sizes (7Fr in small patients or larger in all patients) a surgical cut-down should be performed.
- Long introducer sheaths may reduce the frequency of arterial spasm during intervention.
- A hydrophilic guidewire and a cobra catheter should be advanced up the brachial artery under fluoroscopy.
- It may be difficult to pass the catheter and guidewire into the descending rather than the ascending aorta. If it is not possible, then this is accomplished with a cobra catheter. Unfolding a pigtail catheter in the arch adjacent to the origin of the left subclavian artery, or the use of a reverse curve catheter such as a Sos-Omni or a Simmons catheter usually achieves this outcome.

Radial Artery Access

This is an alternative to the brachial artery route. This route offers advantages in terms of increased safety, although it is more technically difficult. Moreover, the increased distance from the aorta makes interventional procedures in the lower aorta and iliac artery more challenging than from a brachial artery access.

- Advantages of radial artery access:
  - ○ Absence of major neural and vascular structures immediately adjacent to the artery.
  - ○ Good collateral ulnar artery circulation.
  - ○ Superficial position.
  - ○ Easy palpation for puncture.
- Prior to puncturing the artery the Allen test is performed:
  - ○ This involves compressing the radial artery and ulnar artery with the operator's fingers until the hand becomes pale.
  - ○ The ulnar artery is released and the hand is observed to see if the whole hand becomes pink (positive test), or only the half of the hand and fingers supplied by the ulnar artery (negative test).
  - ○ A positive Allen test verifies adequate collateral circulation between the ulnar and the radial arteries and enables safe puncture without the risk of hand ischemia.
  - ○ When the Allen test is clearly negative in one arm, it is often positive in the contralateral arm (less than 10% of patients have a negative Allen test in both arms).
- If the Allen test is not clearly positive, fingertip pulse oximetry during compression of the radial artery may be helpful.

Technique
- If there is a choice, the left radial artery is preferred.
- The arm is placed on an arm board with the elbow and wrist extended, and the arm in supination.
- It is helpful to place the wrist in hyperextension with the aid of a folded sheet placed on the armrest. The hand should be stabilized in position with elastoplast or strapping.
- Local anesthetic cream or nitrate paste can be applied at the puncture site to diminish pain or to dilate the artery.
- The radial artery is punctured at the wrist, 1–2 cm proximal to the styloid process. The puncture angle is 30–45° in relation to the horizontal plane.
- A micropuncture system should be used.
- Alternatively, a 21-gauge sheathed cannula can be inserted followed by passage by an 0.018-inch guidewire.

- After sheath insertion, intrarterial GTN and heparin should be administered.
- After the procedure, the puncture site is closed by manual compression for 10–15 min. Prolonged bed rest is unnecessary. Patients should wait for a period of 1–2 h and can be discharged if there are no complications.
- Clearly, a major benefit of angiography and interventions performed via the radial artery is that these procedures can be performed as outpatient procedures without the need for an overnight stay.

Axillary Artery Access

This route is seldom used nowadays due to the increased risk of complications compared with the brachial or radial artery route:

- The main complication of this access is the significant risk of brachial plexus injury from needle puncture or from compression by hematoma.
- The procedure is uncomfortable for the patient because of the required prolonged immobilization of the arm in abduction.
- The left axillary artery is preferred to minimize the possibility of stroke.

Technique

- The technique is performed with the patient lying supine with the hand positioned behind the head, so that the arm is at right angles to the thorax.
- The mobile axillary artery is fixed firmly at the intended puncture site by the operator's left index and middle fingers on either side.
- The puncture site is at the junction of the anterior third with the middle third of the space between the anterior and posterior folds of the axilla.
- A single-wall puncture technique is preferred.
- US guidance may be helpful.

Puncture Site Complications

Hemorrhage

- Risk factors include hypertension, anticoagulation, low platelet count, large sheath size, heavy vascular calcification, and obesity.
- Puncture above the inguinal ligament increases significantly the danger of post-procedural bleeding.
- However, even an apparently "correct" puncture of the CFA below the inguinal ligament can occasionally be complicated by the development of abdominal wall or retroperitoneal hematoma as a result of bleeding in the femoral sheath tracking superiorly between the fascial planes of the abdominal wall.

Pseudoaneurysm

- May occur secondary to inadequate manual compression during hemostasis or may occur with SFA punctures where the arterial entry site cannot be compressed against bone.
- The main treatment method for femoral artery pseudoaneurysm is US-guided percutaneous injection of thrombin with an overall thrombosis rate of 93–100% (Fig. 2).
- In the majority of cases, a thrombin dose of 500–1,000 IU is adequate to promote complete thrombosis of the pseudoaneurysm.
- Anticoagulation does not seem to affect the efficacy of the procedure.

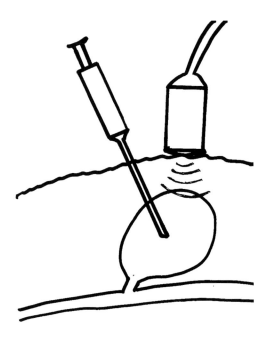

Fig. 2 US-guided percutaneous thrombin injection technique. The thrombin is injected slowly under US guidance into the middle of the pseudoaneurysm cavity away from the neck

Arterial Thrombosis

- Risk factors include a severely diseased access artery, extensive intimal damage, vasospasm, and abnormal coagulation status.

Other Complications

- Arteriovenous fistula
- Nerve damage
- Distal embolization

Key Points

- The common femoral artery is the most frequently used access site.
- A long sheath placed across the aortic bifurcation should be used when performing interventions using the cross-over technique.
- Antegrade femoral artery puncture is preferable to the cross-over technique for infrainguinal interventions unless the lesions are close to the SFA origin.
- Intra-arterial GTN and heparin should be administered routinely for popliteal, pedal, brachial, and radial artery access routes to prevent thrombosis and spasm.

Suggested Readings

1. Lilly MP, Reichman W, Sarazen AA, Carney WI (1990). Anatomic and clinical factors associated with complications of transfemoral arteriography. Annals of Vascular Surgery 4: 264–269
2. Morgan R, Belli AM (2003). Current treatment methods for postcatheterization pseudoaneurysms J Vasc Interv Radiol 14: 697–710
3. Seldinger SI (1953). Catheter replacement of the needle in percutaneous arteriography. Acta Radiologica 39: 368–376
4. Trerotola SO, Kuhlman JE, Fishman EK (1990). Bleeding complications of femoral catheterization. CT evaluation. Radiology 174: 37–40

Venous Access

Clare L. Bent and Matthew Matson

Introduction

Venous access may be peripheral or central and the route taken usually depends on the indication:

- Peripheral venous access is performed if the required access is temporary. Central venous access is undertaken if long-term venous access is required.
- Long-term venous access usually involves the placement of tunneled catheters. These are passed from the site of access into the vein through a subcutaneous tunnel to the skin-exit point. This tunnel aids in fixation and helps to prevent catheter infection.

The indications for long-term venous access are many:

- Acute and chronic renal failure: fluid replacement, hemodialysis, etc.
- Malignancy: chemotherapy, and blood product replacement.
- Parenteral nutrition.
- Access to the central veins is required as a precursor for numerous interventional procedures.

The aim of this chapter is to describe the methods for standard venous access for interventional procedures. Access into upper extremity veins distal to the subclavian vein, e.g., for insertion of vascular cannulae is a generic medical skill and will not be dealt with.

General Principles of Venous Access

The vein to be catheterized may be located either by using anatomical landmarks or by ultrasound.

R.A. Morgan, E. Walser (eds.), *Handbook of Angioplasty and Stenting Procedures*, Techniques in Interventional Radiology, DOI 10.1007/978-1-84800-399-6_5, © Springer-Verlag London Limited 2010

There is evidence that ultrasound-guided venous access is associated with a lower incidence of complications compared with the use of anatomical landmarks. Within the UK, the National Institute of Clinical Excellence has recommended the routine use of ultrasound for venous access (NICE Technology Appraisal Guidance No. 49).

- Either the longitudinal or the transverse image of the vein may be used to guide the puncture. This is generally decided by the personal preference of the operator.
- During venous puncture, it is important to visualize the needle tip as it passes through the subcutaneous tissues to the vein to optimize the chances of successful puncture and to minimize complications.
- With ultrasound guidance, the needle tip can be visualized as it enters the vein. Before the needle enters the vein, it usually deforms the vein wall and sometimes requires a gentle, firm push to pass through the wall into the lumen.
- Unlike arterial puncture, venous blood is at a low pressure and does not generally emerge from the needle in a jet indicating entry into the venous lumen. Therefore, it is advisable to perform venous puncture while applying *gentle* suction via a small saline-filled syringe (e.g., a 2 or a 5 mL syringe). Entry of blood into the syringe confirms the location of the tip within the lumen of the vein.
- Catheterization of a vein utilizes the Seldinger technique:

  ○ The vein is punctured using a single-part needle.
  ○ A standard floppy-tipped guidewire is advanced through the needle into the vein followed by removal of the needle.
  ○ This is followed by insertion of a dilator, a sheath, or a catheter depending on the location of the vein and the reason for the access into the vein.

- Either standard puncture systems or small caliber systems (e.g., micropuncture) may be used (see below).
- It should be noted that veins are thin walled and prone to spasm, particularly smaller veins. Therefore, it is advisable for wire and catheter manipulations to be performed with care.

Equipment

- 10 mL 1% lignocaine local anaesthetic (LA) with 25G or 23G needles for subcutaneous injection
- Standard access:

  ○ 18- or 19-gauge single-part needle
  ○ 0.035 standard floppy-tipped guidewire
  ○ 4F sheath or larger

- Micropuncture access:

  ○ 21- or 22-gauge needle
  ○ 0.018-inch guidewire

- Two- or three-part dilator, which allows the insertion of a 0.035- or 0.038-inch guidewire
- 4F sheath or larger

- 2 or 5 mL syringe containing saline for attachment to the puncture needle during venipuncture
- Small scalpel blade
- Central venous catheter kit
- Ultrasound machine with a high frequency 7.5 or 12 MHz linear transducer

Access into the Femoral Vein

Femoral vein access is usually performed as a prelude to a diagnostic or interventional procedure in the venous system.

It is an important site for temporary and long-term venous access, particularly in children.

The close proximity of the common femoral vein to the perineum has been a cause of concern with regard to infection. However, the published literature has demonstrated no difference in infection rates when comparing femoral venous catheters with subclavian or internal jugular catheters in the pediatric population.

Indications

- Inferior vena cava filter insertion and removal
- Iliac venography, venoplasty, and stenting
- Central venous stenting for benign and malignant venous obstruction
- Cardiac catheterization in children with congenital heart disease
- Testicular or ovarian vein embolization
- Tunneled and non-tunneled central venous catheter insertion (e.g., for dialysis or total parenteral nutrition)

Contraindications

- Venous thrombosis.
- When inserting a long-term tunneled central venous catheter, untreated sepsis is considered a contraindication.

Patient Preparation

- The lower limb should be extended and abducted slightly at the hip.
- Standard antiseptic preparation.

Anatomy

- The femoral vein lies within the femoral triangle, an area of the anterior thigh where several muscles and ligaments cross each other to produce an inverted triangle.
- Lying within the triangle, from lateral to medial, are the femoral nerve, the femoral artery, and the femoral vein (Fig. 1).

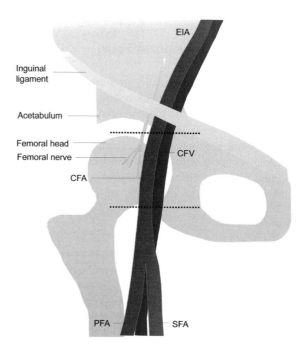

Fig. 1 Anatomy of the right groin. The ideal femoral artery puncture site is shown by the black dotted line, below the inguinal ligament and at a site over which pressure can be exerted to achieve hemostasis (e.g., the femoral head)

Performing the Procedure

a. Without ultrasound guidance:

- The common femoral artery is located by palpation of the pulse.
- Infiltrate the subcutaneous tissues medial to the pulse with local anesthetic.
- Locate the inguinal ligament with anatomical landmarks or by fluoroscopy.
- In practice, the vein is punctured over the femoral head, similar to femoral artery catheterization.
- While keeping fingers over the artery, introduce a vascular access needle attached to 2–5 mL syringe into the skin 1 cm medial to the pulse.

- Slowly advance the needle at a 45° angle cephalad and posteriorly while maintaining gentle suction on the syringe.
- It is helpful to ask the patient to perform a Valsalva maneuver during venous puncture to distend the femoral vein (Fig. 2).

Fig. 2 Transverse ultrasound image of the right common femoral vein (CFV). Note the position of the CFV medial to the common femoral artery (CFA) and the large caliber of the CFV seen during the Valsalva maneuver

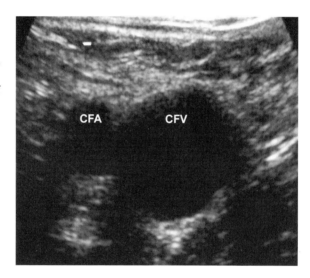

- If blood is aspirated into the syringe, maintain the needle position and insert a guidewire into the vein.
- Sometimes the needle may pass through both walls of the vein, without the appearance of blood in the syringe. If no blood is aspirated, slowly withdraw the needle while maintaining suction.
- Repeat the procedure if the needle pass is unsuccessful.

b. With ultrasound guidance:

- Locate the inguinal ligament.
- Visualize the femoral vein in the transverse or longitudinal plane.
- If the transverse image is to be used, keep the image of the vein in the center of the image and infiltrate the skin at the center of the probe. During this process, it should be possible to visualize the needle and the lignocaine during injection of LA into the subcutaneous tissues.
- The venous puncture needle is advanced through the same track and the vein is punctured under direct vision.
- If the longitudinal image is to be used for guidance, the principle is the same as above. The vein should be kept in vision throughout LA infiltration and passage of the venous puncture needle into the vein.

Complications

- Femoral artery puncture or damage. This is avoided by:

  ○ Ensuring that the arterial pulse is felt lateral to the skin entry site
  ○ Asking the patient to perform a Valsalva maneuver
  ○ Using ultrasound guidance

- Femoral nerve damage: see above.
- Hematoma (including retroperitoneal): following arterial puncture use compression to the achieve hemostasis (for 5–10 min)
- Thrombophlebitis: unusual
- Deep venous thrombosis: may occur after use of large access sheaths
- Pulmonary emboli: uncommon
- Arteriovenous fistula due to puncture of the vein after passage through the artery: this is avoided by the use of ultrasound guidance
- Infection

Access into the Popliteal Vein

Indications

Indications for popliteal venous access are few:

- Antegrade thrombolysis for iliofemoral deep vein thrombosis may be performed by this approach. This procedure may be used in combination with arterial thrombolysis in Phlegmasia Caerulia Dolens.
- If clinically indicated, the popliteal vein may also be accessed to perform common femoral venoplasty.

Contraindications

- Cellulitis
- Inability to lie prone

Patient Preparation

- The patient should be placed in a prone position.
- Standard antiseptic preparation.

Anatomy

- The popliteal fossa is a shallow depression posterior to the knee joint.
- The popliteal vein typically lies posterior to the popliteal artery.

- The popliteal fossa contains the popliteal artery and vein, the short saphenous vein, the tibial, and common peroneal nerves, the lower part of the posterior femoral cutaneous nerve, the articular branch from the obturator nerve, and a few small lymph glands.

Performing the Procedure

- The popliteal vein should be punctured using ultrasound guidance.
- A micropuncture system should be used.
- Care should be taken to avoid puncture of the femoral artery.

Complications

- Arteriovenous fistula: the risk of AV fistula formation is minimized by accurate ultrasound guidance and a single-wall puncture.
- Arterial puncture.
- Nerve damage: the tibial and common peroneal nerves lie lateral to the popliteal vessels. The operator should be aware of the anatomical position of the nerves (which appear as hypoechoic rounded structures) during ultrasound-guided puncture to avoid nerve damage.

Access into the Internal Jugular Vein (IJV)

The vertical orientation and its relationship to the superior and inferior vena cava makes the IJV well suited for the insertion of large caliber catheters for hemodialysis, stiff catheters for caval filter insertion, and for stiff needle assemblies required for procedures such as transjugular liver biopsies.

In addition, a right internal jugular vein route is frequently more suitable than a right femoral vein approach for access and catheterization of the hepatic, gondal, and pelvic veins.

Indications

The internal jugular vein is used as the access route for several interventional procedures, including:

- Tunneled and non-tunneled central venous catheter insertion (e.g., for dialysis or total parenteral nutrition)
- Portacath insertion
- Inferior vena cava filter insertion
- Central venous stenting

- Transjugular liver biopsies
- TIPPS

Contraindications

- Ipsilateral jugular venous thrombosis
- Local sepsis

Patient Preparation

- The patient should be placed supine with the head turned 45° to the contralateral side to enable adequate exposure of the neck.
- If a tilting table is available, the patient should be placed 15° head down to dilate the vein and reduce the risk of air embolism during the procedure.
- Full antiseptic preparation.

Anatomy

- The IJV leaves the skull through the jugular foramen, accompanied by the 9th, 10th, and 11th cranial nerves. The vein runs vertically down the neck inside the carotid sheath along with the carotid artery and vagus nerve. The IJV joins the subclavian vein posterior to the sternoclavicular joint to become the brachiocephalic vein.
- As the IJV descends in the neck, it is located lateral or anterolateral to the carotid artery (Figs. 3 and 4).

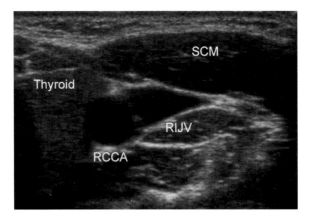

Fig. 3 Transverse ultrasound image of the right internal jugular vein (RIJV). The RIJV lies lateral to both the right common carotid artery (RCCA) and the right lobe of the thyroid gland; and lies inferior to the sternocleidomastoid muscle (SCM). It is essential to maintain visualization of the needle tip throughout the venous puncture (see Fig. 6)

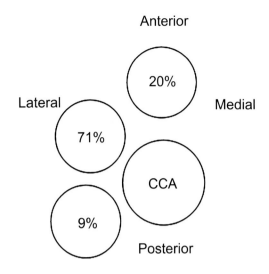

Fig. 4 Diagram illustrating the variations in the RIJV anatomy. The RIJV lies antero-lateral to the right common carotid artery in 71% of cases, lateral in 9%, and anterior in 20% of cases. Anatomical variation reduces the success rate of the landmark method of venous puncture

Performing the Procedure

Using Anatomical Landmarks

Historically, internal jugular access was performed using the landmark method, based on a knowledge of the surface anatomy.

- The carotid artery is palpated and the needle is inserted lateral to the artery at the apex of the triangle formed by the two heads of sternocleidomastoid muscle.
- The needle is aimed laterally, pointing toward the ipsilateral nipple aspirating as the needle is advanced.

Using Ultrasound Guidance

For interventional radiologists, with access to ultrasound, there is no reason to perform IJV access without ultrasound guidance (Figs. 5, 6 and 7).

- The transverse image of the vein is probably preferable to the longitudinal image.
- The vein is usually catheterized in the mid-to-lower neck.
- If available a micropuncture system should be used in all cases. This limits the possibility of severe hemorrhage if the carotid artery is punctured inadvertently.
- Efforts should be made to reduce the possibility of air embolism by using a tilting table and performing catheter exchanges though non-valved sheaths (e.g., peelaway sheaths) with respiration suspended.

Fig. 5 Longitudinal ultrasound image of the RIJV. This orientation allows complete visualization during needle puncture and is preferable for deep venous punctures

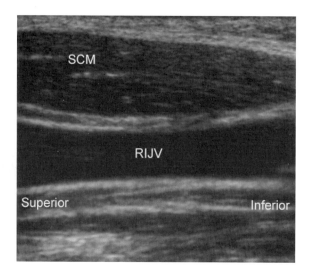

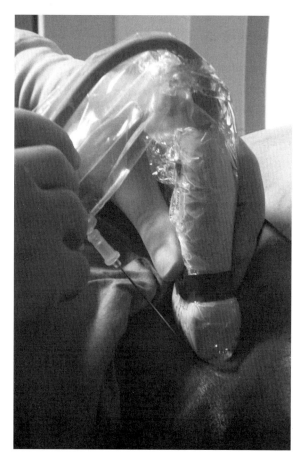

Fig. 6 Ultrasound-guided RIJV puncture. Notice the transverse orientation of the linear 7.5 MHz ultrasound probe. A vascular access needle is used attached to a saline syringe at a 45° angle

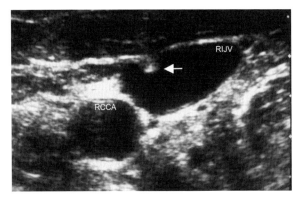

Fig. 7 Transverse ultrasound image of a RIJV needle puncture. As the needle tip (echogenic focus arrowed) enters the RIJV, there is distortion of the anterior vessel wall. Aspiration via the syringe confirms intravascular position

Complications

- Carotid artery puncture and cannulation: an uncommon complication if the operator is experienced in ultrasound-guided venipuncture.
- Pneumothorax (0–2.5%) or hemothorax: this is minimized by ultrasound-guided puncture.
- Air embolism (0.3%): avoid by using a tilting table and place the patient with the head down. Suspend respiration during catheter exchanges if using a peelaway sheath.
- Arrhythmias: avoid passing the guidewire into the right ventricle. Preferable guidewire placement is within the IVC.
- Infection.

Access into the Subclavian Vein

- The subclavian vein is commonly used for central venous catheterization.
- However, it is a poor first choice for venous access, because even with ultrasound guidance, the risk of pneumothorax or hemothorax remains higher than for access via the IJV. Moreover, the risk of long-term stenosis and thrombosis is increased compared with the internal jugular approach, which is particularly relevant in patients with renal failure who require patent subclavian veins for hemodialysis fistula function.
- On a practical level, the left subclavian vein is the preferred side versus the right, due to the longer, straighter course via the left brachiocephalic vein into the right atrium. In contrast, there is a sharp angulation at the junction between the right subclavian vein and the right brachiocephalic vein, which may promote catheter kinking during central venous line insertion.

Indications

- The most frequent indication for subclavian vein access is the insertion of a tunneled central venous catheter (e.g., for dialysis or total parenteral nutrition) when the internal jugular vein route is no longer available.

Contraindications

- Subclavian vein thrombosis
- Local skin sepsis

Patient Preparation

- Similar to IJV puncture, the patient should be supine, in a Trendelenberg position of 15°, with the head turned 45° to the contralateral side to enable adequate exposure of the neck.
- A towel placed between the shoulder blades encourages the clavicles to move posteriorly allowing easier access to the subclavian vein.
- Full antiseptic preparation.

Anatomy

- The subclavian vein begins as a continuation of the axillary vein at the lateral border of the first rib. Here it grooves the first rib immediately anterior and inferior to the scalene tubercle, the insertion site of the scalene anterior, which separates the vein from the subclavian artery.
- The subclavian vein continues behind the medial third of the clavicle where it is immobilized by small attachments to the rib and clavicle.
- At the medial border of the anterior scalene muscle and behind the sternoclavicular joint, the subclavian vein unites with the internal jugular vein to form the brachiocephalic vein.

Performing the Procedure

Using Anatomical Landmarks

- A single-part needle is inserted into the skin two-thirds of the way along the clavicle and 1 cm inferior to its inferior margin.
- The needle is passed deep into the clavicle, aiming toward the head of the clavicle.

Using Ultrasound Guidance

- Subclavian vein access should be performed using ultrasound guidance.
- During ultrasound-guided subclavian vein puncture, the site of needle puncture is determined by the portion of subclavian vein, which is most visible.
- A micropuncture system is sensible and limits hemorrhage and the risk of pneumothorax.

Using Fluoroscopic Guidance

- If the subclavian vein is poorly visible by sonography (this is very unusual if the vein is patent), the vein can be punctured using fluoroscopic guidance.
- A venogram is performed from a peripheral vessel. The subclavian vein may be punctured using either the venographic image and/or a road map.

Complications

- Pneumothorax: this is avoided by using ultrasound guidance for catheterization.
- Hemothorax or local hematoma due to puncture of the subclavian artery: this is avoided by ultrasound guidance.
- Inadvertent access into the subclavian artery: this is avoided by ensuring that all catheter manipulations are performed under fluoroscopic guidance. Ensure that catheters and guidewires follow the appropriate course though the central veins (and not through the arteries!).
- Pseudoaneurysm of the subclavian artery.
- Arteriovenous fistula.
- Air embolism: this is avoided by using tilting tables and suspending respiration if exchanging catheters through peelaway sheaths.
- Arrhythmias: avoid passing the guidewire into the right ventricle.
- Catheter compression between the clavicle and first rib: an unavoidable complication of this access route.
- Phrenic nerve palsy.
- Infection: reported cases of infection are generally lower than for that with internal jugular vein catheters.

Access into the Inferior Vena Cava (IVC)

- Translumbar inferior vena caval access may be used as an access port in patients who require long-term hemodialysis or who require chemotherapy, but have exhausted traditional access sites.
- It is not a common access route because of complications and poor long-term durability.
- It is generally used as an access route of last resort.

Contraindications

- IVC thrombosis
- Local sepsis

Patient Preparation

- The patient is placed prone on the angiography table.
- Full antiseptic preparation.
- If the procedure is going to be performed under fluoroscopic guidance, it is helpful to place a transfemoral guidewire into the IVC, which may act as a target for percutaneous puncture of the IVC.

Anatomy

- The IVC is a retroperitoneal structure and is located on the right side of the anterior margin of the lumbar spine. The renal veins drain into the IVC at the level of L1 or L2 vertebral bodies.

Performing the Procedure

- The procedure may be performed using fluoroscopic or CT guidance.
- Fluoroscopic guidance is probably preferable for most straightforward procedures, and is facilitated by the use of a target such as a transfemoral guidewire or a wire loop snare.
- A puncture site is chosen just cephalic to the right iliac crest and approximately 8–10 cm to the right of the midline.
- Under fluoroscopic guidance, a 21G 15 cm long needle is advanced cephalad and medial to the anterolateral margin of the vertebral bodies aiming to puncture the IVC at the level of L2/L3 below the renal veins.
- A small caliber access system such as an Accustick system (Boston Scientific Corp, Galway, Ireland) is ideal for this procedure.
- A 0.018-inch wire is inserted through the needle, and the needle is exchanged for a three part dilator enabling the insertion of a 0.035-inch very stiff guidewire.
- A 4 or 5F catheter is inserted into the IVC, and contrast medium is injected to confirm entry into the IVC and not the renal vein.
- The track is subsequently dilated to the necessary diameter for the catheter required.
- It should be emphasized that the track is usually quite long and care should be taken during track dilation not to lose access or to buckle the guidewire.

Complications

- Air embolism: care during venous access is vital to prevent air entry into the IVC. Perform catheter exchanges using a peelaway sheath in suspended respiration.
- Right ureteric damage: ensure that the needle is in close proximity to the vertebral bodies to avoid this complication.
- Catheter migration or dislodgment into the subcutaneous tissues or retroperitoneum:

  - A late rather than an acute complication.
  - This is one of the major drawbacks of this access route.
  - Maintaining the position of the catheter tip in the IVC, despite the constant motion of the body, is a real and often insurmountable challenge.

- Venous thrombosis (IVC or renal vein): in view of the high flow within the IVC and its large caliber, thrombosis of the IVC is less common than other routes of access.
- Infection.

Key Points

- Apart from cannulation of superficial veins in the extremities, ultrasound guidance should be used for most procedures to minimize complications.
- Full antiseptic preparation should be performed in all cases.
- Familiarity with standard interventional radiology skills is essential for complicated venous access routes.

General Principles of Angioplasty and Stenting

Elias N. Brountzos and Efthymia Alexopoulou

Pathophysiology of Angioplasty

- Percutaneous transluminal angioplasty (PTA) involves the dilatation of a vascular stenosis or occlusion with a balloon catheter.
- The mode of action of PTA is fracture of the arterial plaque and a localized tear or dissection of the arterial wall. The tear may extend circumferentially or longitudinally in the vessel wall and may extend into the internal elastic lamina or into the media. The adventitial layer remains intact. This mechanism accounts for the majority of luminal increase (>70%).
- Balloon dilatation also causes stretching of the medial layer if the balloon diameter is adequately oversized.
- Microscopic plaque material may become separated and embolize distally. However, this is usually asymptomatic in the peripheral circulation. In carotid artery angioplasty, this phenomenon has potentially more severe consequences.
- Concentric arterial lesions respond well to PTA, because the arterial plaque and the arterial wall layers are dissected in a uniform fashion, which improves the increase in the luminal diameter (Fig. 1 A and B).
- Eccentric arterial lesions may respond less well to balloon dilatation. This is because the wall opposite the plaque is stretched by the balloon rather than the plaque itself (Fig. 1C and D). Once the balloon is deflated, the normal elastic wall may recoil, resulting in an unsatisfactory result.
- Vascular stents provide an internal scaffold for the vessel lumen (Fig. 1 E). The advantages of stents include

  - Rapid, reliable, and sustained increase in the luminal diameter
  - Entrapment of vulnerable plaque material that may cause embolization
  - Elimination of elastic recoil

- A cutting balloon consists of a non-compliant balloon with microblades (atherotomes) mounted longitudinally on its outer surface. The blades are designed to score a lesion during balloon inflation, allowing easier angioplasty at lower pressures. Cutting balloons are used most frequently in hemodialysis patients with graft or fistula-related venous stenoses resistant to standard angioplasty.

R.A. Morgan, E. Walser (eds.), *Handbook of Angioplasty and Stenting Procedures*,
Techniques in Interventional Radiology, DOI 10.1007/978-1-84800-399-6_6,
© Springer-Verlag London Limited 2010

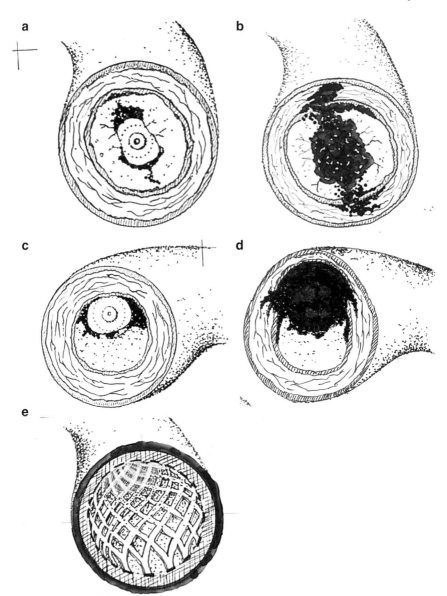

Fig. 1 The mechanism of action of balloon angioplasty in atherosclerotic lesions: (**A**) The balloon catheter is centered in a concentric arterial lesion. (**B**) Balloon dilatation results in uniformly controlled wall dissection with adequate luminal gain. (**C**) The balloon catheter lies within an eccentric arterial lesion. (**D**) After balloon dilatation the wall opposite to the plaque is stretched. (**E**) The stent provides an internal scaffold for the arterial lumen with excellent luminal gain

They may also be used to treat recurrent in-stent stenosis, and peripheral graft anastomotic stenoses if standard PTA is unsuccessful. It is usually necessary to use a conventional balloon after a cutting balloon has been used to achieve the optimal result.

Pre-interventional Work-Up

- A detailed clinical history should be obtained. Information regarding vascular symptoms, relevant comorbidity, (including cardiac disease, renal impairment, diabetes), risk factors for vascular disease, i.e., smoking, hyperlipidemia, and a history of contrast allergy should be ascertained.
- Perform a detailed physical examination. Focus on findings pertinent to vascular disease (palpate pulses, skin temperature, skin lesions, etc).
- Ask about current medication. You may need to stop, change, or modify some medications, e.g., warfarin, insulin, clopidogrel.
- Review all recent vascular imaging studies to decide the optimal site and direction of arterial puncture, i.e., right versus left femoral artery, antegrade versus retrograde puncture.
- Evaluate the morphology of the lesion to select the optimal treatment, i.e., PTA versus stent. As a rule, short stenoses are more likely to respond favorably to PTA, while PTA of long occlusions is associated with lower immediate and long-term success rates. Consider whether a stent would be the better primary treatment instead of PTA.
- If renal insufficiency is present, intravenous hydration should be started the day before the procedure. Consider the use of iso-osmolar contrast agents.
- Consent the patient regarding the alternative treatment modalities, the success and failure rates, and the potential complications.

The Procedure

- The patient is positioned on the angiographic table and draped in a sterile fashion.
- ECG and blood pressure monitoring is commenced before the procedure and is maintained until the patient leaves the interventional suite.
- In some clinical settings, for example in carotid artery stenting, antiplatelet medications such as clopidogrel 75 mg daily, and acetylsalicylic acid 160 mg daily are administered 3–7 days before the procedure, to minimize thrombotic complications and the development of restenosis.

Vascular Access

- The method of vascular access is dependent on the vascular lesion to be treated.
- For arterial interventions cephalad to the inguinal ligament, a retrograde common femoral access is usually employed.
- For infrainguinal arterial interventions, the antegrade common femoral puncture is the preferred access route, although it is also possible to treat these lesions using a cross-over technique from the contralateral femoral artery.
- Other arterial access sites include the axillary artery, the brachial artery, the radial artery, and the popliteal artery. Rarely other arteries, such as the tibial arteries or the radial artery may be used to obtain access.
- Similarly, for the dilatation of venous lesions, i.e., venoplasty, the site of venous access depends on the location of the lesion under treatment.

Crossing of the Lesion

- A vascular sheath is inserted into the access artery.
- The lesion is crossed with a steerable (selective) catheter and an atraumatic guidewire such as a Bentson wire or a hydrophilic guidewire.
- Heparin (3,000–7,000 units) should be administered intravenously or intra-arterially.
- Once the guidewire has crossed the lesion, the catheter is advanced over the guidewire and the guidewire is removed. Care should be taken to always aspirate blood and/or inject contrast medium to confirm that the catheter lies within the lumen of the vessel, as inadvertent subintimal position of the guidewire will jeopardize the success of the intervention.
- Many interventionalists insert a stiff guidewire to provide stability for the insertion of the balloon catheters or for the delivery of stents. In general, angioplasty and stenting are not performed over hydrophilic guidewires, because of the potential for inadvertent movement of these slippery wires, particularly proximally back across the lesion, during exchange of the catheters.
- Care should be taken to make sure that the guidewire is long enough for exchange of the selective catheter and the balloon catheter or stent delivery system. In general, 145 cm long guidewires are seldom long enough. Guidewires of 180- or 260 cm long should be used depending on the distance of the lesion from the point of vascular access.
- Care should also be taken that the guidewire is of the correct diameter for the guidewire lumen of the balloon catheter or stent delivery systems. For example, it is not possible to insert a balloon catheter designed for a 0.018-inch guidewire over a 0.035-inch guidewire.
- A decision regarding whether it would be better to treat the lesion by PTA or stenting may be made before the procedure starts, after angiographic identification of the lesion location and morphology, or in the case of stenting, if PTA fails or makes the lesion worse.

Balloon Angioplasty

- A balloon of appropriate diameter and length should be selected.
- Regarding the balloon diameter, there is little agreement on whether to oversize balloons or not with respect to the native artery diameter. Many interventionalists select balloons 10–20% wider than the native artery diameter.
- Several methods are used for estimation of the vessel diameter:

    ○ Calibrated catheter angiography (Fig. 2).
    ○ Use of the integrated software of the angiography equipment.

- If there is doubt regarding the vessel diameter because the techniques above are not available, it is better to use a balloon of probable smaller diameter than the vessel with the use of a road map. If the balloon is clearly too small, and the post PTA result is unsatisfactory, a larger balloon can be used. This option is better than choosing a balloon that is obviously too large which may cause vessel rupture.
- Many interventionalists select the balloon size using the "Eyeball technique" based on the operator's experience and knowledge of the expected diameter of the vessel to be treated.
- The length of the balloon selected should be adequate to dilate the whole length of the lesion. If a balloon is much longer than the lesion, this will result in dilatation of areas of non-diseased vessel, which should be avoided if possible to minimize

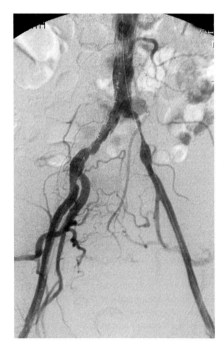

Fig. 2 An aortogram of a patient presenting with disabling left leg claudication depicts a 25-mm long severe stenosis of the left common iliac artery and a mild/moderate stenosis of the right common iliac artery. Bilateral common femoral access has been obtained in order to perform diagnostic angiography and angioplasty at the same setting. A marker pigtail catheter (distance between dots is 1 cm) has been placed from the right groin for accurate measurement of the vessel under treatment

vessel trauma to the normal artery. Conversely, if a short balloon is selected for a much longer lesion, the multiple dilatations required along the entire length of the lesion may be time consuming.

- The location of the balloon on the catheter is indicated by proximal and distal radiopaque markers.
- The balloon catheter is inserted over the guidewire under fluoroscopic guidance. The balloon is centered precisely across the lesion using the radiopaque markers.
- Angioplasty is performed by slow inflation of the balloon with dilute water-soluble contrast.
- The inflation maybe performed using a 5 mL Luer-lock syringe or with a mechanical inflator with or without a pressure gauge. Each technique has its supporters, although there is no evidence that any one method is better or safer than the others.
- With the balloon centered over the lesion, it inflates from the periphery initially, followed by the middle of the balloon as the lesion itself is dilated. Often, the lesion produces a central waist on the balloon causing an hourglass configuration. The elimination of this waist indicates successful dilatation of the stenosis (Fig. 3).
- If the lesion is very narrow and/or fibrotic, the balloon may slip off the lesion during inflation. If this occurs, the balloon catheter shaft should be held firmly where it enters the sheath to prevent it from moving forward or backward.

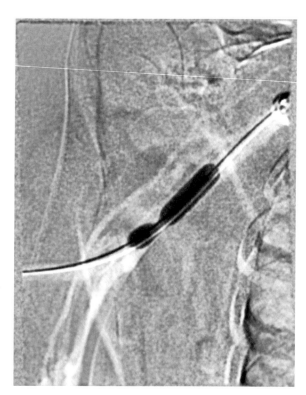

Fig. 3 Balloon angioplasty of a venous stenosis in a patient with dialysis graft. Digital spot image during balloon dilatation depicts the typical hourglass configuration on the balloon caused by the tight venous lesion

- There is no consensus regarding the optimal length of balloon inflation. Inflation times may vary from a few seconds to a minute or more. It is likely that the duration of inflation does not matter in most cases.
- Prolonged inflation times over a minute may be helpful to stabilize vessel dissection after PTA, although there is little evidence to support this.
- The balloon is deflated with a 10–20 mL syringe. If there are air bubbles in the syringe, this will prolong the time to full deflation.
- Once the balloon is fully deflated, it can be moved to the next part of the artery to be dilated.
- It is very important to monitor the pain of the patient during balloon inflation. Usually the balloon inflation causes mild pain caused by stretching of the adventitia. The pain diminishes after balloon deflation. Persistent pain after deflation is very suspicious of vessel rupture (Fig. 4).
- After the entire lesion has been dilated, the balloon catheter should be removed, *while keeping the guidewire across the lesion.* This last point is very important. If the guidewire is removed by mistake back across the lesion, and the lesion requires further treatment because of an inadequate result or a complication (such as distal embolization), it might not be possible to recross the recently treated lesion which might result in procedure failure or a limb-threatening complication.
- After withdrawing the balloon over the guidewire, a post-PTA angiogram should be performed to evaluate the technical result and to check for complications (i.e., arterial rupture, distal embolization) (also see "how to decide the endpoint").
- Angiography should be performed of the run-off vessels as well as the site of PTA, to exclude distal vessel occlusion because of distal embolization of material from the PTA site.
- If the angiogram looks satisfactory, the guidewire can be removed, followed by removal of the sheath, if hemostasis is to be achieved by manual compression. If a closure device is to be used, vessel closure is performed at this time according to the instructions for use of the selected closure device.
- If the lesion involves the origin of an artery just beyond a vessel bifurcation (e.g., right common iliac artery at the aortic bifurcation), there is a theoretical risk of causing an ostial stenosis of the contralateral vessel (i.e., left common iliac artery) by displacement of plaque "across the bifurcation". Some interventionalists advocate protection of the contralateral vessel by placement of a balloon. This is known as the "kissing balloon technique". However, this inevitably involves an additional femoral artery puncture and the potential risk of a complication to the "normal" artery caused by inflation of the "protecting balloon". This practice is controversial and many operators do not use the technique when treating such lesions at bifurcations. If a stent is required to treat a lesion at a bifurcation because the PTA result is suboptimal, many operators opt to place a stent in the opposite artery using the same rationale ("kissing stent technique") (Fig. 5).
- An alternative technique avoiding the risk of trauma to the normal artery is to place a safety wire in the opposite vessel from the contralateral groin until the main lesion has been treated without complication (Fig. 6).

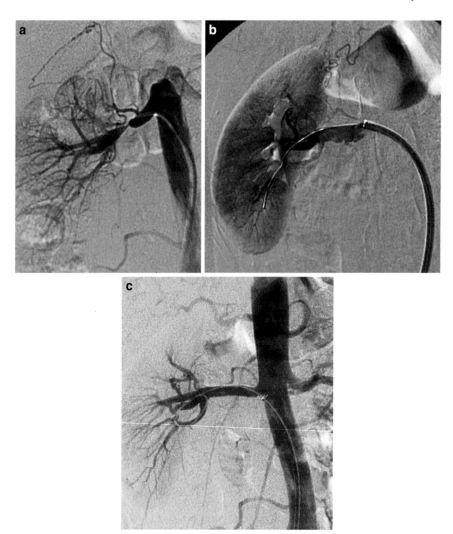

Fig. 4 Rupture of the renal artery during balloon angioplasty of a stenotic lesion in a 27-year-old hypertensive patient. (**A**) Selective DSA of the right renal artery of the patient depicts a tight stenosis suggestive of the intimal type of fibromuscular dysplasia. (**B**) The patient experienced severe persistent pain during and after balloon dilatation using a 6 × 20 mm balloon. Angiography shows extravasation of contrast medium. (**C**) Angiography after placement of a 6 × 25 mm stent graft shows a successful outcome with a patent artery and no evidence of a residual leak

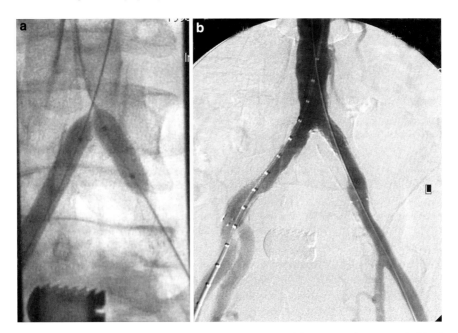

Fig. 5 Use of the kissing balloon technique in the treatment of the same patient shown in Fig. 2 (**A**) Two balloon catheters are simultaneously inflated to treat the severe left common iliac artery lesion and the less severe right common iliac artery lesion. (**B**) DSA after the deployment of two stents, one in each common iliac artery, depicts good patency of both iliac arteries

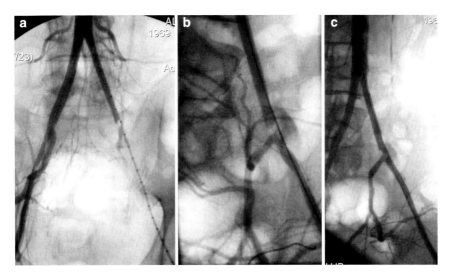

Fig. 6 (**A**) Magnified image of an angiogram of a patient presenting with left leg claudication shows a short common iliac artery lesion involving the origin of the left internal iliac artery. (**B**) A guidewire has been introduced into the left internal iliac artery to protect it against occlusion during stent deployment in the common iliac artery. (**C**) Angiography shows good patency of the left common iliac artery after the deployment of an 8 × 30 mm stent without compromise of the internal iliac artery

How to Decide the Endpoint

- The site of the angioplasty should be carefully examined on the completion angiogram to ensure that the vessel is adequately dilated with no residual stenosis >30%.
- Assessment of the result may involve a visual evaluation of the angiographic result or a combination of angiography and intra-arterial pressure measurements.
- For larger vessels such as the iliac arteries, the majority of interventionalists advocate the measurement of intra-arterial pressures because a reliance on the images alone may be misleading. Pressure measurements in small vessels such as the infrainguinal arteries are less reliable and a visual assessment of the result in this vascular territory is deemed to be adequate.
- Pressure measurements are obtained above and below the site of PTA. This is usually achieved by attaching manometers from a pressure monitor to the side arm of the vascular sheath below the lesion and to a catheter placed across the lesion. In order to enable a pressure reading through the sheath, the catheter should be at least 1F size smaller than the sheath. Alternatively the gradient maybe recorded by withdrawing an end-hole catheter across a lesion.
- Pressure measurements are usually obtained after the intra-arterial injection of a vasodilator such as glyceryl trinitrate (100–150 mcg). A peak-to-peak systolic pressure gradient of 10 mmHg or greater is considered to be hemodynamically significant and an indicator of an inadequate result.

Subintimal Angioplasty

- Stenoses are crossed by passing a guidewire through the lumen of the vessel. In the case of occlusions, it is not always possible to know whether the guidewire has passed though the lumen or within the wall of the vessel. Passage of the guidewire though occlusions within the vessel wall, usually the subintimal space, is known as subintimal angioplasty or percutaneous intentional extraluminal recanalization (PIER).
- There are theoretical benefits of achieving a totally subintimal recanalisation through vessel occlusions because the subintimal space offers a relatively disease-free lumen compared with recanalization of the lumen itself. Thus, many interventionalists aim to intentionally enter the subintimal space proximal to an occlusion to enable subintimal PTA rather than attempt recanalization of the lumen.
- The technique involves the intentional passage of an angled-tip hydrophilic guidewire into the subintimal space proximal to the occlusion by forcibly protruding it through the tip of a catheter (an angled-tip catheter such as a cobra or Berenstein catheter may be helpful), so that it dissects the intima and enters the subintimal space.
- The guidewire is advanced further into the space and a loop is created at the tip. With a loop of approximately 5–10 cm, the guidewire and catheter are advanced

distally until the occlusion is traversed. Once the loop has passed beyond the distal margin of the occlusion, the loop is shortened slightly, and by rapid backward and forwards movements, the guidewire usually easily re-enters the vessel lumen. Re-entry into the lumen is accompanied by a loss of resistance to passage of the guidewire. After re-entry, the dissection plane is dilated with an angioplasty balloon of a suitable size (Fig. 7).

Stents

- The standard indications for stent insertion vary depending on the site of the vascular lesion.
- In many locations, stents are used mainly as a salvage method when the PTA result is unsatisfactory, either as a result of elastic recoil or a flow-limiting dissection of the PTA site. This is known as secondary stenting.
- Primary stenting, without prior PTA, is advocated by many interventionalists in some locations and for some morphological lesions on the basis of evidence of varying quality. For example, ostial renal artery stenosis, iliac artery occlusions, malignant venous obstruction. Some interventionalists treat some lesions by primary stenting in the absence of good supportive evidence, e.g., SFA occlusions. Further discussion regarding the indications for stenting in specific vascular locations will be covered in subsequent chapters.
- Stents may consist of bare metal or may consist of a metallic stent covered with graft material when it is referred to as a stent-graft.
- There are two basic types of stent or stent-graft based on their method of deployment: balloon expandable and self-expanding.
- Although each type of stent may be used in most locations, balloon-expandable stents are useful for treating ostial lesions when a high degree of accuracy is required (i.e., renal ostial lesions).
- Self-expanding stents are often available in longer lengths than balloon-expandable stents, and are useful when long lesions are to be stented. They are also useful if a lesion is very tortuous as they are more flexible, while balloon-expandable stents are usually more rigid.
- Self-expanding stents are resistant to external compression because they re-expand if they are compressed, unlike balloon-expandable stents. Therefore, they are used preferentially to treat lesions in superficial locations.
- Self-expanding stents require dilatation with a balloon of the same diameter after deployment to facilitate their expansion to their full diameter. Clearly, balloon-expandable stents do not require such dilatation as they are fully expanded by balloon dilatation during deployment.
- In general, if a lesion cannot be fully dilated with a balloon because it is so fibrotic, there is no advantage to be gained from placing a stent because there is no guarantee that the stent will be able to expand to its full diameter if the balloon has failed.

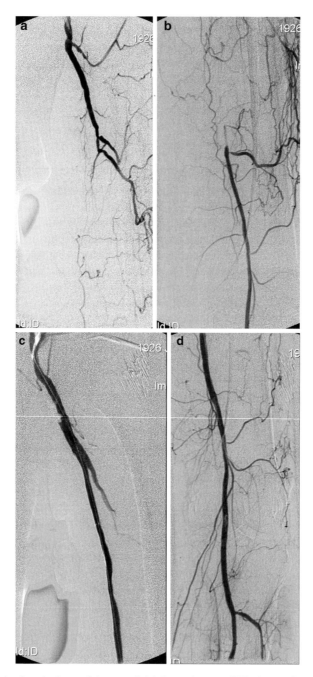

Fig. 7 Subintimal angioplasty of the superficial femoral artery (SFA) in a patient with left leg-disabling claudication. (**A, B**) Selective left leg DSA depicts occlusion of the left SFA with distal reconstitution in the adductor canal. (**C, D**) Selective DSA following subintimal angioplasty depicts successful recanalization of the occluded artery

Complications

- Procedure-related complications occur more often in older patients with acute symptoms, diffuse vascular disease, and concomitant severe illness.

Vessel Rupture

- The most severe complication is vessel rupture (<1%), which is usually self-limiting in the periphery, because the bleeding is subject to tamponade by the surrounding soft tissues.
- However, if the vessel is located in the chest, abdomen, or pelvis where it is not surrounded by muscle and fascia, vessel rupture may be fatal.
- Clinical symptoms suggesting rupture are severe pain experienced by the patient during PTA (which persists after balloon deflation), hypotension, and tachycardia.
- Vessel rupture after PTA of lower extremity arteries usually requires no treatment.
- However, vessel rupture in the chest, abdomen, or pelvis requires treatment in the majority of cases. Immediate balloon re-inflation across the lesion should be performed to stop the bleeding, followed either by placement of a stent-graft to seal the rupture or transfer to the operating theater for surgical repair.
- Every interventional radiologist who performs PTA and stent procedures should keep a selection of stent-grafts to treat vessel rupture if it occurs.

Cholesterol Embolization (CE)

- Cholesterol Embolzation is another severe complication (<1%), which can lead to tissue ischemia and necrosis.
- This may occur if there is a large amount of soft atheromatous plaque lining the walls of the vessel being treated.
- It is likely that some CE occurs in most angioplasty and stent procedures. However, if the volume of cholesterol embolization is high, critical limb ischemia requiring amputation, permanent renal failure, stroke, bowel ischemia, and death may occur.
- Prevention by careful technique and patient selection is the only way to avoid this complication.

Puncture Site Complications

- Hematomas (3–5%)
- Pseudoaneurysms (<0.5%)
- Arteriovenous fistulas (0.05–7.7%)

Stent-Related Complications

Complications related to the use of stents include

- Stent dislodgement during deployment
- Stent migration
- Stent fracture

Restenosis

- Restenosis may occur after PTA alone or may occur within stents (instent restenosis).
- Restenosis may be due to the progression of disease or to the formation of neointimal hyperplasia (NIH).

Key Points

- Eccentric lesions respond less well to PTA.
- Antegrade access is generally preferable to contralateral access for infrainguinal lesions.
- Never withdraw the guidewire back across the lesion before the procedure is finished.
- Always check the run-off vessels at the end of the procedure for distal embolization.
- Stents are indicated if angioplasty fails.
- Primary insertion of stents is indicated in selected cases such as iliac artery occlusions and ostial renal artery stenoses.

Acknowledgements   The authors thank Mr Dimitrios Trakadas M.Arch.NTUA for the preparation of the illustrations.

Suggested Readings

1. Block PC, Myler RK, Stertzer S, et al. (1981) Morphology after transluminal angioplasty in human beings. N Engl J Med 305: 382–385
2. Bolia A (1998) Percutaneous intentional extraluminal (subintimal) recanalization of crural arteries. Eur J Radiol 28: 199–204
3. Bhat R, McBride K, Chakraverty S, Vikram R, Severn A (2007) Primary cutting balloon angioplasty for treatment of venous stenoses in native hemodialysis fistulas: long-term results from three centers. Cardiovasc Intervent Radiol 30: 1166–1170

4. Cole PE, Darcy M (2001) Angioplasty: Pathophysiology and techniques. In: Michael Darcy, Suresh Vedantham, John Kaufman (eds) SCVIR Syllabus: Peripheral vascular interventions 2nd edition, Society of CV and Interventional Radiology, pp. 53–69
5. Kaufman JA (2004) Vascular interventions. In: Kaufman JA, Lee MJ (eds) Vascular & Interventional Radiology: The Requisites, Mosby, Philadelphia, Pennsylvania, pp. 83–118
6. Kinney TB, Rose SC (1996) Intraarterial pressure measurements during angiographic evaluation of peripheral vascular disease: techniques, interpretation, applications, and limitations. Am J Roentgenol 166: 277–284
7. Pentecost MJ, Criqui MH, Dorros G et al. (1994) Guidelines for peripheral percutaneous transluminal angioplasty of the abdominal aorta and lower extremity vessels: a statement for health professionals from a special writing group of the Councils on Cardiovascular Radiology, Arteriosclerosis, Cardio-Thoracic and Vascular Surgery, Clinical Cardiology, and Epidemiology and Prevention, the American Heart Association. Circulation 89: 511–531
8. Reekers JA, Bolia A (1998) Percutaneous intentional extraluminal (subintimal) recanalization: how to do it yourself. Eur J Radiol 28: 192–198
9. Waston HR, Bergqvist D (2000) Antithrombotic agents after peripheral transluminal angioplasty: a review of the studies, methods and evidence for their use. Eur J Vasc Endovasc Surg 19: 445–450

Arterial Closure Devices

Stephen P. D'Souza and Dare M. Seriki

Introduction

- Worldwide, between 7.5 and 8 million catheter-based vascular procedures are performed a year. Only around 20–25% of these procedures utilize a Vascular Closure Device (VCD) for access site hemostasis.
- The use of larger sheaths and the widespread use of periprocedural anticoagulation have increased the risk of bleeding complications, resulting in the need for better methods of hemostasis.
- Complication rates related to hemostasis for diagnostic angiograms range from 0 to 1.1% and increase to 1.3–3.4% for therapeutic procedures.
- While the outcomes of VCD studies have shown increased patient satisfaction, early ambulation and decreased hospital resource utilization, compared with manual compression, there is limited evidence that hemorrhage and other puncture-site complications are reduced by VCDs. Indeed, the use of VCDs is associated with a new group of complications related to the devices themselves.

Manual Compression

- The method considered the gold standard, described by Seldinger et al in 1953, involves manual compression over the puncture site, for 10–30 min, followed by overnight bed rest. This method achieves hemostasis due to the formation of a fibrin and platelet plug following exposure of the blood to the collagen in the arterial wall at the puncture site.
- Traditional bed rest times after manual compression are set arbitrarily.
- The evidence suggests that overnight bed rest is unnecessary. For example, in a study of early mobilization following manual compression of 6F arterial punctures post-angioplasty, 90% of 128 patients were ambulant at 4 h following gradual mobilization after 2 h of supine bed rest. This was achieved with no major puncture-site complications and no delayed complications.

R.A. Morgan, E. Walser (eds.), *Handbook of Angioplasty and Stenting Procedures*, Techniques in Interventional Radiology, DOI 10.1007/978-1-84800-399-6_7, © Springer-Verlag London Limited 2010

Types of Vascular Closure Device

Vascular closure devices fall into two main categories:

1. *Active Devices*
Achieve hemostasis immediately and involve some kind of mechanical seal.

- Suture alone

  ○ Perclose AT and Prostar XL10 (Abbott Vascular, Redwood City, California).

- Extravascular collagen alone
- Suture−collagen combinations

  ○ Angioseal (St. Jude Medical, St. Paul, Minnesota)

- Surgical staple or clip:

  ○ StarClose (Abbott Vascular, Redwood City, California)
  ○ EVS-Angiolink (Medtronic Co., Minneapolis, Minnesota)

2. *Passive Devices*
These do not achieve immediate hemostasis.

- Augmented manual compression:

  ○ External patches with prothrombotic coatings − Syvek Patch, (Marine Polymer Technologies, Danvers, Massacheusetts).
  ○ Wire-stimulated track thrombosis-Boomerang ClosureWire (Cardiva Medical, Mountain View, California).

- Mechanically assisted manual compression − *these will not be discussed further:*

  ○ Femstop − (RADI Medical Systems, Uppsala, Sweden)
  ○ Clamp-ease (Pressure Products, Rancho Palos Verdes, CA)
  ○ Sandbags and pressure dressings

Active Vascular Closure Devices

Prostar XL10 and Perclose A-T

Both are suture-mediated devices and create a purely mechanical seal.

Prostar XL10:

- The device consists of a 10F shaft holding two pairs of needles connected by two braided polyester suture loops and a rotating barrel that is used to facilitate the positioning of the device before needle deployment and to guide the needles during their travel through the subcutaneous tract.

- **Device deployment:**

  1. At the end of the procedure, the sheath is removed and the device is inserted over a standard guidewire.
  2. Dilatation of the subcutaneous tract is needed to accept the oversize barrel.
  3. Correct positioning of the device with the barrel against the arterial wall is confirmed when pulsatile blood exits the marker lumen (this occurs when the distal end of the marker lumen enters the artery).
  4. The needles are deployed, passing from within the device in the arterial lumen through the arterial wall and back into the barrel.
  5. They take the suture ends with them and exit from the top of the device.
  6. The needles are cut from the sutures that are then freed from the device.
  7. The surgical knots are tied using a slipknot. The knots are slipped (pushed) down onto the arterial wall while the device is removed.
  8. The knots are tightened with a knot pusher, achieving hemostasis, and the suture ends are cut short.

- This device can be used to close very large arteriotomies and has been used to perform endovascular aneurysm repair using a totally percutaneous technique without the need for a surgical femoral arteriotomy.
- The availability of the Prostar device varies widely worldwide. At the present time, it is very difficult to acquire the device in the UK.

Perclose A-T (Fig. 1):

- This is a smaller device and is designed to be used to close puncture sites 6–8F in diameter.
- With the Perclose A-T (auto-tie) a slipknot is already created within the device, which enables a more rapid, easier, and single-handed operation.
- The device is inserted over a guidewire, which can be reintroduced during the procedure if a problem is encountered.
- The device can also be used to close larger arteriotomies using the technique known as *predeployment*:

  - Predeployment involves inserting the suture into the arterial wall *at the start of the procedure*.
  - Providing the stitch is not "tied and locked", the puncture site can be dilated to a larger French size.

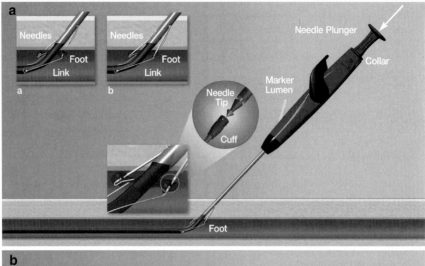

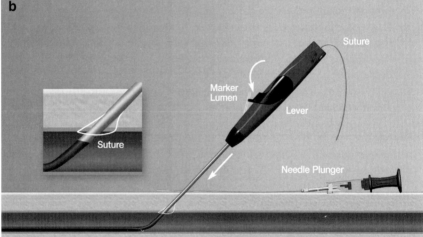

Fig. 1 (**a, b**) Diagrammatic representation of the deployment of a Perclose AT device

  ○ Once the procedure is completed, hemostasis is achieved by the tightening the
     predeployed suture.

• Thus the 6F device can be pre-deployed prior to dilation of an arteriotomy up to
  12F.
• It is also possible to use more than one device at a time in order to close even
  larger arteriotomies.
• Similar to the Prostar XL10, the Perclose A-T can be used to perform endovascular aneurysm repair using a combination of the predeployment technique and
  more than one device.
• Perclose devices have been used successfully to close puncture sites in other
  locations such as the brachial and popliteal arteries.

- The devices have also been used to close inadvertent subclavian artery punctures created during central venous catheter insertion.

Angioseal

This device creates a mechanical seal by sandwiching the arteriotomy between a biodegradable polymer anchor, which remains inside the vessel, and an extravascular collagen sponge. The collagen augments the mechanical seal by inducing platelet adhesiveness and is held in place by a self-tightening suture (Fig. 2).

- The device is available in 6 and 8F versions.
- It consists of a delivery system and three bioabsorbable components.
- The delivery system consists of

  ○ A 0.035-inch guidewire
  ○ An insertion sheath
  ○ A dilator with a marker lumen (which locates the arteriotomy)

- The bioabsorbable components consist of

  ○ A flat 10 mm × 2 mm × 1 mm anchor (footplate)
  ○ A collagen plug
  ○ A suture that maintains tension between these two components

- **Device deployment:**

  1. At the end of the procedure the insertion sheath/dilator combination is inserted over a guide wire.
  2. The sheath is inserted until blood exits from the marker hole at the proximal end of the dilator.

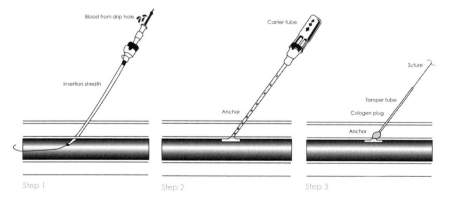

Fig. 2 Diagrammatic representation of the deployment of an Angioseal device

3. The entire system should be gently withdrawn over the guidewire until the passage of blood from the marker hole stops.
4. After this point has been reached, the device should be reinserted 1.5 cm into the artery.
5. The guide wire and dilator are removed.
6. While holding the sheath fixed in position, the carrier tube containing the anchor, plug, and suture is inserted into the sheath.
7. The anchor is deployed into the arterial lumen and is pulled back to abut against the wall of the artery over the arteriotomy site.
8. The carrier tube and the sheath are withdrawn to reveal a tamper tube that is used to tamp the collagen plug against the outer arterial wall and locks into place.
9. The suture is cut below the skin.

- The anchor is reabsorbed in a process that is physically complete at approximately 30 days and chemically complete at approximately 90 days post-procedure.
- Arterial re-puncture within 90 days is not recommended, because of the risk of displacement of the anchor. It may be possible to identify and avoid the anchor using ultrasound, if arterial puncture at the same site is required urgently before this interval.
- The current device is the Angioseal STS PLUS platform.
- A more recent development is the Angioseal VIP (V-twist Integrated Platform). This version features a larger collagen plug that conforms to the vessel by twisting down onto the arterial wall. Apart from this design change the deployment is the same as the STS device.

StarClose

- The StarClose system (Abbott Vascular, Redwood City, California) is designed to deliver a 4 mm diameter nitinol staple onto the outside of the vessel.
- The device can close a 6F puncture site.
- The system is designed for single-operator use and closure time should be less than 60 sec.

Passive VCD

Boomerang ClosureWire

- This is a relatively new device.
- The Boomerang ClosureWire consists of a collapsed nitinol disc on an introducer/deployment wire (Fig. 3).
- Device deployment:

Fig. 3 (**a, b**) Diagrammatic representation of the deployment of a Boomerang CloseWire

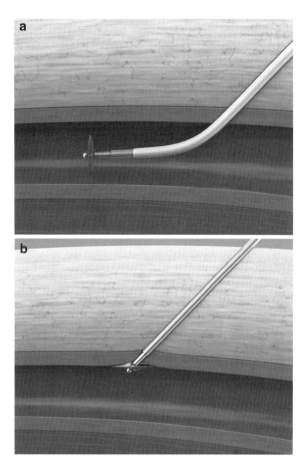

1. The device is introduced into the artery through the sheath at the end of the procedure.
2. Once the wire is in place, the nitinol disc is opened to form a flat, low-profile disc within the vessel.
3. Upon removal of the arterial sheath, the Boomerang disc is positioned against the arterial wall forming a temporary hemostatic seal until the natural elastic recoil of the arteriotomy, known as the Boomerang Effect, returns the arteriotomy to the size of an 18-gauge needle.
4. Following the procedure, the device is completely removed leaving no residual foreign body and minimal scarring.
5. Final hemostasis is achieved by a few minutes of occlusive finger pressure.

- A recent modification of the device, *the Boomerang Catalyst wire*, incorporates an active agent that can initiate hemostasis in the track. The surface of the Boomerang Catalyst wire adjacent to the arteriotomy site has a negatively charged proprietary compound, which activates factor XII thereby promoting hemostasis.

- The device has been used to close arteriotomies up to 10F with only a few minutes of manual compression required following removal of the device.
- The main drawback of the device is that elastic recoil at the arteriotomy site may take 20–30 min and therefore hemostasis may be time consuming, arguably with no tangible benefit versus conventional manual compression.

Patch Technology

In the past there has been some interest in so-called patch technologies which encompass a group of products that augment manual compression:

- They consist of celluloid polymer patches coated with agents that are applied externally and accelerate the coagulation process when blood comes into contact with the patch, along the puncture tract.
- Manual compression is still required.
- However, they have a number of advantages:

  - Ease of use.
  - They can be used in anticoagulated patients.
  - They can be used in patients on anti-platelet therapy.
  - No foreign body is left in situ.
  - There are no stipulations regarding repeat arterial puncture at the same site cf Angioseal.
  - One size fits all.

- At present, there is no clinical evidence that the time to ambulation is reduced with these devices.

Syvec Patch

- The Syvec Patch consists of a celluloid polymer patch coated with poly-N-Acetyl glucosamine (pGlcNAc).
- When it comes into contact with blood, it invokes both clot formation and local vasoconstriction as part of its overall hemostatic effect.
- Following the procedure, the sheath is removed and the saline moistened Syvec Patch is applied and held in place with manual compression for 4 min.
- Manual compression is maintained if blood continues to ooze.
- Once hemostasis is achieved, the patch is left in place with a non-occlusive dressing for 24 h.

D-Stat

- D-Stat uses an adhesive dressing containing thrombin and is available for use in the UK. However, clinical information is limited.
- Application is the same as with the Syvek patch, although the company recommends an initial check after 5 min.
- Once hemostasis is achieved, the patch is left in place with a non-occlusive dressing for 12–24 h.
- The patch can be used for puncture sites up to 8F, and in patients on anticoagulation and/or antiplatelet therapy.

ChitoSeal

- As with the other devices, the ChitoSeal is a topical hemostasis pad. In this case, the active ingredient is Chitosan gel.
- Application is the same as with the other two devices, although the company recommends an initial check after 2–3 min.
- Once hemostasis is established, a dressing is applied and removed within 24 h.

Outcomes

- Published outcome data of closure devices in patients with peripheral vascular disease are relatively limited.
- Published outcomes for passive VCDs are negligible and the limited evidence involves active VCDs.
- Unfortunately, the use of arterial vascular closure devices has not eliminated the occurrence of puncture-site complications.
- In a review of the world literature of VCDs, the minor complication rates are 5.3 and 5.9%, and major complication rates are 1.3 and 4% for Angioseal and Perclose, respectively.
- In a prospective study of 1605 cardiology patients, the major complication rates were 3.2, 2.3, and 1% for Angioseal, Perclose, and manual compression, respectively.
- One of the main problems of such studies is the lack of consistency in the definition of complications, particularly hematoma formation.
- Most of the published data on closure devices relates to cardiology patients. However, complication rates are broadly similar in the few published series of patients with peripheral vascular disease.
- VCD are used in only 20–25% of all catheter-based procedures and the decision to use them is generally based on the potential advantages and disadvantages in each case.

Benefits of VCDS

- Patients with an increased risk of hemorrhage:

  - Large sheath size
  - Long complex procedures
  - Anticoagulation
  - The need for continued anticoagulation immediately post-procedure, e.g., post-carotid stenting.

- Improved catheter laboratory throughput:

  - With the current Perclose, Angioseal, and Starclose devices, hemostasis is usually achieved in minutes.
  - Use of VCDs enables more procedures to be performed on a day-case basis.

- Patient comfort:

  - These devices allow early mobilization and discharge.

Drawbacks of VCDS

- Potentially long learning curve and device/deployment failure:

  - Deployment success rates vary from 86 to 100%, with evidence of increased failure early in the learning curve.
  - Perclose Prostar deployment failure rates vary from 3.6 to 12% of procedures.

- Small vessels (5 mm or less) are unsuitable for active VCDs .
- Non-common femoral artery (CFA) punctures or antegrade CFA punctures may not be suitable for a VCD.
- Peripheral vascular disease (PVD) is a frequent contraindication to use endoluminal components (e.g., Angioseal) as they may promote vessel thrombosis if the native vessel lumen is narrow.
- Device costs.
- Patients may still require bed rest post-closure.
- Impaired or delayed CFA re-puncture with some VCDs.
- Catastrophic complications (1–2%, but may be underreported):

  - Detachment and distal embolization of the footplate of the Angioseal device.
  - The retrograde movement of the needles of the Prostar Perclose devices can result in device entrapment in the heavily scarred groins of patients with prosthetic grafts, requiring surgical removal.

- As all of the collagen plug and suture-mediated closure devices involve leaving a foreign body at the puncture site, there is an increased risk of local infection, especially in the presence of a hematoma.

Conclusions

- As with any situation where there are a number of solutions to a problem, no single method of achieving hemostasis is perfect.
- Without doubt, the most important step in reducing puncture-site complications is good technique and operator experience, both with respect to the initial puncture and the use of the favored closure device.
- The available data make it difficult to recommend the use of closure devices for all patients, but there are certain circumstances and patient types for which their use may be particularly advantageous, such as day-case procedures, patients who are unable to lie flat post-procedure, patients who require immediate post-procedural anticoagulation, and patients who are unable to stop their anti-coagulant medication before a procedure (e.g., patients with prosthetic heart valves).
- Interventional radiologists should become familiar with a few of the available devices and select each device on the basis of each individual patient.

Key Points

- Arterial closure devices have been shown to reduce the time to hemostasis and ambulation. This is associated with reduced length of hospital stay and increased patient satisfaction.
- However, there is no evidence that overall complication rates are reduced compared with manual compression.
- Closure devices are expensive.
- There is a reasonable case for using closure devices for day-case procedures, patients who are unable to lie flat post-procedure, patients who require immediate post-procedural anticoagulation, and patients who are unable to stop their anticoagulant medication before a procedure (e.g., patients with prosthetic heart valves).

Suggested Reading

1. Baim DS, Knopf WD, Hinohara T, et al. Suture-mediated closure of the femoral access site after cardiac catheterization: results of the suture to ambulate and discharge (STAND I and STAND II) trials. Am J Cardiol 2000; 85: 864–869.
2. Berlet MH, Steffen D, Shaughness G, et al. Closure using a surgical closure device of inadvertent subclavian artery punctures during central venous catheter placement. Cardiovasc Intervent Radiol 2001; 24: 122–124.
3. Butterfield JS, Fitzgerald JB, Razzaq R, et al. Early mobilization following angioplasty. Clin Radiol 2000; 55: 874–877.
4. Cooper CL, Miller A. Infectious complications related to the use of the Angio-Seal hemostatic puncture closure device. Cathet Cardiovasc Interv 1999; 48: 301–303.

5. Dauerman HL, Applegate RJ, Cohen DJ. Vascular closure devices: the second decade. J Am Coll Cardiol. 2007; 50: 1617–1626

6. Doyle BJ, Konz BA, Lennon RJ, et al. Ambulation 1 hour after diagnostic cardiac catheterization: a prospective study of 1009 procedures. Mayo Clin Proc 2006; 81: 1537–1540.

7. Duda SH, Wiskirchen J, Erb M, et al. Suture-mediated percutaneous closure of antegrade femoral arterial access sites in patients who have received full anticoagulation therapy. Radiology 1999; 210: 47–52.

8. Eidt JF, Habibipour S, Saucedo JF, et al. Surgical complications from hemostatic puncture closure devices. Am J Surg 1999; 178: 511–516.

9. Gerckens U, Cattelaens N, Lampe EG, et al. Management of arterial puncture site after catheterization procedures: evaluating a suture-mediated closure device. Am J Cardiol 1999; 83: 1658–1663

10. Goyen M, Manz S, Kroger K, et al. Interventional therapy of vascular complications caused by the hemostatic puncture closure device Angio-seal. Catheter Cardiovasc Interv 2000; 49: 142–147.

11. Hoffmann K, Schott U, Erb M, et al. Remote suturing for percutaneous closure of popliteal artery access. Cathet Cardiovasc Diagn 1998; 43: 477–482.

12. Kulick DL, Rediker DE. Use of the Perclose device in the brachial artery after coronary intervention. Catheter Cardiovasc Interv 1999; 46: 111–112.

13. Muller DW, Shamir KJ, Ellis SG, Topol EJ. Peripheral vascular complications after conventional and complex percutaneous coronary interventional procedures. Am J Cardiol 1992; 69: 63–68.

14. O'Sullivan GJ, Buckenham TM, Belli AM. The use of the Angio-Seal hemostatic puncture closure device in high-risk patients. Clin Radiol 1999; 54: 51–55.

15. Rickli H, Unterweger M, Sutsch G, et al. Comparison of costs and safety of a suture-mediated closure device with conventional manual compression after coronary artery interventions. Cathet Cardiovasc Interv 2002; 57: 297–302.

16. Schnyder G, Sawhney N, Whisenant B, et al. Common femoral artery anatomy is influenced by demographics and comorbidity: implications for cardiac and peripheral invasive studies. Cathet Cardiovasc Interv. 2001; 53: 289–295

17. Seldinger SI. Catheter replacement of the needle in percutaneous arteriography. Acta Radiol 1953; 39: 366–376

18. Shrake KL. Comparison of major complication rates associated with four methods of arterial closure. Am J Cardiol 2000; 85: 1024–1025.

19. Silber S, Tofte AJ, Kjellevand TO, et al. Final report of the European multi-center registry using the Duett vascular sealing device. Herz 1999; 24: 620–623.

20. Silber S. 10 years of arterial closure devices: a critical analysis of their use after PTCA. Z Kardiol 2000; 89: 383–389.

21. Strategic growth opportunities in cardiovascular interventional treatment drives cardiology sector. American Health Consultants. BBI Newsletter. 2001; 5: 1–6.

22. Waksman R, Spencer BK III, Douglas JS, et al. Predictors of groin complications after balloon and new device intervention. Am J Cardiol 1995; 75: 886–889

23. Warren BS, Warren SG, Miller SD. Predictors of complications and learning curve using the Angio-Seal closure device following interventional and diagnostic catheterization. Catheter Cardiovasc Interv 1999; 48: 162–166.

Aortoiliac Angioplasty and Stenting

Robert A. Hieb

Diagnostic Evaluation

Clinical

- Aortoiliac occlusive disease often presents as hip, buttock, or thigh claudication. Diminished or absent femoral pulses as well as impotence in men may also be noted. This constellation of findings is known as the "Leriche Syndrome."
- Hypoplastic aortoiliac syndrome is a similar situation often seen in middle-aged women with a significant smoking history and consists of a severe stenosis at the terminal abdominal aorta extending into both common iliac arteries. The syndrome is thought to represent congenital hypoplasia of the distal aorta aggravated by tobacco-induced occlusive disease.
- Aortoiliac disease may also be seen as part of more global atherosclerotic vascular disease in patients with multilevel disease and critical limb ischemia.
- Stigmata of distal embolization in the so-called blue toe syndrome may also be seen even in the absence of significant stenosis. These patients may not describe pre-existing claudication.
- As with peripheral vascular disease in general, the prevalence of aortoiliac occlusive disease increases with age and is more common in men than in women.
- Patients usually describe hip, buttock, and thigh claudication, which may be unilateral or bilateral and occasionally will proceed to calf claudication if challenged.
- Clinical symptoms of peripheral vascular disease can be classified using Fontaine's stages or Rutherford's categories (Table 1).
- Note of the severity and duration of the symptoms, as well as aggravating and alleviating factors should be made. An understanding of the impact of the symptoms on the patient's life is essential.
- A focused history with respect to the patient's risk factors for peripheral arterial disease should also be obtained. Well-known risk factors for peripheral vascular disease include increased age (males over age 60 and females over 70), male gender, family history of peripheral vascular disease, stroke or myocardial infarction, diabetes mellitus, chronic hypertension, tobacco use hypercholesterolemia, and coronary artery disease.

R.A. Morgan, E. Walser (eds.), *Handbook of Angioplasty and Stenting Procedures*,
Techniques in Interventional Radiology, DOI 10.1007/978-1-84800-399-6_8,
© Springer-Verlag London Limited 2010

Table 1 Fontaine's stages and Rutherford's categories of chronic lower limb ischemia

Fontaine		Rutherford		
Stage	Clinical	Grade	Category	Clinical
I	Asymptomatic	O	0	Asymptomatic
IIa	Mild claudication	I	1	Mild claudication
IIb	Moderate to severe claudication	I	2	Moderate claudication
		I	3	Severe claudication
III	Ischemic rest pain	II	4	Ischemic rest pain
IV	Ulceration or gangrene	III	5	Minor tissue loss
		III	6	Major tissue loss

Reprinted from Norgren L. et al. [3].

- Physical examination should include a complete pulse examination as well as auscultation for carotid, abdominal, and femoral bruits. Decreased or absent femoral pulses are commonly found; however, the femoral pulses may be normal or near normal occasionally.
- At a minimum, bedside ankle/brachial indices (ABIs) should be obtained. Ideally, a complete vascular laboratory evaluation with ABIs and segmental limb pressures should be performed. An ABI ≤0.90 is diagnostic of peripheral vascular disease. Treadmill testing is useful in the setting of claudication and relatively normal physical examination and resting ABIs. Post-exercise ABIs demonstrate an abrupt decrease in lower extremity pressures with a prolonged recovery to normal. Exercise ABIs can help separate claudication from other causes of lower extremity symptoms.

Laboratory

- Routine laboratory evaluation as would be obtained prior to any endovascular procedure is all that is required for aortoiliac intervention. Attention should be given to the patient's renal function, coagulation status, and known allergies.

Imaging

- CTA (computed tomographic angiography) and MRA (magnetic resonance angiography) are the preferred modalities for imaging peripheral vascular disease. Both are well suited for aortoiliac disease and are often combined with "runoff" examinations to evaluate the infrainguinal anatomy. Physician preference, institutional expertise or capabilities, as well as patient factors may dictate the modality of choice. In general, MRA is best for calcific disease and for patients with allergy to iodinated contrast material, while CTA is best for arterial aneurysms/dissections and in patients with pacemakers or claustrophobia.

- Catheter angiography is rarely used for diagnostic imaging unless combined with an intervention or in those rare cases where all contrast must be avoided necessitating CO_2 angiography (i.e., severe renal dysfunction).

Endovascular Treatment of Aortoiliac Occlusive Disease

Indications

- The primary indication for aortoiliac intervention is significant lifestyle limiting claudication or limb salvage in the setting of critical limb ischemia and multi-level disease.
- Mild claudication symptoms may require no therapy, but rather optimal medical management and reduction of the patient's general cardiovascular risk factors. The overall health and activity level of the patient should also be considered.
- Another indication is stent placement over complex/ulcerated aortoiliac atheromata responsible for distal embolization in the "blue toe syndrome"
- Endovascular treatment of aortoiliac stenosis as an inflow procedure for either extra anatomic or femoral bypass is also appropriate. Treatment of so-called inflow lesions prior to bypass are often performed as a "hybrid" procedure at the same setting.
- Aortoiliac intervention may also be performed either preoperatively for renal transplant surgery or postoperatively in the setting of stenosis proximal to a transplant renal artery mimicking renal artery stenosis.

Contraindications

- Most contraindications for aortoiliac interventions are relative. However, as with any endovascular procedure, the risk/benefit ratio must be evaluated with clear benefit anticipated for the patient.
- Life-threatening contrast allergy, severe renal insufficiency in a patient not yet on dialysis, as well as uncorrectable coagulopathies can be considered medical contraindications.
- Relative anatomic contraindications include ipsilateral common femoral artery occlusion, severe aneurysmal disease, or the lack of appropriate, safe arterial access.

Alternative Therapies

- Monitored exercise program such as daily walking or treadmill programs.
- Risk factor reduction such as smoking cessation (with or without pharmacologic adjuncts), glycemic and blood lipid control, as well as hypertension management

are recommended for all patients with symptomatic peripheral vascular disease. Antiplatelet therapy in the simple form of one aspirin per day is indicated for all patients tolerant of this. For patients who are only mildly symptomatic, such risk factor modification may be all that is indicated. Pletal (Cilostazol) has been shown to improve walking distances in claudicants, especially when coupled with a supervised exercise program.

- Despite the excellent 3- and 5-year primary patencies for endovascular interventions, young patients who have severe bilateral iliac occlusive disease and who are healthy enough to undergo surgery may benefit from consideration for aortobifemoral bypass. This is especially true if there is significant concomitant common femoral artery disease – also easily corrected during open surgical bypass.
- Combined open surgical and endovascular procedures (so-called hybrid procedures) such as a common femoral endarterectomy and an iliac intervention are often performed in the setting of significant common femoral disease.
- Extra-anatomic bypasses such as axillofemoral and crossed femoral bypasses have acceptable 5-year patencies (50–75%) and may be the best option for patients without endovascular or other surgical options.

Patient Preparation

- Full-informed consent from the patient regarding the nature of the procedure, the intended outcome, as well as the potential risks and complications should be obtained. Alternative forms of therapy should be discussed.
- Both groins should be sterilely prepared, as bilateral retrograde femoral artery access is frequently needed.
- Placement of a urinary bladder catheter should be considered, especially if the procedure is expected to be lengthy. A large amount of excreted contrast in the bladder may interfere with imaging and increase pelvic radiation exposure.

Relevant Anatomy

Normal Anatomy

- The aorta enters the abdominal cavity at the level of T12 through the diaphragmatic hiatus. It continues along the left anterolateral aspect of the spine until approximately the L4 vertebral level, where it bifurcates into the common iliac arteries. The common iliac arteries subsequently divide into the internal iliac arteries, which supply the pelvis and the external iliac arteries, which continue to the level of the inguinal ligament, where they become the common femoral arteries.

- Disease in the abdominal aorta is typically found in the infrarenal segment. The pattern of occlusive disease may either be focal or diffuse with involvement of the entire aorta and iliac system. Occasionally, both aneurysmal and occlusive disease are seen in the same patient.

Aberrant Anatomy

- Aberrant anatomy is usually not a factor in treatment of aortoiliac occlusive disease. Rarely, however, absent or very short common iliac artery segments may be seen. Other rare anatomic variants exist, such as a persistent sciatic artery (runoff to the popliteal artery originates as a branch of the internal iliac artery) with an absent or hypoplastic external iliac artery.

Equipment

- The importance of adequate imaging in treating aortoiliac disease cannot be overstated. The relative depth of the anatomy in question, as well as the frequent presence of overlying bowel gas can be challenging with suboptimal equipment. A large field of view image intensifier or flat panel system is desirable for complete evaluation of the aortoiliac system. Digital subtraction capabilities as well as the ability to perform carbon dioxide angiography are also useful.
- Multi side-hole catheters ("pigtails") are useful for complete angiographic evaluation as well as for accurate measurement of pressure gradients. Complex, long-segment stenoses, and occlusions may require hydrophilic torqueable wires, directable catheters of various shapes, or chronic total occlusion (CTO) devices for successful recanalization. Occasionally re-entry devices to regain access to the true lumen may be necessary after inadvertent subintimal passage.
- In addition, longer sheaths (25 cm), as well as flexible sheaths for contralateral interventions are essential. Radiopaque distal markers on sheaths are most useful.

Pre-procedure Medications

- There is no consensus (or data) regarding pre procedural antiplatelet therapy for patients undergoing aortoiliac intervention. However, many patients are already on some form of antiplatelet therapy either as part of medical management of their vascular disease or because of a prior endovascular intervention. There is no need to withhold these medications prior to angiographic evaluation or intervention.

- Occasionally, pre procedural anxiolysis with oral benzodiazepines is helpful for patients who are overly anxious.
- Routine antibiotic prophylaxis is not warranted. Some advocate prophylactic use of antibiotics for especially long cases with multiple catheter exchanges, for patients receiving overnight catheter-directed thrombolysis, or when puncturing a prosthetic graft.

Procedure

Access

- Use of the patient's history, physical examination findings, noninvasive testing, and pre procedural imaging is mandatory in order to best plan the approach for aortoiliac revascularization.
- Ipsilateral retrograde common femoral artery access is often the easiest and most convenient, provided that the pre-procedural imaging is adequate. If such imaging is inadequate or unavailable, the standard practice of retrograde access on the side of absent or reduced symptoms is favored for thorough diagnostic arteriographic evaluation and subsequent intervention. Bilateral common femoral access is frequently needed when treating long segment occlusions.
- Fluoroscopic marking of the puncture site is helpful to prevent access related complication. The use of ultrasound guidance may also be beneficial.
- Arterial access from other than the common femoral artery (CFA) approach, such as the brachial or axillary arteries is occasionally needed but should be done carefully due to the increased risk of access related complication.

Angiography

- Flush aortic evaluation with a pigtail or other multi side-hole catheter positioned above the level of the renal arteries is essential for complete evaluation of the abdominal aorta. Digital subtraction technique and rapid filming (3–4 frames per second) is routine.
- Conventional iodinated contrast and/or carbon dioxide angiographic techniques may be used depending on the clinical scenario.
- In the setting of aortic stenosis, lateral aortography may be useful to better profile the extent and severity of the lesion.
- Bilateral oblique pelvic angiography allows for complete evaluation of the distal aorta, the iliac, and femoral arteries, as well as their respective bifurcations. The importance of the appearance of the common femoral arteries when contemplating or performing an aortoiliac intervention cannot be overstated. These vessels not only serve as the runoff for the intervention, but if highly diseased, are also much better addressed surgically.

Intra-procedural Medications

- Diagnostic and therapeutic catheter-based procedures are typically performed with local anesthesia at the puncture site and mild conscious sedation with monitoring of blood pressure, heart rate, ECG, and oxygen saturation.
- Generally, once the lesion has been crossed or the interventional sheath has been placed, systemic heparinization is performed with a weight-based IV bolus of heparin (generally 80 units per kilogram). Occasionally for straightforward lesions, empiric heparin dosing of 2,000–4,000 units may be administered. The routine use of anticoagulants with other agents such as glycoprotein IIb/IIIa receptor antagonists is not indicated.
- If acute or subacute thrombus complicates an underlying lesion, thrombolytic therapy may be indicated prior to definitive angioplasty or stent placement.
- Vasospasm in the aortoiliac segments requiring vasodilator therapy is rare.

Lesion Characterization and Location

Morphology

- Aortoiliac lesions cover the spectrum from short-segment focal concentric lesions to long-segment irregular complex stenoses or occlusions.
- The Trans-Atlantic Inter-Society Consensus Document on Management of Peripheral Arterial Disease (TASC) was first published in 2000. This multispecialty document made recommendations regarding the treatment of chronic iliac lesions based on outcomes data. It was revised in 2007; (TASC II − Intersociety Consensus for the management of PAD) (Fig. 1).

Location

- Aortoiliac occlusive disease can be seen anywhere from the renal arteries to the level of the common femoral arteries. Disease involving multiple levels is not unusual, nor is bilateral disease.
- FMD (fibromuscular dysplasia) is typically limited to the external iliac arteries.

Hemodynamics

- Pressure measurements are exceedingly useful when evaluating an area of stenosis.
- Commonly used criteria for determining a significant pressure gradient is a resting gradient of 10 mmHg peak systolic pressure or 5 mmHg mean pressure gradient across a lesion. Others consider a 10% systolic pressure drop across a lesion as significant.

Type A lesions

· Unilateral or bilateral stenoses of CIA
· Unilateral or bilateral single short (≤3 cm) stenosis of EIA

Type B lesions:

· Short (≤3cm) stenosis of infrarenal aorta
· Unilateral CIA occlusion
· Single or multiple stenosis totaling 3–10 cm involving the EIA not extending into the CFA
· Unilateral EIA occlusion not involving the origins of internal iliac or CFA

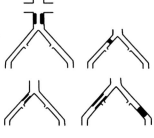

Type C lesions

· Bilateral CIA occlusions
· Bilateral EIA stenoses 3–10 cm long not extending into the CFA
· Unilateral EIA stenosis extending into the CFA
· Unilateral EIA occlusion that involves the origins of internal iliac and/or CFA
· Heavily calcified unilateral EIA occlusion with or without involvement of origins of internal iliac and/or CFA

Type D lesions

· Infra-renal aortoiliac occlusion
· Diffuse disease involving the aorta and both iliac arteries requiring treatment
· Diffuse multiple stenoses involving the unilateral CIA, EIA, and CFA
· Unilateral occlusions of both CIA and EIA
· Bilateral occlusions of EIA
· Iliac stenoses in patients with AAA requiring treatment and not amenable to endograft placement or other lesions requiring open aortic or iliac surgery

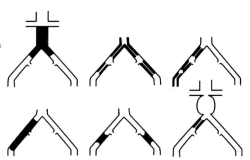

Fig. 1 TASC classification of aorto-iliac lesions. CIA-Common iliac artery; EIA-external iliac artery; CFA-common femoral artery; AAA-abdominal aortic aneurysm. (Reprinted from Norgren et al. [3], with permission from Elsevier.)

• When simultaneously measuring pressures, there should ideally be a 2 Fr size difference between the catheter and sheath for reliable pressure gradient assessment.
• A confounding factor when evaluating pressure gradients may be severely diseased outflow, especially at the level of the common femoral artery.
• Augmentation of the pressure gradient to simulate changes in blood flow with exercise can be done by the intra-arterial administration of a vasodilator.

Nitroglycerine 100 mcg or papaverine 25 mg may be used. A peak systolic pressure gradient of 10–15 mmHg post-vasodilator administration is significant.

Choice of Percutaneous Transluminal Angioplasty (PTA) or Stent Placement

- Lesion morphology will largely determine the optimal treatment. Overall, stenting provides for better initial technical results and may provide for better long-term outcome. Some practitioners prefer selected stenting for suboptimal PTA rather than routine primary stenting.
- Dense calcification and aortic bifurcation lesions may be better treated with balloon-expandable stents due to their resistance to recoil and superior accuracy in deployment. In general a 1:1 sizing ratio is used.
- Self-expanding stents require less precise sizing and are typically slightly oversized. They are superior in areas of size discrepancy over the length of the treated segment such as in post-stenotic dilatation or combined mild aneurysmal and occlusive disease.
- Self-expanding stents may also be favored in excessively tortuous anatomy, such as the external iliac artery, which may be more prone to dissection.
- Covered stents are rarely needed with the exception of combined aneurysmal and occlusive disease, in the setting of arterial rupture, or in the setting of arterial fistulae.

Endovascular Procedure

Crossing the Lesion

- Use of reference images or road-mapping guidance in the projection which best profiles the lesion is helpful.
- Complex, long-segment stenoses, and occlusions require torqueable wires or hydrophilic wires along with a directional catheter to help steer or direct the wire in the desired path. Recanalization of occlusions is typically in an ipsilateral retrograde fashion followed by a contralateral antegrade approach if necessary.
- Specialized chronic total occlusion (CTO) devices as well as re-entry catheters are occasionally needed to cross the occlusion and to re-enter the true lumen.

Deploying the Stent/Balloon

- Confirmatory angiography and use of bony or other landmarks is helpful for accurate positioning of the stent
- An insufflation device is used with angioplasty, stent deployment, or post-stent dilatation to accurately monitor inflation pressures. Resolution of the waist is

desired, but care should be taken with inflation pressures >10 atmospheres, especially in heavily calcified lesions.

- Pain is unusual and can be a sign of stretching of the artery and impending rupture. Pain should resolve on balloon deflation.
- While "kissing stent" techniques (bilateral common iliac stents extending into the aorta) are often needed for bifurcation lesions, care should be taken not to extend the stents any farther than necessary into the aorta as this negatively influences long-term patency.
- Additionally, except in unusual circumstances, one should avoid placing stents across the inguinal ligament.

Endpoint

- Complete to near complete effacement of the lesion is desired. Mild residual stenosis, <30% is acceptable in densely calcified lesions. Pressures are often useful to confirm resolution of the trans-stenotic gradient.
- Angiographic evaluation of the more distal runoff is desirable to exclude complications such as distal embolization.

Post-procedure Care

Immediate

- Establishing safe, reliable hemostasis following the procedure is paramount, whether by manual compression or with the use of one of any number of available closure devices.
- While the use of vascular closure devices has become commonplace, familiarity with the device(s) and their limitations is essential to avoid complications.
- As these procedures are typically performed in an outpatient setting, recovery in a post-procedure care unit from 2–6 h is routine. There should be a low threshold for admission for observation in the case of suspected complication or in a patient with significant co-morbidities.

Follow-up and Post-procedure Medications

- Patients should be seen in follow up within approximately 2 weeks after intervention. Post intervention physical examination and ABIs are important as a new baseline. Over the course of longitudinal follow up, a decrease of >0.15 in the ABI is typically used to suggest restenosis.

- Most patients are placed on aspirin (81 mg daily) or Plavix (75 mg daily) after aortoiliac intervention. This is done in the absence of specific data, but is recommended as part of optimal medical therapy to reduce the overall risk of in-stent restenosis or thrombosis

Results

- Both the initial and long-term results of aortoiliac intervention are excellent. Initial technical success in general is approximately 95–100%. Primary patencies and 3 and 5 years have been reported in the 70–85% range.
- Numerous studies have been performed to look at PTA, primary stenting as well as selective stenting for PTA failures. In general, the results favor stenting compared to PTA alone. There is also less re-intervention required with stenting than with PTA alone. Approximately 30–45% of lesions treated with PTA alone will require stenting either initially due to suboptimal result or over time due to restenosis.
- Factors which negatively influence patency include critical limb ischemia, poor runoff, long segment disease, smoking and chronic renal failure with hemodialysis. Women who are taking hormone replacement therapy also have reduced primary patency rates.

Complications

- Significant complications, especially those requiring operative intervention are uncommon (<2%), with major complication rates approaching 6%. Many complications are access-site related and can be avoided with meticulous attention to both the arterial puncture and obtaining hemostasis at the end of the procedure.
- Puncture-site-related hematomas require close monitoring of the affected limb and the patient's vital signs. With large hematomas, serial measurement of hemoglobin and hematocrit is indicated.
- As many as 90% of puncture-related pseudoaneurysms <3 cm in size will resolve spontaneously. Follow-up ultrasound to ensure resolution is warranted. For those pseudoaneurysms that are large, symptomatic, or do not resolve spontaneously, ultrasound-guided thrombin injection (approximately 1000 units) is a safe and very effective method of treatment.
- Distal embolization occurs rarely but can be a devastating complication. An attempt at catheter or device aspiration should be made. Thrombolytic therapy is probably of little benefit unless a significant thrombotic component is suspected. Meticulous attention to careful wire and catheter manipulation, as well as appropriate anticoagulation can reduce this risk.

- Arterial rupture occurs rarely, but may have catastrophic consequences. Thankfully in the era of modern endograft availability, these can usually be treated endovascularly without serious sequelae. Maintaining wire access across the lesion is obviously paramount until completion angiography demonstrates no evidence of such complication.

Key Points

- Attention to the patient's symptoms, physical examination, and pre procedural imaging is necessary for successful aortoiliac intervention.
- Safe appropriate access and complete arteriographic evaluation with the use of pressure measurements of all significant lesions will improve success and reduce the risk of complication.
- Adequate anticoagulation, especially in the setting of complex recanalizations is essential.
- Follow up of patients with post-procedural examination and new baseline ABIs is mandatory for objective follow up of the intervention. Although the initial and long-term results of aortoiliac interventions are excellent, restenosis can occur. As most of these lesions are amenable to re-intervention, patients deserve longitudinal follow up to ensure the best long-term outcome.

Suggested Reading

1. Klein WM, van der Graaf Y, Seegers J, et al. Dutch iliac stent trial: log-term results in patients randomized for primary or selective stent placement. Radiology, 2006 Feb; 238(2):734–744, Epub 2005 Dec 21.
2. Kudo T, Chandra FA, Ahn SS. Long-term outcomes and predictors of iliac angioplasty with selective stenting. J Vasc Surg, 2005 Sep; 42(3), 466–475.
3. Norgren L, Hiatt WR, Dormandy JA, et al. Inter-Society Consensus for the Management of Peripheral Arterial Disease (TASC II). J Vasc Surg, 2007; 45(1), Supplement S.
4. Park KB, So YS, Kim DI, et al. The transatlantic intersociety consensus (TASC) classification of system in iliac arterial sent placement: long-term patency and clinical limitations. J Vasc Inter Radiol, 2007; 18, 193–201.

Angioplasty and Stenting of the Superficial Femoral Artery and Popliteal Artery

Anna-Maria Belli

Clinical Features

Disease in the superficial femoral artery (SFA) and popliteal artery (PA) may be isolated to a short segment or may involve the whole length of both vessels:

- The clinical symptoms should be taken into account when considering whether or not to treat the disease.
- Long occlusions in one or both of these arteries should only be treated when clinical symptoms are severe, and not when symptoms are relatively mild.
- Occlusions involving the entire SFA and PA can be treated by endovascular treatment, although these lesions are more commonly treated surgically.
- It is important to ensure that significant inflow disease (aortoiliac disease) has been excluded or treated before a lesion in the femoropopliteal segment is treated.
- Long-term patency after intervention depends on the quality of the outflow. At least one continuous artery to the foot is required.
- Technical failure is more likely in heavily calcified arteries. Therefore, treatment of lesions in heavily calcified vessels should only be considered if symptoms are very severe.

Diagnostic Evaluation

Clinical

- Ensure that during the consent process, the patient understands the aim of the treatment and possible adverse outcomes (including limb loss), and has realistic expectations of the potential benefits of intervention.
- If you are treating a claudicant, ensure that they are on best medical therapy (see Chapter "Drugs – Pre-, Peri- and Post-intervention"), have stopped smoking, and have failed conservative measures such as a program of exercise, before proceeding to intervention.
- Ensure that there is no history of contrast allergy.

R.A. Morgan, E. Walser (eds.), *Handbook of Angioplasty and Stenting Procedures*,
Techniques in Interventional Radiology, DOI 10.1007/978-1-84800-399-6_9,
© Springer-Verlag London Limited 2010

Laboratory

The following should be obtained before intervention:

- Hb
- Platelets
- INR
- Serum urea and creatinine

Imaging

- The pre-procedural imaging should be reviewed to plan the intervention, e.g., the site of access.
- Duplex ultrasound is the main method of imaging used by most centers.
- CTA and MRA are being increasingly used as the first non-invasive imaging test.

Indications

- TASC 2 categories A–D (Fig. 1):
- Critical limb ischemia
- Lifestyle-limiting claudication

Contraindications

Absolute:

- There are no absolute contraindications.
- However, it would be unusual for claudicants to be treated if their claudication distance was greater than 200 yards.

Relative contraindications include:

- Allergy to iodinated contrast medium:

  - Carbon dioxide and MR contrast agents can be used instead.
  - Depending on the severity of disease and local expertise, ultrasound can be used to guide intervention.

- Severe renal impairment:

  - Contrast-induced nephrotoxocity can be avoided by ensuring that the patient is hydrated, by minimizing iodinated contrast volume and the use of carbon dioxide.

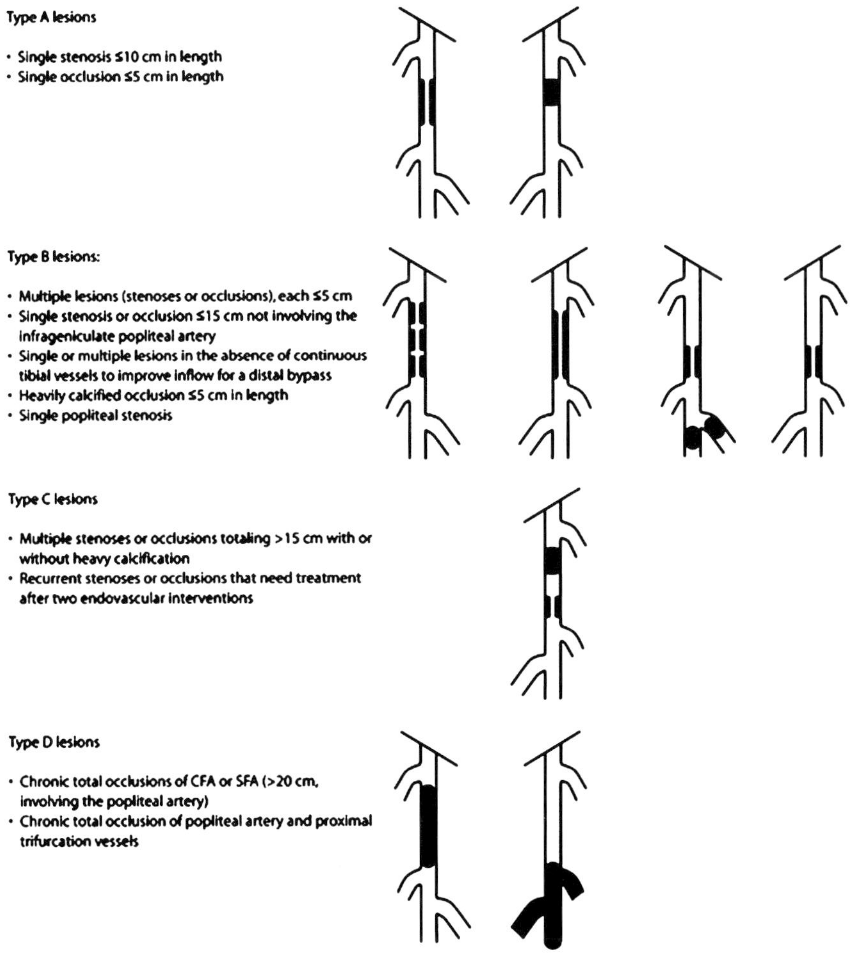

Type A lesions

- Single stenosis ≤10 cm in length
- Single occlusion ≤5 cm in length

Type B lesions:

- Multiple lesions (stenoses or occlusions), each ≤5 cm
- Single stenosis or occlusion ≤15 cm not involving the infragenkulate popliteal artery
- Single or multiple lesions in the absence of continuous tibial vessels to improve inflow for a distal bypass
- Heavily calcified occlusion ≤5 cm in length
- Single popliteal stenosis

Type C lesions

- Multiple stenoses or occlusions totaling >15 cm with or without heavy calcification
- Recurrent stenoses or occlusions that need treatment after two endovascular interventions

Type D lesions

- Chronic total occlusions of CFA or SFA (>20 cm, involving the popliteal artery)
- Chronic total occlusion of popliteal artery and proximal trifurcation vessels

Fig. 1 TASC classification of femoral and popliteal lesions. "Reprinted from Norgren et al. [2], with permission from Elsevier."

Patient Preparation

- Patients should be hydrated and allowed to drink clear fluids up to the time of the procedure, but should have had no solid food for 6 h before the procedure.
- They should have been given a patient information leaflet and consented by a member of the team familiar with the technique, its aims, and potential complications with plenty of time for consideration and questions before the time of the procedure.
- They should be aware of alternative therapies and understand why they are undergoing PTA as opposed to an alternative therapy.

- A venous line should be established. An 18-gauge (green) cannula in a peripheral vein is required for rapid delivery of fluids or blood in the event of a hemorrhagic complication.
- If the patient is taking warfarin, it should be discontinued 72 h before an elective PTA.

  ○ If PTA is urgent, warfarin can be reversed by Vitamin K or fresh frozen plasma. It is safe to proceed if the INR is 2.5 or less.
  ○ If continuous anticoagulation is required, heparin should be given.
  ○ Heparin should be stopped 3 h before PTA and the activated clotting time (ACT) checked.

Relevant Anatomy

Normal Anatomy

- The common femoral artery runs across the medial half of the femoral head, and usually bifurcates into the profunda femoris and superficial femoral artery at the level of the lower half of the femoral head.
- The superficial femoral artery (SFA) does not have any major branches. Collateral vessels occur above the site of occlusive disease.
- The SFA becomes the popliteal artery as it passes through the adductor canal, just above the level at which the vessel crosses the cortex of the lower femur on AP fluoroscopy.
- The PA terminates below the knee joint where it usually divides into the anterior tibial artery and the tibioperoneal trunk (aka common peroneal artery).

Aberrant Anatomy

- The femoral bifurcation can be high, leaving no room to access the common femoral artery below the inguinal ligament. In this case direct, puncture of the SFA, or a contralateral femoral puncture is required.
- Occasionally, a persistent sciatic artery is the main supply to the leg. This occurs when the embryonic supply fails to regress and the femoral system fails to develop. The sciatic artery arises from the internal iliac artery, leaving the pelvic cavity through the lower part of the greater sciatic foramen. It passes to the posterior compartment of the thigh where it continues as the popliteal artery.
- The popliteal artery may terminate in a true trifurcation where it divides into the anterior tibial, the peroneal, and the posterior tibial arteries.
- There may be anomalous high origins of any of the infrapopliteal arteries from the proximal popliteal artery.

Equipment

The equipment required is the standard equipment required for any invasive vascular procedure:

- 18/19-gauge arterial puncture needle.
- Guidewires – a standard 0.035-inch guidewire and a 0.035-inch hydrophilic guidewire are usually the only guidewires required.
- A 180 cm long stiff guidewire (e.g., Amplatzerstiff) for support if access is from the contralateral femoral artery.
- Introducer sheath: 4–6F.
- Selective catheters to guide and support the wire, e.g., cobra or Berenstein. A straight catheter may also be useful.
- Balloon catheters – usually 5 or 6 mm diameter for the SFA and 4 or 5 mm diameter for the PA. Balloon lengths of at least 4 cm should be used. Longer balloons can be used for long lesions, although they should not be much longer than the length of the lesion as dilatation of normal segments of vessel is undesirable.
- For balloon inflation, use a 5 cc Luer lock syringe with half strength contrast medium.
- High-pressure balloons may be required in resistant, calcified, or restenotic lesions. Cutting balloons may also be of value in these resistant lesions.
- An inflation device with a pressure gauge is used to inflate the balloon to the required pressure when using a high-pressure or cutting balloon.
- If stenting is required, select a self-expanding stent 1 mm diameter greater than the diameter of the artery and long enough to avoid placing more than 2 stents.
- Self-expanding and not balloon expandable stents should be used in the SFA and the PA.
- Examples of stents for use in the femoropopliteal segment include the Smart stent (Cordis, Hamburg, Germany), Luminexx stent (Bard Angiomed, Karlsruhe, Germany), Absolute stent (Abbott Vascular, UK).
- Distal embolization may occur as a complication of PTA or stenting, and equipment for aspiration thrombecomy should be readily available:
  - Wide bore 5–8F aspiration catheters
  - 6–8F sheaths with removable hubs
  - 50 mL Luer lock syringe.

Preprocedure Medications

- Patients should already be on antiplatelet therapy and this does not need to be stopped.
- Patients on warfarin (see section "Patient Preparation" above).
- If patients have CLI, they should already be taking adequate analgesia before they arrive at the angiography suite.

- Premedication is generally not required.
- In patients at high risk of contrast allergy, steroids may be given prophylactically.
- If there are any prosthetic grafts or valves, appropriate prophylactic antibiotics should be administered intravenously immediately prior to the intervention.

Procedure

Arterial Access

This should be planned after review of the pre-operative imaging:

- Antegrade, ipsilateral common femoral artery puncture is preferred unless the lesion is very close to the SFA origin.
- If the common femoral bifurcation is high, select one of the following options:

  ○ Contralateral femoral puncture and perform PTA over the aortic bifurcation
  ○ Ipsilateral antegrade SFA puncture under ultrasound guidance
  ○ Retrograde ipsilateral puncture of the popliteal artery
  ○ Access from the upper limb (usually the lower brachial artery)

  The choice out of the above three options will usually depend on the anatomy and operator preference.

- If there is an SFA occlusion flush with the vessel origin and the popliteal artery is patent, an ipsilateral, retrograde popliteal artery puncture is a useful access for these lesions.

Angiography

Angiography is generally performed using hand injections of 5–10 cc of contrast medium through the side arm of the sheath, or through the selective/straight catheters used to traverse the arterial lesion. A pump injector is not required:

- Angiographic runs are obtained with sufficient overlap to cover the whole leg:

  ○ In claudicants, it is sufficient to image down to the mid calf.
  ○ In critically ischemic limbs, angiographic runs should include a lateral view of the foot to assess the pedal arch.

- Oblique views may be necessary to distinguish the course of the SFA from overlying collaterals or to better identify the lesion.
- Lateral or oblique views may be required if there is a metal prosthesis such as a total hip or knee replacement (Fig. 2).

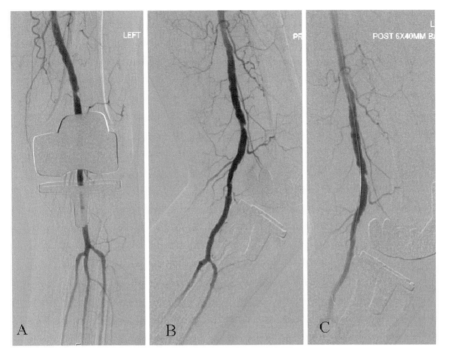

Fig. 2 (**A**) Distal SFA and popliteal artery obscured by total knee replacement. (**B**) Lateral projection shows the previously obscured segment and the stenosis more clearly. (**C**) Post-PTA angiogram

Intra-procedural Medications

- Intravenous sedation relieves patient anxiety, e.g., Midazolam 1–2.5 mg.
- Intravenous analgesia is not generally required, unless the patient is in a great deal of pain from CLI.
- A bolus of 3000–5000 units of heparin is given by intra-arterial injection once the lesion has been crossed.
- Antispasmodic drugs are not required routinely unless spasm occurs. Prophylactic antispasmodic drugs (e.g., Glyceryl trinitrate 100–150 mcg) are administered when the popliteal artery is used for access.

Assessing the Lesion

- The site of the lesion is confirmed by angiography.
- If an occlusion is present, the site of reconstitution of the artery is established.
- Eccentric, calcified plaques may not respond to PTA.

- Angiographic views should be performed in two or more projections if there is any doubt regarding the significance of a lesion or to unravel overlying collaterals.
- A decision regarding whether a moderate stenosis (approximately 45–55% in severity) is significant or not, is generally made from the visual appearances alone.

Pressure Measurements

- Intra-arterial pressure measurements are rarely used in the femoral arteries to assess whether a borderline stenosis is significant or not, in contrast to the iliac arteries.

Performing the Procedure

Crossing the Lesion

- The standard tools for recanalization of stenoses and occlusions consist of a hydrophilic guidewire and an angled-tip catheter, e.g., cobra, Berenstein.
- Stenoses are usually recanalized intraluminally using a roadmap to direct passage of the guidewire.
- Occlusions are usually recanalized subintimally.
- A roadmap is very useful for the recanalization of stenoses and occlusions. In occlusions, it is very useful to identify when distal passage of the catheter/wire beyond the site of reconstitution of the artery has occurred.
- Once the lesion has been crossed, the catheter should be advanced beyond the lesion, the wire removed and contrast injected to ensure that the catheter is within the lumen.
- The hydrophilic or standard wire should be re-introduced. The wire tip should be maintained in the popliteal artery around the level of the knee joint to avoid inducing spasm in the distal vessels.
- If possible, the tip of the guidewire should always be kept in the field of view during the intervention to prevent it advancing into the distal vessels and inadvertently causing trauma.
- The catheter should be withdrawn, ensuring that the wire remains across the treated site

Deploying the Balloon/Stent

Angioplasty

- A balloon catheter, selected for appropriate diameter and length, is advanced over the wire to the distal extent of the lesion (or proximal lesion if the approach is via the popliteal artery).

- The balloon is inflated until any waist on the balloon has been abolished. The inflation time is not standardized. Inflation times vary from a few seconds to a few minutes.
- Prior to inflation of the balloon, the patient should be warned that they may experience pain, although this should not be excessive.
- As the balloon inflates, assessment of the roadmap image should confirm that the balloon catheter is appropriately sized. If there is excessive pain or the balloon looks too big, the balloon should be exchanged for a smaller diameter balloon.
- After balloon deflation, the balloon catheter is withdrawn slightly and the balloon catheter should be reinflated with overlaps until the whole lesion has been covered.
- The balloon catheter is withdrawn completely, while keeping the guidewire in place across the lesion so that re-insertion of the balloon catheter or a stent delivery system can be performed if required.
- Angiography to assess the result is performed by injecting contrast medium through the side arm of the sheath. .
- There should be rapid forward flow through the treated segment with no residual stenoses greater than 30%.
- Dissections in the wall of the artery are expected and do not imply a poor result unless they are flow limiting.
- If there are residual stenoses, the balloon catheter should be re-inserted and reinflated at the site of stenosis.
- If the balloon will not inflate fully, a high-pressure balloon or a cutting balloon may be required:

  o If using a cutting balloon, a smaller diameter than that used for the ordinary balloon inflation should be selected to avoid arterial rupture. After cutting balloon PTA, angioplasty with the conventional balloon is performed again to the full arterial diameter (Fig. 3).

Stent Insertion

- If the balloon inflates fully, but the stenosis persists, indicating elastic recoil, insertion of a stent is indicated.
- If there is a flow-limiting dissection, prolonged balloon inflation can be performed to tack the flap back. In this case the balloon is kept inflated for up to 5 min. If this fails, a stent is indicated.
- Thus, recognized indications for stent insertion in the femoropopliteal segment are

  o Elastic recoil
  o Flow-limiting dissection

- Other presentations such as recurrent lesions after a recent PTA, long segment occlusions, and long segment stenotic disease are not recognized standard indications for a stent.

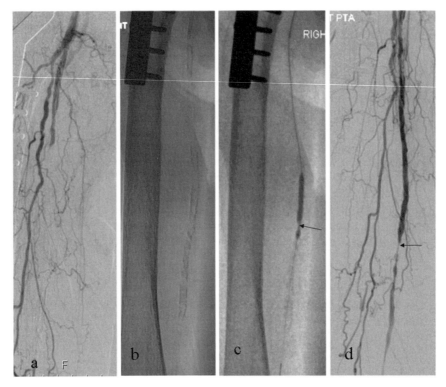

Fig. 3 (**a**) SFA occlusion in calcified artery. (**b**) Non-subtracted image showing the calcified wall of the artery. (**c**) Very tight stenosis. Balloon catheter shows residual waisting (black arrow). (**d**) CBPTA also failed to dilate the lesion and post-procedural angiography shows a residual tight stenosis

- If a stent is indicated, a self-expanding stent should be used. This is because balloon-expandable stents are subject to external pressure and will not re-expand if they are compressed. Stents in the SFA and PA are subject to external compression and therefore balloon-expandable stents should not be used in these locations.
- The stent should be oversized by 1 mm relative to the diameter of the SFA. The stent should be long enough to cover the lesion with 5–10 mm coverage of the normal artery either side of the lesion.
- Manufacturers generally recommend that no more than two stents should be inserted. However, more stents may be inserted if necessary, to cover the extent of a lesion. The manufacturers' guidelines should be followed for the recommended amount of overlap between stents. This may differ between manufacturers.

Endpoint

- The endpoint of the procedure is unrestricted forward flow of contrast with no evidence of significant (>30%) residual stenosis.

- The run-off should be assessed at the end of the procedure for the occurrence of distal embolization caused by the PTA or stent insertion.
- If the patient is being treated for critical ischemia, PTA of any relevant tibial lesions should be performed during the same procedure.
- When the procedure is completed, the arterial access sheath should be removed and hemostasis achieved by manual compression or the use of an arterial closure device.

Immediate Post-procedure Care

- The pulse and blood pressure should be monitored to detect hemorrhage.
- The arterial puncture site should be observed according to a standard protocol for signs of bleeding or hematoma.
- There should be clear nursing instructions regarding the required length of bed rest.

Follow-Up and Post-procedure Medications

- If the procedure was performed as a day case, a post-procedural visit to the patient prior to discharge is essential:
  - This is generally around 6 h following the procedure, but could be earlier if a closure device has been used.
  - The patient should be instructed as to how soon they can return to normal activities, drive, and who to call in case of emergency.

- If patient was an inpatient, a visit to the ward should be performed at the end of the working day.
- Follow-up of the patient in a clinic is undertaken at 6 weeks, either by the physician who performed the intervention or by the referring clinician, depending on local circumstances.
- Best medical therapy is continued as before the angioplasty. If a stent has been inserted, the patient should be commenced on clopidogrel.

Results

The results of femoropopliteal PTA/stenting depend on the severity of symptoms, the lesion length, and the extent of outflow disease. Pooled data from the TASC 11 document show the following:

- The technical and clinical success of PTA/stenting exceeds 95% in stenoses and 85% in occlusions.

- The 1-, 3-, and 5-year patency rates for PTA of femoral stenoses are 77%, 61%, and 55%, respectively.
- The 1-, 3-, and 5-year patency rates for PTA of femoral occlusions are 65%, 48%, and 42%, respectively.
- The 1- and 3-year patency rates for stenting of femoral stenoses are 75% and 66%, respectively.
- The 1- and 3-year patency rates for stenting of femoral occlusions are 73% and 64%, respectively.
- Although the patency rates for femoral stenting compared with PTA in occlusions are superior, cost effectiveness has not yet been demonstrated.

Alternative Therapies

- For claudicants, the alternative to PTA is continued best medical therapy with supervised exercise.
- For patients with critical limb ischemia, the alternative is bypass surgery, preferably using a vein. Bypass surgery requires good inflow into the graft and a patent artery onto which the graft can be attached. SFA bypass can be performed to the popliteal artery above or below the knee joint. If the popliteal artery is occluded, then a femorodistal graft onto a patent tibial artery may be performed.
- If bypass surgery is not feasible, fails, or gangrene is present, amputation may be necessary. This can be minor, with amputation of a digit or forefoot, or major, with either above or below knee amputation.

Complications

Most complications are common to all angioplasty procedures. These may occur at the puncture site, the site of angioplasty, or they may occur distal to the treatment site:

- *Rupture* of the artery at the site of angioplasty can occur if a balloon size too large for the artery is selected, or if there is eccentric calcified plaque, which can be pushed through the arterial wall by PTA. Rupture may also occur with very resistant stenoses requiring a high-pressure or cutting balloon. Rupture is treated by balloon tamponade, extrinsic compression with a thigh cuff, or by placement of a covered stent. In most instances, any bleeding related to the rupture is self-limiting because the developing hematoma tamponades the site of hemorrhage. However, if rupture follows cutting balloon PTA, there may be a linear tear. This may result in a pseudoaneurysm, if the rupture is left untreated, and in this situation, placement of a covered stent is recommended.
- *Immediate occlusion* of the treated site may occur either due to elastic recoil or due to flow-limiting dissection. This may also occur if the outflow has been

occluded by distal embolization (see next paragraph). Immediate reocclusion can be treated by a combination of thrombolysis and repeat PTA or stenting. If this complication occurs within days of the PTA, local administration of 1–3 boluses of a thrombolytic agent will usually suffice to restore patency of the vessel. If thrombolysis is contraindicated, immediate stenting can be performed (Fig. 4).

• *Embolization* to the tibial trifurcation or more distally may occur. A check angiogram of the run-off should always be performed at the end of a procedure. Suction thrombectomy using a wide bore catheter, a 50-cc Luer lock syringe, a sheath with a removable valve, and antispasmodic drugs are recommended first. If the emboli are in the distal tibial arteries, a 5F Berenstein or cobra catheter can be used to aspirate the emboli. If this fails, thrombolysis may be performed.

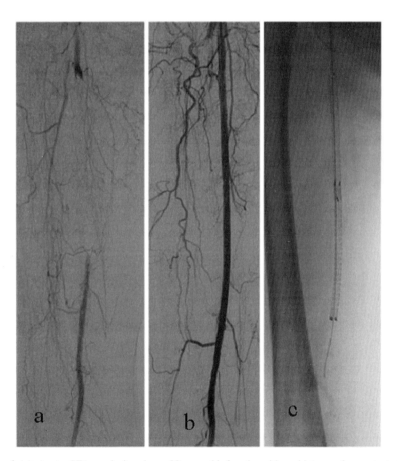

Fig. 4 (a) Acute SFA occlusion in a 90-year-old female with a history of recent stroke. **(b)** Stenting of SFA. **(c)** Non-subtracted image showing two self-expanding stents in situ

Key Points

- Obtain and review the pre-procedural imaging to plan the intervention.
- Treat any inflow problems first.
- Use the most direct and simplest approach. This may require more than one arterial access site.
- Ensure that there is good forward flow at the end of the procedure.
- Deal with outflow problems during the same procedure in patients with CLI to produce continuous arterial flow to the foot.
- Check run-off at the end of the procedure.
- If uncertain, discuss the problem with a colleague or stop the procedure. It is always possible to bring the patient back another day.

Suggested Reading

1. Adam DJ, Beard JD, Cleveland T, Bell J, Bradbury AW, Forbes JF, Fowkes FG, Gillespie I, Ruckley CV, Raab G, Storkey H (2005) Bypass versus angioplasty in severe ischaemia of the leg (BASIL): multicentre, randomised controlled trial. Lancet 366:1925–1934
2. Norgren L, Hiatt WR, Dormandy JA, Nehler MR, Harris KA, Fowkes FGR (2007) Inter-Society Consensus for the Management of Peripheral Arterial Disease (TASC11). European Journal of Vascular and Endovascular Surgery 33(Suppl 1):S1–S75
3. Schillinger M, Sabeti S, Loewe C, Dick P, Amighi J, Mleckusch W, Schlager O, Cejna M, Lammer J, Minar E (2006) Balloon Angioplasty versus Implantation of nitinol Stents in the superficial Femoral Artery. The New England Journal of Medicine 354:1879–1888
4. Tsetis D, Belli A-M (2004) Guidelines for Stenting in Infrainguinal Arterial Disease. Cardiovascular & Interventional Radiology 27:198–203

Subintimal Angioplasty

Guy Fishwick

Clinical Features

- In most centers in the UK, the majority of patients treated by subintimal angioplasty have critical limb ischemia (CLI):
  - Rest pain
  - Ulceration
  - Gangrene
- Occasionally patients with short-distance intermittent claudication are considered for treatment.

Diagnostic Evaluation

The aims of diagnostic evaluation are

- To establish ischemia as the cause of the symptoms and signs
- To establish the extent and level of the vascular occlusion
- To establish the proximal and distal extent of the lesion

Clinical

The following should be assessed:

- Risk factors:
  - Diabetes
  - Smoking
  - Hypertension
  - Duration of symptoms
  - Previous circulatory problems/investigations/surgery

R.A. Morgan, E. Walser (eds.), *Handbook of Angioplasty and Stenting Procedures*, Techniques in Interventional Radiology, DOI 10.1007/978-1-84800-399-6_10, © Springer-Verlag London Limited 2010

- The degree of ischemia:

  - Presence/absence of pulses
  - Skin changes
  - Tissue loss
  - Concomitant venous problems
  - Capillary circulation in the foot
  - ABPI

Laboratory

The following should be assessed:

- Hb
- INR
- Renal function
- Glucose
- (Thrombophilia screen in selected cases)

Imaging

One of the following (or a combination) should be performed:

- Duplex ultrasound:

  - This is the main initial imaging method performed in most vascular departments in the UK.
  - Adequate information regarding the femoropopliteal segment and tibial arteries can be obtained in the vast majority of patients.
  - Although duplex ultrasound is reasonably good in the assessment of the iliac arteries, excessive abdominal wall fat or bowel gas can obscure these vessels in such patients.

- CT angiography:

  - This is being increasingly used as a non-invasive alternative to conventional angiography.
  - The advantage over duplex is the provision of a series of images of the arterial tree in an "angiographic format."

- The requirement for ionising radiation and iodinated contrast medium are obvious disadvantages.
- Heavy vascular calcification may obscure the view of the vessel lumen and reduce the usefulness of this modality in such patients.

- MR angiography

  - Also used more and more as an alternative to conventional angiography.
  - A moving table is required for peripheral MRA.
  - The disadvantages of heavy calcification, ionizing radiation, and iodinated contrast medium are not seen with MRA.
  - However, due to the recently recognized syndrome of renal nephrosclerosis related to MR contrast media, MRA is not suitable for patients with marked renal dysfunction.

- Catheter angiography

  - Remains the gold standard for peripheral vascular imaging.
  - The main disadvantage, apart from ionizing radiation and iodinated contrast media, is the invasive nature of the procedure.

Indications

- Critical limb ischemia due to occlusive arterial disease or long diffuse stenotic arterial disease.
- A relative indication is short-distance intermittent claudication due to occlusive or long-segment stenotic arterial disease. However, the management of claudication in most cases should be conservative i.e., advice regarding lifestyle change and a program of exercise.

Contraindications

- Recent arterial occlusion.
- Popliteal aneurysm.
- A relative contraindication is the presence of significant common femoral artery disease in the affected leg.

Patient Preparation

- Standard skin preparation.
- If the patient has renal impairment, preangiographic hydration should be provided (+/– N-acetyl cysteine).

- It is important that the patient is able to lie still for the duration of the procedure.
- Standard aseptic preparation should be used.

Relevant Anatomy

Symptoms are produced by arterial disease at any level from the aorta to the crural (tibial) vessels.

- As a rule, the more proximal lesions should be treated before distal lesions.
- If a distal lesion is treated in isolation (ignoring a proximal lesion), the result will not be durable.
- Common femoral artery access is usual and preferable.
- Brachial artery access is an option, but is not a good access route for lower limb subintimal angioplasty.

  ○ A very long relatively rigid sheath will be required; even then getting adequate "push" through a lesion will be difficult.

Aberrant Anatomy

The following variants of normal anatomy are noteworthy for IRs undertaking lower limb subintimal angioplasty:

- A high bifurcation of the femoral artery above the inguinal ligament − which causes difficulties in antegrade common femoral artery puncture
- A high origin of the posterior tibial artery from the popliteal artery
- A hypoplastic anterior tibial artery with the dorsalis pedis artery supplied from the peroneal artery

Specific Equipment

The following are the basic tools required to perform subintimal angioplasty and to deal with complications:

- A 0.035-inch guidewire with a relatively short tip, which can be shaped
- Short length angled-tip catheter (approximately 15–30-cm long)
- Sheaths with removable hemostatic valves
- Angioplasty balloons (over-the-wire balloons, 0.035 inch) of a range of appropriate sizes
- A re-entry catheter (e.g., Outback (Cordis, Europe))

- Wide bore straight aspiration catheters
- Stents and stent grafts

Pre-procedure Medication

- None specific to this procedure.
- Patients on warfarin should be converted to heparin until their INR is at an appropriate level – usually below 1.5.
- For patients on clopidogrel – review the indication for the prescription and discontinue if appropriate.
- Continue antihypertensive agents and medication for diabetes (metformin should be stopped at the time of the angioplasty and should not be restarted until the renal function has been checked post-procedure)

Procedure

Access

The following are suggestions for optimal access to approach lesions in different anatomical locations:

- Ipsilateral antegrade common femoral artery puncture for superficial femoral, popliteal, and crural artery lesions.
- Ipsilateral retrograde or contralateral retrograde common femoral artery puncture for iliac artery access.
- Contralateral retrograde common femoral artery puncture for superficial femoral, popliteal, and crural lesions in obese patients.
- Ipsilateral retrograde popliteal artery access is also an option for superficial femoral artery (SFA) lesions in obese patients or for problematic flush SFA occlusions.
- Ipsilateral retrograde popliteal artery access is also an option if recanalization from the antegrade direction fails.

Angiography

- Digital subtraction angiography (DSA) is used to confirm the pre-procedural imaging findings.
- This is usually achieved by hand injection, unless the lesion involved is a common iliac artery occlusion to be recanalized from the aorta.
- Be sure to check that there is no fresh occlusion of arteries that were patent on pre-procedure imaging.

Intra-procedural Medication

- Heparin is given prior to creating a dissection i.e., the subintimal track (approximately 50 IU/kg).
- GTN 100–150 mcg given intra-arterially by bolus injections may be given into any vessel that goes into spasm during the procedure. However, arterial spasm is rare in this group of patients with generalized arterial disease.

Assessing the Lesion

The following questions should run through the interventionalist's mind before beginning the recanalization:

- Where is the most proximal point of the occlusion?
- Is the vessel diseased proximal to the occlusion?
- Is there disease distal to the occlusion? – This will likely affect the level of re-entry into the lumen from the dissection.
- Is there multi-level disease?
- What is the quality of the run-off to the foot?

  ○ How many vessels?
  ○ Are they diseased?

- If the SFA is diseased throughout its length, is there any indication where the SFA origin is located? The SFA origin may be visualized with approximately 30° oblique angulation (LAO for left, RAO for right).

Performing the Procedure

Crossing the Lesion

Antegrade Approach for the SFA, and Distal Vessels but Not Involving the SFA Origin

- Set up the image intensifier over the lower half of the femoral head, tightly coned, just showing the needle tip at the top of the image, so that the operator's fingers are excluded.
- Perform antegrade CFA puncture.
- Inject contrast through the needle (Fig. 1).
- Identify the SFA origin and confirm that the puncture is sufficiently proximal to the origin to manipulate either the guidewire or an angled-tip catheter into the SFA.
- Direct the guidewire into the origin and insert a sheath over the wire.

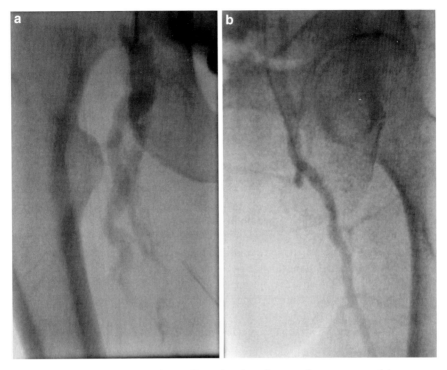

Fig. 1 Contrast injected through the needle or short introducer confirms puncture of the common femoral artery above its bifurcation and the location of the SFA origin

- If the SFA origin is not easily accessed with the guidewire, the wire should be passed into the profunda femoris artery.

  ○ An angled-tip catheter should be passed into the profunda.
  ○ The angled-tip catheter should be pulled back almost to the profunda origin.
  ○ Perform a roadmap through the angled-tip catheter to define the location of the CFA bifurcation and the course of the SFA.
  ○ Using the roadmap, and by rotating the catheter, select and advance a hydrophilic guidewire into the SFA
  ○ Advance the catheter over the wire into the SFA.

- Perform selective angiography as above.
- Select the point of origin of dissection.

Select the preferred segment of vessel distal to the occlusion i.e., where to end the dissection

  ○ This segment should ideally be disease free.

- Initiate the dissection channel above the occlusion, by pushing the wire tip and/or the tip of the angled-tip catheter into the vessel wall.
- If this is difficult (not common), intimal tears can also be created by inflation of a balloon in the artery above the occlusion.
- Introduce the catheter tip into/under the tear. The location in the subintimal space can be confirmed by injection of a very small (0.5 mL) injection of contrast medium, although this is seldom necessary (Fig. 2).

A dissection is seen as a linear contrast blush in the arterial wall, often with contrast medium washed away in small rete veins in the wall, and then into the venae commitantes.

- Introduce the hydrophilic guidewire tip further into the dissection.
- Push the tip forward until it curls into a loop.
- Using a gentle forward and backward (nudging) action, advance the loop of the wire down the vessel alongside the occlusion.
- The wire will tend to advance in a spiral in the artery wall (Fig. 3).
- Support the wire with a catheter (or a balloon catheter) advanced behind the loop.
- If the balloon catheter/guidewire fails to advance in any area, the balloon can be inflated in the area to facilitate passage.

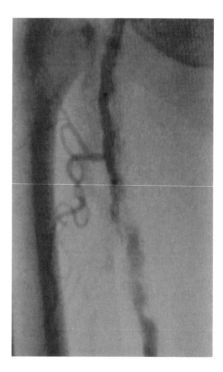

Fig. 2 Contrast injection to confirm creation of a dissection

Fig. 3 Wire supported by
balloon catheter, looped and
advanced, spiraling around
the intimal calcification

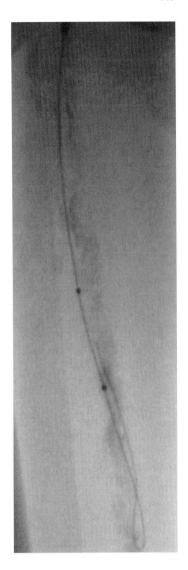

Re-entry

- When the loop reaches the preferred area for re-entry into the lumen, advance the catheter to this area.
- Remove the wire and inject a small volume of contrast to see whether:

    a   The catheter tip is still within the dissection (no flow).
    b   The catheter tip is in the vessel lumen (rapid flow away in normal vessel).

   c   The catheter tip is still within the dissection, but there is communication with the lumen (lingering contrast around the catheter tip, which rapidly flows away into the normal vessel nearby).

- If the situation is scenario c, the wire tip should be introduced into the vessel lumen using the roadmap facility.
- If the situation is scenario b, with no communication demonstrated from the dissection to the lumen, recreate the loop on the guidewire but only with the floppy portion of the wire.

  - Using the same nudging movement, advance the wire a little further down the dissection.
  - While advancing and withdrawing the loop, roll the wire between the thumb and forefinger to spin the looped tip.
  - If re-entry to the lumen is still not achieved, a decision is needed as to whether to continue the dissection distally, or to use a re-entry catheter to limit the length of the dissection (see below).

- When re-entry occurs, the guidewire will move freely in the arterial lumen and the guidewire loop may also appear smaller as it is now constrained within the smaller arterial lumen.

Re-entry Catheters

Two catheters are available to facilitate re-entry into the lumen below an occlusion.

- The Outback catheter − Cordis, Europe.
- The Pioneer catheter − Medtronic, Santa Rosa, CA.

Both catheters have a curved needle near the tip, which can be advanced out of the side of the tip of the catheter and then retracted. These catheters are introduced over a 0.014″ guidewire.

- The Outback catheter relies on a shaped marker at the tip to show the needle position and orientation on fluoroscopy.
- The Pioneer catheter has an IVUS probe within the tip to visualize the vessel lumen and to guide the advance of the needle tip.

Once the retractable needle has been advanced into the lumen, the guidewire is advanced and the catheter is exchanged for the balloon catheter.

The dissection channel is angioplastied as before.

Contralateral Retrograde Approach

This is useful in large patients where antegrade access over the femoral head is compromised due to the bulk of abdominal wall fat.

- With this approach, controlled advance of the guidewire is more difficult. Even if the wire can be advanced relatively easily through the occlusion, it can be difficult to follow the wire with the catheter.
- To overcome these potential problems, the use of a balloon catheter as a predilating catheter is recommended.
- Difficulties are increased if there is tortuous iliac artery anatomy, or there is a steeply angled aortic bifurcation.
- Sheaths specifically designed for "cross-over" may be useful.
- Re-entry catheters can still be used from this approach.

Popliteal Artery Approach

This access is useful if antegrade access fails and if there is a true "flush" occlusion of the SFA origin and it is not possible to know where the SFA origin is.

- A disease-free segment of above knee popliteal artery is required.
- The patient must be capable of lying prone.
- The puncture should be ultrasound guided to avoid the partially overlying popliteal vein.

Subintimal Angioplasty for Below Knee Occlusions

The basic technique is similar to that for the SFA and popliteal artery.

- If the occlusion starts in the popliteal artery, decide which of the crural arteries are the best vessels to recanalize.
- The looped guidewire has a tendency to follow the peroneal or the posterior tibial artery, so if you want to access the anterior tibial artery, an angled-tip catheter is usually required.
- A J tip "semi- stiff" hydrophilic guidewire (Terumo) is a very useful wire in the crural vessels, since it can be difficult to reform a loop in an angled-tip wire in these small vessels.
- It can be difficult to make a catheter track over the wire through long crural vessel occlusions, so it is often better to use a small (3 mm) balloon, which may need to be inflated and deflated to advance it distally.
- Re-entry catheters are not appropriate in these arteries but fortunately re-entry to the lumen is rarely a problem through the thin intima of these vessels.

- As with SFA recanalization, re-entry to the lumen is only usually achieved where the artery becomes relatively disease free, since it is at this location that the intima becomes thin enabling re-entry.

Subintimal Angioplasty in Iliac Artery Occlusions

Intraluminal angioplasty and stenting via an ipsilateral retrograde approach is the preferred technique for iliac artery occlusions.

Where the occlusion cannot be crossed through the lumen (i.e., intraluminal recanalization), subintimal recanalization is appropriate.

- This can be achieved from a contralateral, ipsilateral, or a combined approach.
- From a contralateral approach, a wire is advanced to the occlusion, supported by a catheter.

  ○ The wire is advanced into the occlusion and will either cross the lesion via the lumen (in which case the lesion can be treated by angioplasty and stented), or it will dissect through the subintimal space, will form a loop and can be advanced subintimally.
  ○ If the wire does not break back into the lumen immediately below the occlusion, the length of the dissection can be controlled by creating a dissection from below using an ipsilateral retrograde approach. The dissection plane is usually (though not invariably) the same from below and above.
  ○ Once a wire is established back into the lumen from either below or above, the occlusion can be treated by angioplasty.

- With the ipsilateral approach, the catheter and guidewire are advanced subintimally retrogradely, with the hope that the wire will re-enter the lumen in the patent iliac artery above the occlusion, or at the aortic bifurcation if the occlusion extends to the common iliac artery origin

  ○ However, it is not possible to predict the location of re-entry. Although re-entry at the aortic bifurcation occurs sometimes, the wire often continues to dissect up the aorta, which usually signals a failure of this approach, unless the vessel is also recanalized from above (see above).

- An alternative approach when using an ipsilateral retrograde approach is to use a re-entry catheter when the catheter and wire are located in a dissection and to puncture the intima above the dissection to re-enter the lumen.
- If the ipsilateral retrograde approach is used, it is still necessary to have access from the contralateral femoral artery to image the re-entry point.

Performing the Angioplasty

- When the wire tip has re-entered the vessel lumen below the occlusion, the catheter is exchanged for a balloon of appropriate size (usually 4–6-mm diameter in the SFA/popliteal segment).
- Long balloon lengths are best (10–12 cm).
- Rapid inflation/deflation is performed with a Kimal inflation syringe along the length of the subintimal channel.
- Taking care not to lose the wire position, the entire length of the occlusion is balloon angioplastied once or twice.

Endpoint

- The recanalized segment is examined by angiography for

    ○ Patency – often ribbon like and spiraling (Fig. 4).

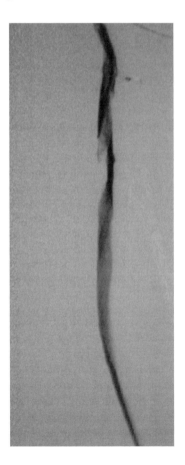

Fig. 4 Patent, spiraling post-angioplasty channel

- ○ Rapid flow – the main determinant of procedure completion.
- ○ Patent run-off below the occlusion.
- ○ Stents are occasionally required at the proximal and distal ends of the subintimal channel to achieve rapid flow. Specific self-expanding SFA stents are now available.

- The foot should also be examined to confirm improved capillary return.
- If the above three angiographic features are present and the foot is improved, the procedure is deemed a success.

Immediate Post-procedure Care

- The groin puncture site is closed either with a closure device (if appropriate), or by manual pressure.
- The duration of prescribed bed rest will depend on whether or not a closure device is used.
- There is no specific post-procedure medication.
- Medication stopped prior to angioplasty can be restarted as appropriate.

Follow-Up and Post-procedure Care

- Patients are followed up initially either in the interventional radiology clinic or in the vascular surgical clinic.
- If the patients' symptoms resolve, they can be discharged back to their primary care physician.
- If symptoms recur or do not respond to the procedure, they should be assessed by duplex ultrasound to evaluate whether the lesions have recurred.

Results

These are technically difficult procedures with an approximate 10% failure rate to achieve the desired endpoint. Technical failure may be due to

- Failure to create a dissection channel (usually due to heavy calcification in the vessel walls).
- Perforation of the channel with failure to bypass the perforation.
- The channel is created, but there is poor flow or thrombosis in the channel.
- Thrombus in the channel can be aspirated via a wide-bore catheter.
- An underlying focal abnormality causing poor flow and thrombosis may need "spot" stenting, e.g., a flow-limiting dissection flap, or more commonly a densely calcified segment of vessel wall.

Fig. 5 Perforation in popliteal segment excluded by new dissection

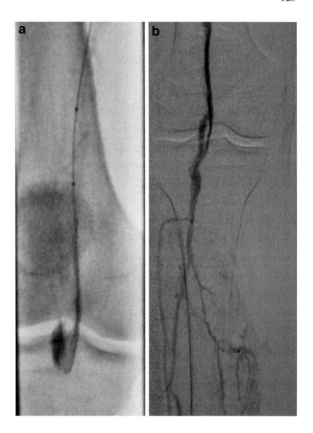

- Perforation in the channel can sometimes be bypassed by recreating a new dissection channel (Fig. 5).
- Around 15% of patients undergoing this procedure fail to gain relief from CLI and its symptoms, and subsequently require bypass surgery.
- Of the procedures undertaken, only 50% of the femoropopliteal segment channels and 40% of the channels extending into the tibial arteries are patent at 2 years.

    - The fact that only 15% of patients require bypass surgery (including initial technical failures) means that even with this relatively low 2-year patency rate, there is considerable relief from CLI even for many of the patients in whom the recanalized vessel subsequently reoccludes.

- Long-term patency is inversely related to the length of the occlusion and is directly related to the number of patent run-off vessels.
- Bypass surgery is rarely compromised by prior subintimal angioplasty.

Alternative Therapies

The alternative to subintimal angioplasty in these patients is bypass surgery.

- Aortofemoral bypass
- Iliofemoral bypass
- Ilio- or femorofemoral cross-over
- Axillofemoral bypass
- Femoropopliteal bypass
- Femorodistal. bypass

In some cases bypass surgery is relatively straightforward, and in many centers it is the preferred option. However, in centers offering subintimal angioplasty, bypass surgery is generally reserved for failed angioplasty.

Where there is significant (particularly eccentric) common femoral artery disease, common femoral endarterectomy is the preferred treatment. This can be done in conjunction with subintimal angioplasty as a combined procedure to try to avoid more extensive bypass surgery.

Complications of Subintimal Angioplasty

Distal Embolization

- The most significant complication of subintimal angioplasty.
- This requires aspiration, usually via a 7 or 8F catheter, if the embolus is in the popliteal artery, or via a 5 or 6F catheter if the embolus is in the crural arteries.

  - The catheter is directed into the embolus and aspiration is performed by suction with a 50-mL Luer-lock syringe.
  - The embolus is usually sucked onto the catheter tip rather than aspirated up the catheter lumen, in which case it is withdrawn into the sheath on the end of the catheter (while still applying suction).
  - It is necessary to have a removable cap on the sheath as emboli will rarely pass through the hemostatic valve and are usually trapped within it.

- Most emboli can be removed by aspiration thrombectomy, although occasionally large emboli may require surgical embolectomy for their extraction.

Vessel Perforation

This is usually a complication of the creation of the dissection caused by the wire, rather than a sequel of balloon dilaton of a channel, which has been successfully created.

- The successful creation of a new dissection channel usually excludes the perforation, in which case no further treatment is necessary.
- Failure to create a new channel usually leads to termination of the procedure.
- Most perforations are self-limiting and require no further treatment.
- Occasionally, vessel perforation is associated with persistent pain and continued extravasation. In this situation, the channel to the perforation may need to be occluded either with gelfoam or by coil embolization.
- Perforation of a successfully created dissection channel due to PTA is very uncommon. Similar to the previous section, it is usually self-limiting. Rarely, a covered stent is required.
- Perforation into a vein creating an A−V fistula occurs occasionally. This is usually around the trifurcation area and is managed in the same way as other perforations.
- A perforation can be recognized as it occurs, due to deviation and expansion of the loop of the wire.

Other Complications

More general complications, not related to the subintimal technique but to the arterial puncture and the use of contrast agents, should be managed appropriately.

The most significant complication related to the puncture site, which must be recognized and treated, is hemorrhage from a high puncture.

- If the femoral artery is punctured above the midpoint of the femoral head, hemorrhage may track superiorly to the retro-peritoneum behind the inguinal ligament, rather than presenting as hematoma in the groin.
- This should be suspected in any patient who becomes hypotensive following antegrade femoral puncture.
- It is a potentially fatal complication if it goes unrecognized.
- Puncture of the femoral artery below the midpoint of the femoral head avoids this complication.

Key Points

- Use a careful and consistent puncture technique.
- Create the dissection precisely and proximal to the occlusion.
- Identify the area where re-entry to the lumen is anticipated.
- Be bold and extend the dissection to the level of the normal artery.
- Work quickly, but without rushing. This reduces the likelihood of thrombosis of the dissection channel.
- Be prepared for, recognize, and treat appropriately any complications that occur.
- There is usually a surgical option − do not compromise this option.

Suggested Further Reading

1. Abdelsalam H, Markose G, Bolia A. Revascularization strategies in below the knee interventions. J Cardiovasc Surg (Torino) 2008 Apr; 49(2):187–91. Review.
2. Ascher E, Hingorani A. Subintimal angioplasty. J Cardiovasc Surg (Torino) 2007 Feb; 48(1): 45–8. Review.
3. Bolia A, Miles KA, Brennan J, Bell PR. Percutaneous transluminal angioplasty of occlusions of the femoral and popliteal arteries by subintimal dissection. Cardiovasc Intervent Radiol 1990 Dec; 13(6): 357–63
4. Bolia A. Subintimal angioplasty in lower limb ischaemia. J Cardiovasc Surg (Torino) 2005 Aug; 46(4): 385–94. Review.
5. Met R, Van Lienden KP, Koelemay MJ, Bipat S, Legemate DA, Reekers JA. Subintimal angioplasty for peripheral arterial occlusive disease: a systematic review. Cardiovasc Intervent Radiol 2008 Jul–Aug; 31(4): 687–97. Epub 2008 Apr 15. Review.
6. Reekers JA, Bolia A. Percutaneous intentional extraluminal (subintimal) recanalization: how to do it yourself. Eur J Radiol 1998 Oct; 28(3): 192–8.
7. Treiman GS. Subintimal angioplasty for infrainguinal occlusive disease. Surg Clin North Am 2004 Oct; 84(5): 1365–80, viii. Review.

Infrapopliteal Angioplasty and Stenting

Marc Sapoval, Olivier Pellerin, and Laurent Bellmann

Clinical Features

- Only patients with critical limb ischemia (CLI) should undergo angioplasty or stenting distal to the popliteal artery.
- CLI is defined as arterial ulceration, gangrene, or rest pain of longer duration than 2 weeks, with hemodynamic evidence of arterial disease (distal blood pressure <50 mmHg or a toe pressure <30 mmHg).
- This subgroup of patients is at a high risk of amputation if revascularization is not performed within a short time period.
- CLI is not acute limb ischemia where immediate limb loss is a major risk.
- Risk factors for CLI include smoking, renal failure, and diabetes mellitus. Diabetic patients have a high incidence of distal arterial disease.

Diagnostic Evaluation

Clinical

- Regarding CLI, the Rutherford classification differentiates between rest pain, minor ulcer, and major ulcer.
- Careful vascular examination is required with examination of the foot especially in diabetic patients.
- Arterial ulcers are painful, and usually occur at the level of the ankle, often at the lateral malleolus. The underlying skin is dry and cold, as opposed to venous ulcers.
- Wound infection and cellulitis in patients with CLI may cause a rapid deterioration in the distal circulation, which may lead to amputation, especially in diabetic patients.

R.A. Morgan, E. Walser (eds.), *Handbook of Angioplasty and Stenting Procedures*,
Techniques in Interventional Radiology, DOI 10.1007/978-1-84800-399-6_11,
© Springer-Verlag London Limited 2010

Laboratory

- Standard preoperative biochemical and hematological workup is necessary. The serum ESR and CRP, in addition to the WBC, are important to rule out possible underlying infection.
- The serum creatinine (and in some patients creatinine clearance) should be assessed, in case measures are required to prevent contrast-mediated nephrotoxicity. Such measures include intravenous hydration and carbon dioxide angiography.
- The ABI and toes pressures are useful non-invasive tests for peripheral arterial disease. A normal ABI is >0.9. If the ABI is >1.2, the arteries are deemed to be non-compressible due to the presence of calcification. This is often the case in diabetic patients, and in such patients, infrapopliteal arterial lesions should be suspected.

Imaging

The aim of imaging is to define the anatomy, to indicate whether the circulation can be improved by intervention, either endovascular or surgical, and to define the locations which require treatment.

- Conventional DSA remains the best imaging method to define the infrapopliteal and pedal vessels in patients with CLI, to enable the optimal strategy for revascularization.
- All three infrapopliteal run-off vessels should be analyzed carefully, as well as the dorsalis pedis artery, the plantar arteries, and the plantar arch.
- Duplex in very experienced hands can be accurate for the assessment of the infrapopliteal vessels.
- MRA in experienced hands can visualize the pedal arteries and the infrapopliteal vessels. However, a poorly performed MRA often provides negligible useful information.
- CTA is less useful in CLI, because there is often heavy calcification in the infrapopliteal vessels.

Indications

- The presence of critical limb ischemia, i.e., rest pain, ulceration, or gangrene indicates intervention.

Contraindications

These are few:

- Occlusion of all three infrapopliteal vessels with no visible vessels either in the distal calf or the foot
- Fixed flexion contractures of the knee, which would makes the procedure technically very difficult
- Inability of the patient to remain immobile
- Acute septicemia related to wet gangrene of the foot requiring emergent amputation

Patient Preparation

- Standard skin preparation.
- If there is impaired renal function, intravenous hydration should be provided (+/– *N*-acetyl cysteine).
- Careful assessment of the patient's capacity to undertake a 2-h intervention on an uncomfortable angiographic table.
- If there is a risk that the patient may be unable to lie still because of confusion or agitation, consideration should be given to performing the examination with the help of an anesthetist who can administer an appropriate sedation protocol or general anesthesia in selected cases.
- Analgesia should be administered for the patient's comfort. The analgesic drugs should be strong enough to provide adequate pain relief.
- Standard aseptic preparation should be used and the affected foot should be protected in padding for patient comfort.
- These complex interventions should preferably be performed in the morning when all resources are available for optimal management. Performing a complex infrapopliteal intervention on an ill elderly patient at the end of the day or out of hours should be avoided, if possible.

Relevant Anatomy

Normal Anatomy

The vast majority of interventions involve antegrade access, which makes the procedure easier than if a contralateral access is used. This is because the access is closer to the point of intervention, and shorter catheters and guidewires can be used compared to the contralateral approach, when longer devices are required.

- The level of the common femoral bifurcation is variable. If the bifurcation is very high, it may be necessary to use a contralateral access or more commonly to puncture the SFA directly.
- The most common anatomy involves the popliteal artery bifurcating into the anterior tibial artery and the tibioperoneal trunk. The tibioperoneal trunk divides a few centimeters later into the peroneal and posterior tibial arteries.
- A minority of patients with CLI also have a popliteal aneurysm, which may be the underlying cause of the CLI because of distal microembolization.
- The anterior tibial artery continues into the foot as the dorsalis pedis artery.
- The posterior tibial artery continues into the foot and divides into the lateral or external (larger of the two) plantar artery and the medial or internal (smaller) plantar artery.
- The lateral plantar artery anastomoses with the dorsalis pedis artery via the pedal arch.
- The peroneal artery bifurcates into anterior and posterior perforating arteries just above the ankle. These may provide collateral flow to the dorsalis pedis or the distal posterior tibial artery if these latter vessels are diseased more proximally.

Aberrant Anatomy

There are anatomic variants for each of the three infrapopliteal vessels.

- There may be a high origin of the posterior tibial artery (it can originate above the knee joint articulation).
- There may be a congenital absence of the posterior tibial artery.
- There are several variants of the pedal arteries.

Equipment Required for Infrapopliteal Intervention

High-quality angiographic images are essential.

- Therefore, these procedures should only be performed using dedicated angiographic units.
- Mobile C-arm image intensifiers do not provide adequate image quality for these complex procedures and should not be used for this purpose.
- Hemodynamic monitoring including pulse oximetry .
- A functioning IV access.
- Balloons and stents of small diameter for use in the tibial vessels. In general, these systems are 0.018- or 0.014-inch platforms.

Pre-procedure Medication

- Anticoagulant medication such as warfarin (coumadine) should be discontinued 4–5 days before the procedure.
- Consider subcutaneous heparin if the patient was previously on oral anticoagulant medication.
- Maintain hydration, either oral or IV.
- Regular fasting policy as stated by the local anesthesiology department is necessary. In general, the patient's oral medication should be taken as usual especially cardiovascular and pain management drugs.
- Consider intravenous hydration and N-acetyl cysteine if the patient has renal failure.
- If the patient has insulin-dependent diabetes, the patient's insulin regime should be altered slightly on the morning of the procedure. In general, patients should be scheduled first on the list. The insulin dose should be reduced, usually by half. The patient should take a light breakfast and a 5% Dextrose IV infusion should be commenced. The blood sugar should be measured at regular intervals.

Procedure

Access

- Ipsilateral anterograde access is preferable to a retrograde contralateral access.
- Relative indications for a retrograde contralateral approach include

  ○ Obese patients
  ○ A very scarred groin
  ○ A high bifurcation of the common femoral artery

However, even in these situations, direct puncture of the SFA is possible and arguably preferable to a contralateral access.

- The contralateral (cross-over technique) can be difficult if there is calcification and tortuosity of the iliac arteries, or if the aortic bifurcation has an acute angle.
- In general, it is sensible to have a sheath size 1Fr larger than the device to be used, to enable control angiography without removal of the device (balloon, stent, etc).
- With antegrade access, a 5Fr sheath enables control angiography when working with a 0.018- or a 0.014-inch platform.
- A 6Fr sheath enables control angiography when workng with 0.035-inch platform.
- Be careful that after sheath insertion, the sheath does not occlude the SFA because of the presence of a narrow proximal stenosis.

Angiography

High-quality, high-resolution angiographic images are essential.

- Use selective injections to assess carefully all stenoses and occlusions.
- Even if the pre-procedural images (CTA, MRA, Duplex) are of very good quality, it is essential to perform initial lower limb angiography to check that the angiographic findings are consistent with the pre-procedural imaging, or that the previous findings have not changed.
- The initial angiogram should include detailed images of the pedal circulation (dorsalis pedis, plantar arteries, and pedal arch).

Intra-procedural Medications

- IA heparin as a bolus (usually 5000 IU for a standard-sized person of approximately 70 Kg). The Activated Clotting Time (ACT) may be used to monitor heparinization during prolonged procedures, although this is seldom measured in practice.
- An arterial vasodilator such as tolozoline, papaverine, or glyceryl trinitrate (e.g., 100–150 mcg).
- Adequate analgesia (Fentanyl i.v. in 25–50 mcg amounts by slow injection).
- Sedation is optional (midazolam 1–2.5 mg i.v. by slow injection).
- For example 5 min evaluation: measurements of Pulse oxymetry, Blood pressure, respiration and consciousness by a dedicated nurse.

Assessing the Lesion

Morphology

- The aim of the procedure is to reopen straight-line flow to the foot.
- If there is extensive mural calcification involving the tibial arteries, subintimal recanalization is unlikely to be successful.

Pressure Measurements

- Pressure measurements are of no proven benefit at this level.

Choosing a Balloon or Stent

In general, PTA is the first-line treatment for lesions below the knee. Most interventionalists reserve stents only for salvage of failed angioplasty or do not use them at all below the knee in view of the paucity of scientific evidence for their use.

With increased experience of stents, some interventionalists have reduced their threshold for placing stents despite little evidence.

PTA

- The balloons used in the infrapopliteal segment are usually designed for use with 0.018-inch platforms.
- Typical balloon diameters used for the tibial vessels are 2.5- and 3-mm diameter.
- Typical balloon sizes for the tibioperoneal trunk are 3-, 3.5-, and exceptionally 4-mm diameter.
- The balloon length chosen is usually 40 mm, although longer balloons are available.
- Coaxial or rapid exchange balloons may be used.
- Cutting balloons may be used for lesions resistant to conventional balloons, although there is no supportive evidence.

Stents

- Self-expanding stents are better for long lesions and dissections. Balloon-expandable stents should be used for shorter lesions.
- Avoid stenting long segments as the patency is inevitably reduces with long stented lengths of infrapopliteal vessels.
- A wide variety of 0.018- and 0.014-inch guidewires are required. Long wire, e.g., 300 cm long may be required if you are treating lesions close to the ankle from the contralateral groin.
- There are several types of stent available, which include carbon-coated stents (Datascope/Maquet), drug-eluting stents (Cordis), and self-expandable stents (Xpert Abbott) and regular dedicated balloon expandable stents (Biotronik).

Reasonable indications for stent placement:

- Severe residual dissection (flow limiting) after failure of prolonged low-pressure inflation
- Recoil
- Residual thrombus not removable by aspiration

Performing the Procedure

Crossing the Lesion

- For proximal infrageniculate lesions, a 4–5Fr Cobra or Berenstein catheter combined with an angled-tip 0.035-inch hydrophilic guidewire (e.g., Terumo, Tokyo, Japan) is a useful combination to cross most stenoses and occlusions. Once the lesion has been traversed, the 0.035-inch guidewire can be exchanged for a smaller caliber guidewire prior to PTA.
- For more distal lesions, the 0.035-inch catheter and guidewire will likely be too large. The combination of the 0.018- or 0.014-inch balloon catheter and a0.018-inch hydrophilic guidewire will be successful in most cases for these distal lesions. The balloon is advanced as the guidewire dissects through the occlusion or is manipulated through the stenosis(es).

- It may be difficult to push catheters through occluded infrageniculate vessels, despite the use of relatively stiff supporting guidewires. A new balloon (Reekross, Clearstream) has been designed for this problem.
- For long occlusions (>40 mm), recanalization is inevitably subintimal.
- Consider an intentional subintimal recanalization for long occlusions. That is, advance a hydrophilic guidewire into the occlusion, form a loop with the wire, and advance the wire until it re-enters the lumen.
- If it is not possible to recanalize occlusions antegradely, consider retrograde recanalization.

  ○ This involves recanalization of the occlusion from a distal access at the foot – either the dorsalis pedis or the posterior tibial artery.
  ○ The basic tools are a 4Fr Cobra and a0.018- or 0.035-inch hydrophilic guidewire.
  ○ If recanalization is successful, PTA can be performed from this distal access via a 4Fr sheath.
  ○ Alternatively, to avoid the use of the 4Fr sheath, after manipulating the guidewire through the occlusion, it can be snared from above via the antegrade access. Subsequent PTA and/or stenting can be performed from the antegrade access. This is the so-called SAFARI technique.

Deploying the Balloon/Stent

- Balloon inflation should be performed with a 5-cc Luer-lock syringe.
- Inflation times are not standardized and vary from a few seconds to a few minutes per segment. Usually around 10–15 sec is adequate.
- If there is a persistent waist on the balloon, the inflation pressure should be increased.
- If there is evidence of dissection, this should be treated by a prolonged low-pressure inflation (3 atm; 3 min). This may improve appearances and flow and avoid the need for a stent.

Endpoint

As previously stated, the overall aim of intervention is to produce straight-line flow to the foot. Increasing collateral flow by treating proximal lesions without producing straight-line flow to the foot is rarely adequate to relieve symptoms and to promote healing of ulcers.

- Although optimal, there is generally no need to reconstruct the three infrapopliteal arteries to relieve CLI.

Brisk flow is a good indication of the success of subintimal recanalization, even if there is evidence of residual stenosis (see Fig. 1).

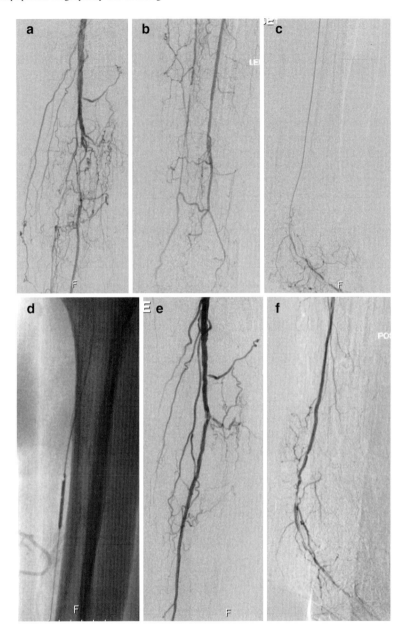

Fig. 1 (**a, b**) This 76-year-old patient presented with ulceration of the left foot. Figure 1a and b show the pre-procedural findings. There is an occlusion of the tibioperoneal trunk. Below this, the anterior tibial artery is occluded throughout its length. The peroneal artery refills in the upper calf and is patent to the distal calf. The posterior tibial artery reconstitutes in the mid-calf and supplies the plantar circulation, which appears to be of reasonable quality. (**c, d**) It was possible using a subintimal technique to recanalize the tibioperoneal trunk and continue the recanalization down the posterior tibial artery to the ankle. The entire length of the lesion was treated by balloon angioplasty with a 3 × 40-mm balloon (**e, f**) Show the final result. There is now straight-line flow to the foot. The patient's ulcer subsequently healed by 6 weeks follow-up

Immediate Post-procedure Care

This consists of standard care after any intra-arterial intervention and specific measures after intervention in CLI. These latter measures include

- Adequate analgesia
- Management and dressing of any arterial ulceration or gangrene
- Surgical debridement of toe/forefoot amputation if required
- Drug therapy (see next section)

Follow-Up and Post-procedure Medications

- Patients are followed up in the clinic to assess for relief of rest pain and healing of ulceration or gangrene.
- Risk factors should be managed including the provision of advice regarding the cessation of smoking.
- There should be interaction with a multidisciplinary team to improve local wound care.
- In general, duplex examination is not performed routinely and is reserved for recurrence of symptoms, failure of symptoms to resolve after the intervention, or a failure of the ulceration/gangrene to heal.
- Recurrent lesions detected by arterial duplex can be treated again.
- Antiplatelet therapy in the form of aspirin 75 mg o.d. for life is standard.
- The place of Clopidogrel in the management of patients following infrapopliteal intervention is not established.

  - Clopidogrel 75 mg/day may be taken for 3 months after stenting.
  - Some interventionalists treat all patients with Clopidogrel for 3 months after all infrapopliteal PTA procedures.
  - Clopidogrel may be continued indefinitely.

Results

The results of infrageniculate intervention should be assessed in terms of limb salvage rather than primary patency.

- Most series of infrapopliteal angioplasty report 24-month limb salvage rates of 70%.
- Patency rates are generally less than limb salvage rates by around 20%.
- The main aim in CLI is to improve the distal blood flow for a period of time long enough for the ulcer to heal or to relieve symptoms. In many cases, if the

angioplastied lesion recurs, new collaterals will have formed, which resists the onset of recurrent symptoms.
- Outcomes data from stents are limited at the time of publication.
- There are early data suggesting favorable outcomes of drug-eluting stents in the infrapopliteal circulation.

Alternative Therapies

These consist of distal surgical bypass or conservative management with a variety of experimental drug therapies.

- Distal bypass should be performed using autologous vein as the graft material.
- Distal bypass is complex arterial surgery requiring considerable surgical skill and patience.
- Distal bypass is not always possible because of the presence of poor distal vessels-infected ulcers or a lack of autologous vein for use as a graft.
- The outcomes of distal bypass are dependent on the patient selection. Five-year "assisted" patency rates using vein approach 60%.
- The results after bypass using prosthetic graft material are dismal.
- Non-surgical therapies, which are tried for the treatment/palliation of CLI, when there is no other alternative, include prostacyclin analogues and gene therapy.

Complications

How to Treat

Complications may be related to treatment of the lesion itself, the puncture site, or to the administration of contrast medium.
    Complications related to treatment of the lesion include:

- Spasm – treat by the intra-arterial administration of a vasodilator, e.g., glyceryl trinitrate in 100–150 mcg bolus injections.
- Dissection – treat by repeat dilation or a stent.
- Distal embolization – treat by aspiration thrombectomy although this is technically difficult because of the small caliber of the vessels.
- Vessel rupture – this seldom requires treatment and is usually self-limiting, although may necessitate the termination of the procedure.

How to Avoid

Apart from the prophylactic administration of a vasodilator to prevent spasm, the other complications related to treatment of the lesion listed above are difficult to prevent.

Key Points

- High-quality imaging is essential.
- The patient must be able to lie still. Therefore, treat any rest pain with adequate analgesia.
- Antegrade access makes the procedure much easier for the operator and increases the chance of success.
- Prevent and treat arterial spasm by the intra-arterial administration of vasodilators.
- There is no evidence in favor of primary stenting versus conventional angioplasty.

Suggested Reading

1. Adam DJ, Beard JD, Cleveland T, Bell J, Bradbury AW, Forbes JF, Fowkes FG, Gillepsie I, Ruckley CV, Raab G, Storkey H, BASIL trial participants. Bypass versus angioplasty in severe ischaemia of the leg (BASIL): multicentre,randomised controlled trial. Lancet 2005 Dec 3; 366(9501): 1925–34.
2. Norgren L, Hiatt WR, Dormandy JA, Nehler MR, Harris KA, Fowkes FG, TASC II Working Group. Inter-Society Consensus for the Management of Peripheral Arterial Disease (TASC II). J Vasc Surg 2007 Jan; 45 Suppl S: S5–S67.
3. Schmehl J, Tepe G. Current status of bare and drug-eluting stents in infrainguinal peripheral vascular disease. Expert Rev Cardiovasc Ther 2008 Apr; 6(4): 531–8.

Renal Artery Angioplasty and Stenting

Sanjay Misra

Clinical Features

- Patients with uncontrolled hypertension will often present with headaches, palpitations, chest pain, and blurry vision.
- Young women with hypertension who are not on oral contraceptives often have fibromuscular dysplasia (FMD).
- Patients with renal artery stenosis (RAS) in the sixties, seventies, and eighties have typically atherosclerotic renal artery stenosis.
- On physical examination, patients with renal artery stenosis will often have a flank or lateral epigastric bruit over the affected kidney.
- Suspect RAS in patients who

  - Develop renal insufficiency while on angiotensin-converting enzyme (ACE) inhibitors
  - Patients with malignant hypertension
  - Patients with long-standing hypertension which accelerates without cause
  - Patients with flash pulmonary edema (usually due to bilateral RAS)

Diagnostic Evaluation

Laboratory

- Kidney function should be assessed prior to intervention with serum blood urea nitrogen, creatinine, and an estimated glomerular filtration rate calculated using Modification of Diet in Renal Disease (MDRD) formula or a short clearance.
- Blood pressure evaluation should be performed. A 24-h blood pressure monitor may be useful.
- Anti-hypertensive medications need to be optimized. Most patients should be on an ACE inhibitor, a beta-blocker, and a diuretic. This should be managed by a physician who is familiar with these medications and can optimally manage them.

R.A. Morgan, E. Walser (eds.), *Handbook of Angioplasty and Stenting Procedures*,
Techniques in Interventional Radiology, DOI 10.1007/978-1-84800-399-6_12,
© Springer-Verlag London Limited 2010

Imaging

- Non-invasive imaging of the renal arteries can be performed using computed tomographic analysis, magnetic resonance angiography, or ultrasound:

Ultrasound

- One advantage of ultrasound is that it is a non-invasive test, which can be performed in patients with normal and abnormal kidney function.
- Sometimes difficult to determine if patient has FMD and limited by body habitus and bowel gas.
- Resistive indices (RIs) should be determined in both kidneys prior to intervention. Resistive indices are used to predict a successful outcome in patients with hypertension, typically an RI of less than 0.7 is favorable for a successful outcome after treatment.
- The velocity measurement of blood in the renal artery can predict the likelihood of a stenosis. Usually a peak systolic velocity of greater than 180 cm/s is predictive of a stenosis. In addition, a ratio between the blood velocity in the aorta to renal artery of >3.5 is suggestive of a stenosis. For restenosis after angioplasty or stent placement, similar blood velocities in the stented artery can predict restenosis.
- The size of the kidney is important by ultrasound and 8-cm or larger kidneys should be stented or angioplastied.

  - Conversely, small kidneys (<6–7 cm) respond poorly to renal artery intervention.

Computed tomographic angiography (CTA)

- One advantage of CTA is that it is a non-invasive test which can be performed in patients with pacemakers and provides anatomical information with regard to the presence of aortoiliac arterial occlusive disease.
- CTA is sensitive for detecting FMD.
- Stenosis determination hindered in the presence of exuberant vascular calcifications

Magnetic resonance imaging/magnetic resonance angiography

- One advantage of MRI/MRA is that it is a non-invasive test which can be performed in patients and provides anatomical information with regard to the presence of aortoiliac arterial occlusive disease.
- One disadvantage of MRI/MRA is that gadolinium has been associated with nephrogenic sytemic fibrosis in patients with decreased glomerular filtration rate (GFR less than or equal to 30) and is contraindicated in these patients.
- MR performs better in the presence of calcification.
- Newer MR sequences actually allow MR angiography without the use of contrast agents.

- Promising new method, which avoids risks of iodinated contrast and gadolinium and ionizing radiation

Digital Subtraction Angiography
- "gold standard" for accurate evaluation of RAS
- Enables hemodynamic measurements to determine significance of RAS
- In case of contrast allergy or renal failure, alternative contrast agents are available:
  - Carbon dioxide for renal dysfunction
  - Gadolinium for iodinated contrast allergy
  - Modern fluoroscopic units have the ability to optimize imaging for alternative contrast agents

Indications

- Renal artery angioplasty or stent placement is performed in patients with
  - Uncontrolled hypertension
    - In young patients
    - In older patients who previously had well-controlled hypertension
  - Worsening renal function
  - Cardiac destabilization syndromes – sudden episodes of
    - Congestive heart failure
    - Flash pulmonary edema
    - Unstable or refractory angina pectoris
- Fibromuscular dysplasia (FMD) responds well to angioplasty of the renal artery and stenting is reserved for flow-limiting dissections.
  - In the event of restenosis with FMD, repeat angioplasty remains effective
- Atherosclerotic renal artery stenoses respond best to primary stenting.

Contraindications

- Abnormal coagulation studies with elevated INR (>1.8), PTT (>60 msec), or decreased platelets ($<50 \times 10^3$ mm^3).
- Severe iodinated contrast allergies
  - Consider CO_2 or gadolinium angiography
- Renal failure with GFR <40
  - Pre treat with *N*-acetylcysteine, intravenous hydration
  - Consider CO_2 angiography

Patient Preparation

- The patient is encouraged to take his normal medications on the date of the procedure, but otherwise is kept fasting (NPO) for 8 h.
- Laboratory investigations include hemoglobin, prothrombin time (PT), international normalized ratio (INR), partial thromboplastin time (PTT), platelets, and serum creatinine prior to the procedure.
- Consider checking the hemoglobin and serum creatinine 48 h after the renal artery procedure to assess for bleeding and contrast medium-induced nephropathy.

Relevant Anatomy

Normal Anatomy

- The renal arteries typically arise immediately inferior to the superior mesenteric artery near the L_1–L_2 intervertebral disk space.
- Typically, 70% of the patients have one renal artery supplying each kidney. In 20–35% of the patients, there is more than one renal artery supplying each kidney.

Aberrant Anatomy

- There may be an early bifurcation of the renal artery.
- The renal artery may uncommonly arise from the common iliac artery, external iliac artery, superior or inferior mesenteric arteries.

Renal Artery Angioplasty and Stent Equipment

- The original description of renal artery angioplasty was described using a 0.035″ wire and balloon. Today, renal artery stents and angioplasty are typically performed using 0.014–0.018″ compatatible catheters and wires.
- The balloons and stents are monorail for 0.014″ or over the wire for 0.018″ systems, many of which require the use of a guiding catheter.
- The guiding catheter shape is based on the orientation of the renal artery origin. Multiple different types of guiding catheter shapes are available with different wires of different stiffness and torqueability.
- One popular option is a 6F (IM) guide catheter (Boston Scientific, Natick, MA) used to engage the renal orgin.

  - A 0.014″ Reflex (Cordis Endovascular, Miami, FLA) or Sparta Core (Abbott Vascular, Redmond, CA) wire is used to cross the renal artery stenosis.
  - The tip of the wire should not prolapse as this may cause a subintimal dissection.

Pre-procedure Medications

- Except those with contraindications such as fluid overload and asthma, patients with glomerular filtration rate less than 30 check in to the hospital 1 day before the procedure for

  - Overnight prehydration with oral fluids and/or intravenous crystalloids ± *N*-acetylcysteine (Mucomyst) to prevent the potential nephrotoxic effects of the contrast.

    - *N*-acetylcysteine 600 mg orally every 12 h for four doses (two before and two after angiography).
    - One method for intravenous hydration is Dextrose 5% in water (850 mL) with 154 milliequivalents sodium bicarbonate administered at 3 mL/kg/h for 1 h before procedure and 1 mL/kg/h for 6 h post-procedure.

Procedure

Access

- Patients receive moderate sedation using a combination of midazolam hydrochloride (Versed, Abraxis Pharmaceutical Products, Schaumburg, IL) and fentanyl citrate (Hospira, Inc, Lake Forrest, IL) for pain as needed administered through a peripheral intravenous line by a registered nurse. The common femoral artery is typically used and anesthetized using 5–10 mL of 2% lidocaine hydrochloride (Hospira Inc, Lake Forrest, IL). The brachial artery or radial artery can be used. The common femoral artery is accessed using a Seldinger technique. A 6F sheath is placed and an IM guide catheter is used to engage the renal orgin (Figs. 1 and 2).

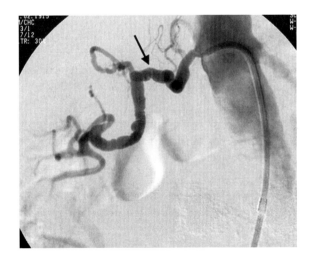

Fig. 1 Renal angiogram showing "string of beads" appearance in a patient with fibromuscular dysplasia (*arrow*)

Fig. 2 Atherosclerotic ostial
renal artery stenosis (*arrow*)

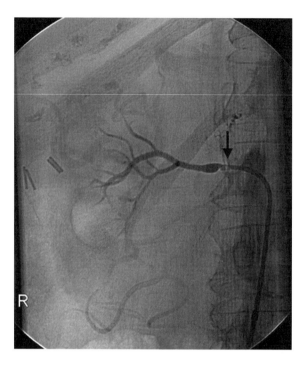

Angiography

- A renal angiogram is performed in the appropriate oblique to image the renal
  origin "en face." Typically, a 15–25° LAO projection using 4–8 mL of contrast
  infused at 4 mL/sec is performed

Assessing the Lesion

- Renal artery stenosis is defined as a diameter reduction of greater than 50% by
  visual estimate when compared to its immediate, distal non-dilated main renal
  arterial segment. A pressure gradient is obtained if there is a question of lesion
  severity.

  ○ A mean pressure gradient measured between the aorta to distal renal artery
    of 10 mm of Hg or a systolic gradient of more than 20 mm of Hg is
    hemodynamically significant.

- Renal artery stenosis are classified into "ostial" if it is located less than or equal
  to 5-mm distance away from renal artery origin from the aorta and "non-ostial"
  if it is located more than 5-mm away from renal artery origin.

- Fibromuscular dysplasia has a "string of beads" appearance, which can involve the main renal arteries and its branches. It typically affects women in their forties and sixties with 80% incidence of bilaterality (Fig. 1). There are three types of FMD:

  ○ Medial fibroplasia (most common, 70% of the patients) – string of beads most common angiographic appearance
  ○ Intimal fibroplasia (20%) – younger patients (often infants). Tubular, concentric stenoses are characteristic
  ○ Subadventitial fibroplasia (10%)

- Atherosclerotic renal artery stenosis is characterized by ostial disease, which has dense calcification (Fig. 2). In 6–10% of the patients, there can be atherosclerotic RAS with FMD.

Intra-procedural Medications

- Before stent placement or angioplasty, one should administer

  ○ Bolus of unfractionated heparin intravenously (50 units per kilogram of body weight).
  ○ Nitroglycerin in 50–100 μg aliquots to prevent guidewire-induced spasm in the peripheral renal arteries.

Performing the Procedure

Crossing the Lesion

- First, a floppy (soft-tipped) wire or glide wire carefully traverses the renal artery lesion. It is important to keep the guidewire within the lumen of the vessel as a subintimal dissection can occur very easily.
- To select the renal artery, some use a cobra-type catheter, while others use a Shepard's hook catheter (Simmons type). Regardless of the catheter used, the operator must use extreme care to pass the guidewire through and not underneath the renal occlusive lesion in question.
- Two methods exist to measure the length and diameter of the renal artery stenosis

  ○ Visual estimation – using the field of view and guide catheter size as markers to estimate distances
  ○ arker catheter – use to calibrate the length of the stenosis and diameter of the non-diseased renal artery using the software provided with the angiographic suite.

Angioplasty/Deploying the Stent

- Atherosclerotic RAS requires the radial force of balloon-expandable stents, the choice of which is based on the preference of the interventionalist as there are many different types available.
- Typically, appropriate renal artery stent diameters are 5–8 mm with a length of 12–15-mm based on the length of the stenosis and diameter of the non-diseased renal artery. The diameter of the stent should not be larger than the diameter of the non-diseased renal artery since this can lead to dissection or rupture.
- If the stent cannot cross the renal artery stenosis, consider a 3–4-mm predilation of the renal artery stenosis to allow easier passage of the stent.
- Deploy the renal artery stent to its nominal diameter based on the pressure chart supplied with the stent from the manufacturer.
- Perform follow-up angiography after stent deployment to the stent to ensure that there is no renal artery dissection, rupture, or spasm (Fig. 3).
- Carefully assess the peripheral renal arteries for embolization, which can occur in 10–20% of renal artery stent placement procedures.
- FMD almost always responds to angioplasty alone with a balloon diameter of 1.1–1.2 greater than that of the non-diseased renal artery.

  ○ Consider a renal stent only if there is a dissection limiting renal artery blood flow.

- Endpoints:

  ○ "Technical success" – less than 30% residual stenosis after deployment of the stent on follow-up angiogram.

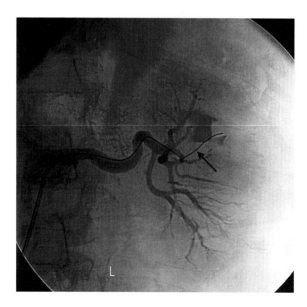

Fig. 3 *Arrow* showing spasm caused by the wire after renal artey stent placement

  ○ Systolic pressure gradient <10 mmHg or mean pressure gradient <5 mmHg

- The sheath and catheter are removed once the activated clotting time has decreased below 200.

Immediate Post-procedure Care

- Patients recover as after any vascular procedure with femoral access with the following additional considerations:

  ○ Hydration post-procedure – oral and intravenous
  ○ Precautions for orthostatic hypotension

    ■ Patients are instructed to avoid standing quickly and to have assistance when standing for the first day.

  ○ Patients should keep a more detailed log of their blood pressure (3–4 times daily) and present to the physician treating their hypertension so that he can modify drug regimens accordingly.
  ○ Some recommend checking serum creatinine and GFR in 1–2 weeks to look for evidence of cholesterol embolization syndrome.

    ■ Delayed presentation of renal dysfunction due to the slow time course of multiple peripheral and segmental areas of renal ischemia.

Follow-Up and Post-procedure Medications

- Six-week course of dual antiplatelet therapy using a loading dose of ClopidogrelPlavix 300 mg by mouth (Bristol-Myers Squibb/Sanofi Pharmaceuticals Partnership, Bridgewater, NJ) and then 75 mg once daily. In adddition, patients take one baby aspirin (81 mg) every day.
- Patients are followed with serial duplex ultrasound to evaluate for restenosis. Restenosis typically occurs in 15–20% of the patients at 9 months.
- Periodic serum BUN, creatinine, and blood pressure measurement to evaluate for functional outcome.
- Restenosis of renal arteries is retreated with a number of different approaches including

  ○ Repeat angioplasty
  ○ Cutting balloon angioplasty
  ○ Cryoplasty
  ○ Placement of a new stent
  ○ Covered or drug-eluting stent placement.

Alternative Therapies

- **Embolic protection devices:** Embolic protection devices (EPDs) have been used to prevent atheroembolism during treatment of stenosis involving saphenous vein bypass grafts used as arterial conduits for coronary artery disease and in conjunction with the placement of a carotid artery stent. Recently, several reports have described the use of these devices to prevent atheroembolism during renal artery stent placement. It has been hypothesized that these devices may help prevent atheroembolism during renal artery stent procedures. There are several papers now describing the role of EPDs with renal artery stent placement in patients with chronic renal insufficiency but no level 1 evidence to support their use.
- **Drug-eluting stents:** Renal arteries with diameters measuring less than 4 mm have a lower patency rate after angioplasty and stent placement because of higher incidence of in-stent restenosis and have typically been not stented. Drug-eluting stents (DESs) have been used for the treatment of stenosis involving the coronary arteries with lower restenosis rates, and may offer a potential alternative to BMS in renal arteries with diameters less than 4 mm. There have been several case reports of the use of DES for treating de novo RAS involving the bifurcation of the renal artery or in-stent restenosis. In a small series from the Mayo Clinic, DES were used to renal artery stenosis with good technical results and low restenosis rates when compared to bare metal stents despite the DES group having significantly smaller diameter renal arteries when compared to bare metal stents.

Results of RAS Angioplasty and Stenting

- Percutaneous renal artery angioplasty with stent placement has become the cornerstone therapy for the treatment of atherosclerotic renal artery stenosis.
- Reported technical results are excellent with a 98–100% procedural success rate.
- The effect on renal function is difficult to predict.

  - Improves in only 30–40% of patients
  - Stabilizes in another 30–40%
  - Deteriorates in 20–30%

- Angioplasty performed for FMD has better results with improvement in blood pressure in as many as 90% of patients.

  - This success rate applies for repeat angioplasty in FMD as well.

Complications and Their Treatment

- There are many different types of complications which can occur during a renal artery stent placement.

- Renal artery dissection.

  - Occurs when the wire used to cross the stenosis tracks under the intimal surface. These often will resolve after the stent has been placed but care must be taken to ensure that the wire is in the true lumen proximal and distal to the dissection.
  - Prolonged inflation of 3 min or longer can be used to tack down the dissection.

- Renal artery rupture occurs when the renal artery is over-dilated either during predilation or stent deployment.

  - This can be treated with prolonged balloon dilation or covered stent.
  - Rarely may result in gross rupture requiring balloon tamponade of the renal artery stump or aorta and emergent surgical repair.

- Renal artery spasm is caused by introduction of the wire into a tiny intrarenal artery.

  - Treated with infusion of 100-μg nitroglycerin.
  - Check for resolution with follow-up angiogram in 3–5 min.
  - If the spasm does not resolve, one must consider the possibility of a dissection or atheroembolism.

- Aggressive distal wire placement can lead to renal capsular perforation and perirenal hematoma

  - Clue is significant flank pain during/after procedure.
  - CT may show perirenal/pararenal hemorrhage.
  - Treat conservatively – rarely requires embolotherapy.

- Renal atheroembolism

  - If possible, treat with suction thrombectomy using a microcatheter.
  - Consider infusion of thrombolytic agent such as Alteplase (Genetech, San Francisco, CA). This is typically infused using a bolus of 4–8 mg over 5–10 min.

    - Alternative, use a short infusion of thrombolytic therapy for 4–8 h using 0.5–1.0 mg/h of Alteplase.

Key Points

- Select patients carefully for optimum outcomes

  - Renal artery intervention is good for patients with non-invasive imaging exams positive for RAS and:

    - Severe, new, or worsening hypertension
    - Cardiac destabilization syndromes

○ Questionable indications for renal dysfunction

■ Little evidence exists to support stenting/angioplasty to improve renal function except in patients with a single kidney and severe RAS.

• Avoid renal artery dissection and rupture:

○ Carefully select renal artery and keep the guidewire in the lumen and avoid wire prolapse.
○ Appropriately size the renal artery.

• Dilate/stent renal artery to 6 mm or more if at all possible.

○ Improved long-term results and less restenosis.

• FMD responds to angioplasty alone.

○ Stents used only for complicating dissection with limitation to forward flow.

Suggested Reading

1. Baum SA and Pentecost MJ. Abrams' Angiography Volume 3 1997.
2. Blum U, Krumme B, Flugel P, et al. Treatment of ostial renal-artery stenoses with vascular endoprostheses after unsuccessful balloon angioplasty. N Engl J Med 1997; 336: 459–465.
3. Misra S, Gomes M, Matthews V, et al. Embolic protection devices in patients with renal artery stenosis with chronic renal insufficiency: A clinical study. J Vasc Interv Radiol 2008 in press.
4. Misra S, Sturludottir M, Matthews V, et al. Treatment of Complex Stenoses Involving Renal Artery Bifurcations using Drug-eluting Stents. J Vasc Interv Radiol 2008; 19(2): 272–278.
5. Misra S, Thatipelli MR, Howe PW, et al. Preliminary study of the use of drug-eluting stents in atherosclerotic renal artery stenoses 4 mm in diameter or smaller. J Vasc Interv Radiol. 2008 Nov; 19(11): 1639–45. Epub 2008 Sep 12.
6. Radermacher J, Chavan A, Bleck J, et al. Use of Doppler ultrasonography to predict the outcome of therapy for renal-artery stenosis. N Engl J Med 2001; 344: 410–417.

Angioplasty/Stenting of Mesenteric Arteries

Stefan Müller-Hülsbeck

Clinical Features

- Chronic mesenteric ischemia (CMI), first described as "abdominal angina" by Goodman in 1918 and as a distinct entity by Dunphy in 1936, is a rare disorder.
- CMI is usually diagnosed late after the initial presentation usually after several investigations have ruled out other causes of the patient's symptoms.
- The number of arteries that must be involved before symptoms of ischemia occur is still debated. Most agree that at least two of the celiac artery (CA), the superior mesenteric artery (SMA), or the inferior mesenteric artery (IMA) should be stenosed or occluded for a diagnosis of CMI to be made. A stenosis or occlusion of a single visceral vessel is usually asymptomatic because of preservation of flow to the gastrointestinal tract via collateral vessels.
- CMI is caused by intermittent episodes of intestinal ischemia, usually associated with the increased metabolic demand caused by digestion.
- Symptoms due to CMI include chronic postprandial pain, nausea, diarrhea, and obvious weight loss. Patients often describe a "fear of food."
- Atherosclerosis is the most common cause of CMI. Vasculitis and Takayasu disease are other less likely causes of this condition.

Diagnostic Evaluation

Clinical

Clinical signs are uncommon.

- Abdominal bruit due to a stenosis is rare.
- Weight loss with no obvious cause.
- The most important factor in the diagnosis of CMI is a suspicion of the condition in the presence of appropriate symptoms and no other obvious cause.

R.A. Morgan, E. Walser (eds.), *Handbook of Angioplasty and Stenting Procedures*, 153
Techniques in Interventional Radiology, DOI 10.1007/978-1-84800-399-6_13,

Laboratory

- There is no laboratory test for the diagnosis of CMI.

Imaging

- Non-invasive imaging has replaced angiography as the main initial imaging method for the evaluation of patients with suspected CMI.
- Color duplex sonography (CDS) is effective for the detection of stenoses at the origins of the visceral vessels.

  ○ A hemodynamically significant lesion is confirmed by Aliasing on color flow Doppler ultrasound and a peak systolic velocity of >1.8 m/s.

- CTA and MRA are also effective for the diagnosis of occlusive disease at the origins of the visceral vessels (Fig. 1).
- All three modalities are of variable accuracy in the diagnosis of more peripheral stenoses or occlusions beyond the vessel origins.
- The aim of imaging is to

  ○ Assess the origins of the CA, the SMA, and the IMA.
  ○ Assess for the presence of a prominent collateral vessel such as the Arc of Riolan or a prominent pancreaticoduodenal arcade.

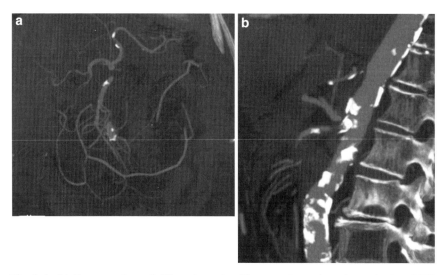

Fig. 1 (a, b) Contrast-enhanced CT angiography. These maximum intensity projection (MIP) images indicate calcified plaque close to the origin of a severely stenosed SMA in the coronal and sagittal planes

- ○ Demonstrate the exact location of any stenoses or occlusions.
- ○ Target subsequent treatment.

Indications

- Symptoms consistent with CMI, i.e., chronic postprandial pain, nausea, diarrhea, and obvious weight loss.
- Diagnosis by imaging of stenoses or occlusions of two or more of the CA, SMA, or IMA.

Contraindications

- Median Arcuate Ligament Syndrome (MALS)

  - ○ This causes a functional stenosis of the CA, occurs in young patients and is rare.
  - ○ MALS may lead to considerable abdominal pain and weight loss.
  - ○ Diagnosis is by color duplex sonography and/or CTA and/or MRA.
  - ○ The condition may be difficult to distinguish from atherosclerotic disease. The absence of atheroma elsewhere, the absence of calcification, symptoms in a relatively young patient, and the characteristic imaging findings of the ligament on CT or MR imaging are helpful indicators of the diagnosis.
  - ○ The treatment of MALS is surgery, not angioplasty or stenting.

- Allergy to iodinated contrast medium is a relative contraindication. Although angioplasty/stenting of the visceral vessels is very difficult if an alternative contrast medium such as carbon dioxide is used.

Patient Preparation

- Standard sterile preparation as for other vascular interventions.

Relevant Anatomy

- Normal anatomy:

  - ○ The SMA rises at the level of L1.
  - ○ The origin of the IMA arises at the level of L3.
  - ○ The origins of the SMA and the IMA are stable.

- Aberrant anatomy: The variable origin of the hepatic arteries is well known from pathological and angiographic studies. These variants are not of concern for this procedure.

- The common hepatic artery arising from the celiac artery is the most common type found in 70% of subjects.

Equipment Required

- The equipment required is similar to other visceral vascular interventions.
- Cannulation of the CA, SMA, and IMA is usually achieved with a cobra catheter or a reversed-curve catheter such as a sidewinder, a Sos Omni, or a Rim catheter.
- Either standard 0.035-inch or better smaller caliber 0.018-inch and 0.014-inch systems can be used for PTA and stenting.

Pre-procedure Medications

- Most patients also have cardiovascular disease elsewhere, and are generally already taking Aspirin +/− Statin medication.
- It is not a requirement of this procedure for patients to be on specific pre-procedural medications.

Procedure

Arterial/Venous Access

- As usual, peripheral venous access is required for the administration of medications during the procedure.
- Procedures are performed usually from a femoral artery access, either the right or the left.
- A standard 6F 10 cm sheath may be used. However, a longer sheath 35–45-cm long is preferable, because it enables peri-procedural angiography through the sheath with catheters, guidewires, or stent delivery systems in situ in the target vessel.
- It may be problematic to pass catheters into vessels that curve inferiorly. In these cases, a transbrachial access may be chosen, either initially after evaluation of the vessel orientation from the imaging or if access into the target vessel from a femoral access fails.
- In general, access is from the femoral artery in more than 90% of patients.

Angiography

- Flush aortography is usually performed before selective cannulation of the target vessel to provide angiographic correlation of the pre-procedural imaging findings.

- Angiography should be performed using an aortic flush catheter, a power injector, and a standard volume and rate of injection suitable for aortography, e.g., 20 mL of contrast medium at 10 mL/sec.
- Aortography should be performed in the anteroposterior and lateral projections to identify the origins of the visceral vessels.

Intra-procedural Medications

- 5,000 units of intra-arterial heparin.
- 20-mg intravenous Buscopan – if there is significant image impairment because of bowel movement.

Assessing the Lesion

- The vast majority of lesions are at the origins of the vessels. More distal stenoses are unusual.
- The vast majority of stenoses can be traversed.
- Occlusions are very difficult to traverse. Most interventionalists would not attempt to recanalize an occluded CA, SMA, or IMA.
- If more than one vessel is stenosed, the SMA or CA should be treated preferentially to the IMA. The IMA is usually a small vessel and any benefit from treating an IMA stenosis is generally less than revascularization of lesions involving the CA or SMA.

Pressure Measurements

- Pressure measurements are usually not necessary and are only warranted in lesions where there is uncertainty regarding whether the stenosis is significant or not. A systolic pressure drop of more than 20 mmHg is an indication for treatment.

Choosing a Balloon or a Stent

- Although there is no convincing evidence regarding angioplasty versus stenting, most operators would select a stent for the treatment of an ostial stenosis or a lesion within 10 mm of the vessel origin.
- For more distal lesions, PTA alone is usually performed.

Performing the Procedure

Crossing the Lesion

- A long sheath or guiding catheter is advanced into the upper abdominal aorta.
- The ostium of the vessel is cannulated with a cobra or a Sidewinder-shaped catheter (if the approach is from the groin), or a multipurpose catheter (if a transbrachial route has been used).
- With the catheter tip located close to the stenosis, the lesion is usually crossed with a 0.035-inch hydrophilic guidewire. Some operators prefer to cross the lesion with a smaller caliber guidewire, in which case a 0.018- or a 0.014-inch guidewire, (either hydrophilic or with a hydrophilic tip) may be used.
- After the guidewire has traversed the lesion, the catheter is advanced across the lesion followed by exchange of the hydrophilic guidewire for a stiffer guidewire (0.035 or 0.018 inch). The Amplatz superstiff or Rosen guidewires are popular guidewires for this purpose.

Deploying the Balloon or Stent

- Most interventionalists perform primary stenting.

  - For tight stenoses, predilation prior to stent insertion may be helpful to enable the stent on its delivery catheter to be advanced across the lesion (e.g., 4 mm balloon).
  - Either over the wire or rapid exchange (monorail) balloons may be used.
  - Predilation is advisable for very narrow, calcified stenoses.

- If PTA is the planned definitive therapy, the diameter of the balloon should be chosen based on the size of the vessel to be stented.

  - This measurement can be obtained from previous CT images or using the measuring facility on the angiographic equipment.
  - Although the diameters of the vessels vary widely from patient to patient, suggested balloon diameters are as follows: Celiac trunk and SMA 6–7 mm; IMA 4 mm.

- Inflation of the balloon using a manometer to limit excessive inflation pressures may prevent the rare complication of vessel rupture.
- Self-expanding or balloon-expandable stents may be used. Short balloon-expandable stents are most commonly used for ostial lesions, because of their improved deployment accuracy in this type of location compared with self-expanding stents.
- In general, balloon-expandable stents are used for ostial lesions. Self-expanding stents are usually reserved more distal lesions, if PTA fails for these latter lesions.

Self-expanding stents are also used occasionally for the treatment of dissection involving the splanchnic vessels.

- Once the stent is in place, angiography is performed to confirm that the stent is in the correct location prior to deployment. For ostial lesions, the stent should protrude by 2–3 mm into the aorta.
- All PTA and stenting procedures should be performed in the appropriate projection at 90° to the lesion, usually the full lateral position. If the proximal end of the stent protrudes into the aorta, the proximal end may be flared by a larger balloon after deployment.

Endpoint

- Completion angiography should indicate a fully expanded stent in the correct location across the lesion.
- A widely patent vessel at completion angiography indicated success.

Examples of three cases are provided in Figs. 2, 3, and 4.

Immediate Post-procedure Care

- If possible, a closure device should be used.
- The arterial puncture site should be monitored in the standard manner.

Follow-Up and Post-procedure Medications

- There is no standard follow-up protocol.
- Color duplex sonography to confirm patency may be performed before discharge.
- Some operators administer intravenous heparin for 24 h or low-molecular heparin until discharge.
- Low-dose aspirin is usually prescribed to be continued indefinitely.
- Most operators would also administer Clopidogrel 75 mg daily for 6 weeks (Fig. 5).

Results

- The outcomes of endovascular therapy are very respectable and compare favorably with surgery with mean primary patency rates of 76% at 15 months,

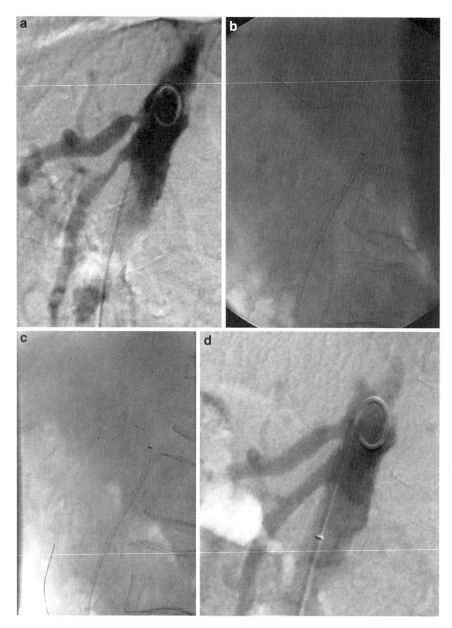

Fig. 2 (**a**) This angiogram, obtained in a lateral 90° projection, shows a high-grade ostial stenosis of the celiac trunk and a moderate stenosis of the SMA main trunk. (**b**) This image shows a 6×18-mm stent deployed in celiac trunk, a 0.014-inch guidewire is still in place, and a 6F sheath is placed below the origin. (**c**) Shows a second stent, 6×18 mm, implanted in the SMA during the same procedure. (**d**) Final angiography after completing the intervention shows a widely patent celiac trunk and SMA with no residual stenosis

Fig. 3 (**a**) Selective angiography of the celiac trunk through a cobra catheter showing a sufficient supply of splenic, liver, and pancreatico-duodenal branches without any large collateral vessels visible to the SMA. (**b, c**) High-grade ostial stenosis of the IMA, which is responsible for the entire bowel supply. (**d, e**)The stenosis has been crossed with an 0.014-inch wire, guided by a Sidewinder catheter. The lesion is predilated with a 5-mm balloon. (**f, g**) After predilation, a 7×19 mm is stent positioned and deployed. Completion angiography shows a good result

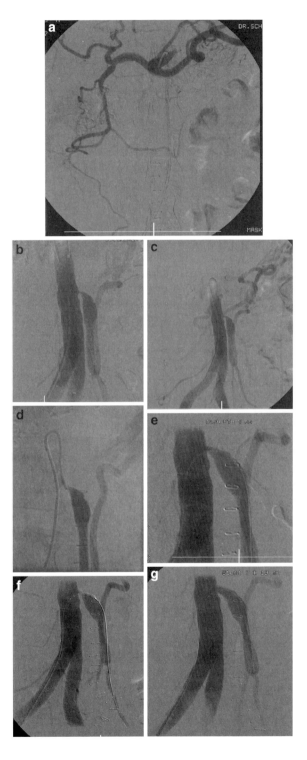

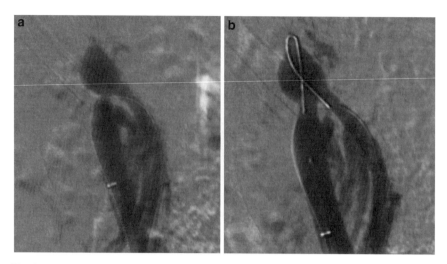

Fig. 4 (**a, b**) A severely stenosed aortomesenteric venous bypass graft. The images show the distal anastomosis before and after PTA using a 5 and 7×20-mm balloon in a 35-year-old young lady (heavy smoker and Takayasu arteritis). There is a residual mild stenosis. N.B. A 0.014-inch buddy wire was placed distal to the stenosis in the proximal part of the SMA. If there is recurrent restenosis, cutting balloon angioplasty using a 6×20-mm balloon might be an appropriate treatment method. Insertion of a stent is also an option, although should be avoided if possible in young patients

a technical success rate close to 100%, a peri-procedural major and minor complication rate of less than 10%, and mortality of below 4%.
- Percutaneous intervention for CMI is safe with durable early and mid-term clinical success. However, repeated intervention may be required for improved primary assisted patency, particularly if PTA rather than stenting was originally performed.
- The symptom-free rates are around 95, 90, 72, and 54% at 0, 1, 24, and 30 months, respectively.
- Complication rates are very low.

Alternative Therapies

- The main alternative treatment is surgery. Surgical procedures include endarterectomy and surgical bypass (e.g., aortoceliac and aortomesenteric bypass).
- Surgery may still be preferred in patients with long occlusions and a low operative risk.
- Retrograde mesenteric stenting during laparotomy for acute occlusive mesenteric ischemia is a potential hybrid endovascular and surgical option.

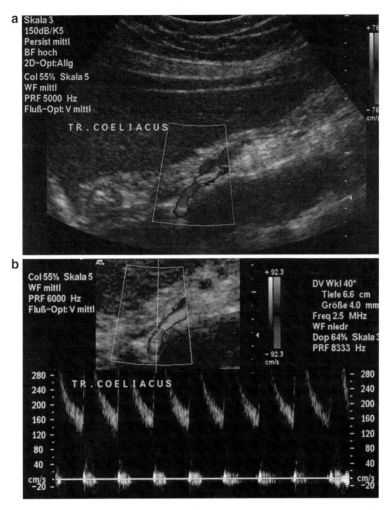

Fig. 5 (a, b) Color duplex sonography during follow-up after previous stenting of a celiac trunk stenosis indicates increased peak velocities within the stent. Repeat PTA is the treatment of choice

Complications

How to Treat

- Stent dislodgement:

  ○ If the stent is displaced behind the lesion and is still in the target vessel, the stent should be deployed in the vessel. A second stent should be subsequently advanced across the lesion and deployed in the correct location.

- ○ If the stent is partially in the aorta and is still partially mounted on the balloon, the balloon and stent combination can be withdrawn into the iliac artery and fully deployed in this location. A new stent can be deployed in the correct location.
- ○ If the stent has become detached from the balloon, it will be necessary to snare the stent using a snare introduced from the ipsilateral femoral artery.

  - ■ This is best achieved by passing the snare catheter through the same sheath as the stent.
  - ■ It is essential to maintain the guidewire in place so that the stent does not become detached from the guidewire.
  - ■ If the sheath is too small for the snare catheter and the guidewire, the sheath should be exchanged for a larger sheath.
  - ■ The snare should be passed through the sheath with the loop over the guidewire until the snare loop is at the level of the stent.
  - ■ The lower end of the stent is snared by closing the loop and is withdrawn in a collapsed state through the sheath.

- Malposition of the stent: The stent should be deployed completely followed by insertion of a second stent to cover the entire lesion.
- Vessel perforation: This is a rare complication. If it occurs, the first maneuver to try is a prolonged low-pressure balloon inflation (for 3 min or longer). If this fails to prevent contrast extravasation, a covered stent should be implanted. If this is not possible or a covered stent is not available, the balloon should be kept inflated across the lesion and a surgeon should be called.

How to Avoid

- Stent dislodgement: If it is not possible to pass the stent across the lesion, the device should be removed carefully. After removal of the device, the lesion should be predilated using a 4×20 mm balloon.
- Stent malpositioning:

  a. This is avoided by performing repeat angiography until the stent is in the correct position. When the correct position is achieved, the shaft of the balloon catheter should be supported by hand pressure at the exit point from the sheath, and a second operator can be asked to inflate the balloon to deploy the stent.

  b. The stent should be centered on the middle of the target lesion. If you are not sure about the correct stent length that may be required, a longer stent should be selected than one that might be too short.

- Vessel perforation: This is very rare.

  - ○ This can be avoided by using stents and balloons that are not too large for the vessel.

   ◦ The use of a manometer during inflation of the balloon avoids excessive inflation pressures and may prevent vessel rupture.

   ◦ If the patient experiences pain during balloon inflation, the PTA should be stopped and a larger balloon should definitely not be used.

Key Points

- Careful case selection is mandatory. Avoid treating patients with stenoses of single vessels.
- Use the transbrachial approach if catheterization from the femoral route is problematic.
- Use predilatation in severe stenoses to avoid plaque embolization and stent dislodgement.
- Perform PTA and stent deployment under manometer control in order to avoid overdilation and vessel perforation.
- Use balloon-expandable stents for ostial lesions.
- Perform repeat check angiograms in the appropriate projection (usually lateral or close to lateral) to visualize the origin of the vessel to confirm that the stent is in the correct location before deployment.

Suggested Reading

1. AbuRahma AF, Stone PA, Bates MC, Welch CA. Angioplasty/stenting of the superior mesenteric artery and celiac trunk: early and late outcomes. J Endovasc Ther 2003; 10:1046–1053.
2. Brandt LJ, Boley SJ. AGA technical review on intestinal ischemia. American Gastrointestinal Association. Gastroenterology 2000; 118:954–968.
3. Cognet F, Ben Salem D, Dranssart M, et al. Chronic mesenteric ischemia: imaging and percutaneous treatment. Radiographics 2002; 22:863–879.
4. Dunphy JF. Abdominal pain of vascular origin. Am J Med Sci 1936; 192:109–112.
5. Goodman GH. Angina abdominis. Am J Med Sci 1918; 155:524–528.
6. Landis MS, Rajan DK, Simons ME, Hayeems EB, Kachura JR, Sniderman KW. Percutaneous management of chronic mesenteric ischemia: outcomes after intervention. J Vasc Interv Radiol 2005 Oct; 16(10):1319–1325.
7. McShane MD, Proctor A, Spencer P, Cumberland DC, Welsh CL. Mesenteric angioplasty for chronic intestinal ischaemia. Eur J Vasc Surg 1992; 6:333–336.
8. Nyman U, Ivancev K, Lindh M, Uher P. Endovascular treatment of chronic mesenteric ischemia: report of five cases. Cardiovasc Intervent Radiol 1998 Jul–Aug; 21(4):305–313.
9. Resch T, Lindh M, Dias N, Sonesson B, Uher P, Malina M, Ivancev K. Endovascular recanalisation in occlusive mesenteric ischemia–feasibility and early results. Eur J Vasc Endovasc Surg 2005 Feb; 29(2):199–203.
10. Schaefer PJ, Schaefer FK, Hinrichsen H, Jahnke T, Charalambous N, Heller M, Mueller-Huelsbeck S. Stent placement with the monorail technique for treatment of mesenteric artery stenosis. J Vasc Interv Radiol 2006 Apr; 17(4):637–643.

11. Schuler A, Dirks K, Claussnitzer R, Blank W, Braun B. Ligamentum arcuatum syndrome: color doppler ultrasound diagnosis in abdominal pain of unknown origin in young patients. Ultraschall Med 1998 Aug; 19(4):157–163.

12. Wyers MC, Powell RJ, Nolan BW, Cronenwett JL. Retrograde mesenteric stenting during laparotomy for acute occlusive mesenteric ischemia. J Vasc Surg 2007 Feb; 45(2):269–275.

Carotid Stenting and Angioplasty

Gerald Wyse and Kieran J. Murphy

Introduction

- Ischemic stroke is a leading cause of death and disability in the developed world. The costs in term of healthcare and lost productivity are enormous but do not adequately reflect the human cost of such significant disability. Ischemic strokes are commonly caused by cardiac emboli, small vessel arterial disease, and atherosclerotic plaque at the carotid bifurcation. Carotid artery stenting (CAS) is a minimally invasive endovascular procedure for the prevention of ischemic stroke in patients with underlying carotid atherosclerosis.
- The development of new techniques and technology has made CAS an attractive alternative to Carotid Endarterectomy (CEA). As a minimally invasive procedure it has clear advantages in terms of the lack of a surgical incision, shorter procedure time, and shorter hospital stay. The procedure can be performed under conscious sedation avoiding general anesthesia with clear advantages for those with underlying medical co-morbidities. In addition, the temporary proximal carotid occlusion of a CEA is avoided.

Clinical Features

Carotid Atherosclerosis

- The underlying mechanism of ischemic stroke from carotid disease is plaque rupture with ulceration. The exposed vascular wall leads to clot formation within the lumen of the vessel. Embolization of clot leads to distal vessel occlusion and resultant ischemia. Although uncommon in the carotid artery, plaque rupture may result in thrombosis and occlusion at the site of rupture. The majority of atherosclerotic disease in the carotids occurs at the carotid bifurcation and extends into the proximal internal carotid artery. The flow dynamics at the carotid bifurcation result in reduced flow velocity and sheer stress at the lateral aspect of the flow divider leading to plaque formation (Fig. 1).

R.A. Morgan, E. Walser (eds.), *Handbook of Angioplasty and Stenting Procedures*,
Techniques in Interventional Radiology, DOI 10.1007/978-1-84800-399-6_14,
© Springer-Verlag London Limited 2010

- Atherosclerotic formation is associated with the usual vascular risk factors:

  ○ Hypertension
  ○ Hyperlipidemia
  ○ Smoking
  ○ Diabetes

- The underlying pathological progression is similar to that of coronary artery disease. The initial lesion is the intimal xanthoma, the so-called fatty streak. This progresses to intimal thickening and an overlying fibrous cap, which can cause luminal narrowing. Further progression leads to a high-risk plaque with a thin fibrous cap. Thinning and weakening of the fibrous cap leads to fissures and eventually plaque rupture.

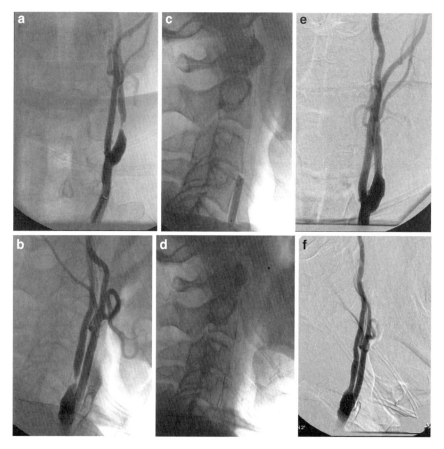

Fig. 1 (**a, b**) AP and lateral angiograms reveal a tight atherosclerotic stenosis in the proximal internal carotid artery. (**c**) A lateral radiograph demonstrating angioplasty of this atherosclerotic lesion. (**d**) A lateral radiograph post stent deployment. (**e, f**) AP and lateral digital subtraction angiograms post angioplasty and stenting of this symptomatic carotid atherosclerotic lesion

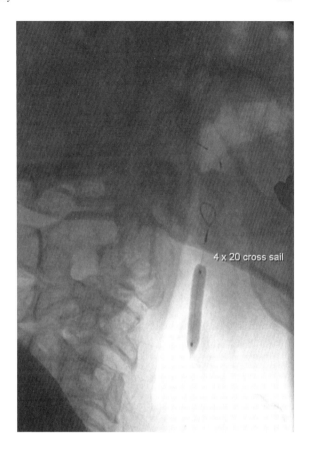

Fig. 2 A lateral radiograph demonstrating primary angioplasty of the internal carotid artery with a distal embolic filter

Angioplasty and Stenting

- Large surgical trials have shown a clear benefit in terms of risk reduction from stroke with CEA in the setting of significant atherosclerotic narrowing.
- CAS is a minimally invasive alternative to CEA for the prevention of ischemic stroke:

  - Angioplasty expands the lumen of the vessel increasing antegrade flow. The stent prevents recoil and plaque from projecting into the lumen.
  - Stenting effectively covers the underlying plaque, sealing the diseased vessel surface and resulting in a neo-intima and endothelialization of the stent.
  - Angioplasty without stenting was commonly performed in the past. Retenosis rates are high with this technique, in the 20–30% range in the coronary arteries.
  - Stents avoid these problems but issues do exist with acute stent thrombosis and delayed endothelialization which can take about 3–4 months to heal.

Medical Management

- Since the large surgical endarterectomy trials, there have been considerable advances in the medical management of carotid atherosclerotic disease:

  ○ Aspirin
  ○ New lipid-lower agents (statins)
  ○ Newer antiplatelet agents (Clopidogrel)
  ○ Aggressive management of blood pressure and blood glucose

Diagnostic Evaluation

Clinical

- Symptoms of hemispheric cerebral ischemia

  ○ Transient ischemic attacks (TIAs)

- Amaurosis Fugax (monocular temporary blindness or visual defects)
- Reversible ischemic neurologic deficits (RINDs)
- Ischemic stroke events lasting >24 h and resulting in non-disabling cerebral infarct:

  ○ Severe, disabling strokes not considered for CAS/CEA

- Sex/age − octogenarians may do worse with CAS versus CEA possibly due to small and/or tortuous aortas and carotid arteries
- Cardiac disease − High risk for CEA:

  ○ Left ventricular ejection fraction (LVEF) <30%
  ○ Congestive heart failure (CHF) Class III/IV
  ○ Unstable angina, recent myocardial infarction (MI)
  ○ Multi-vessel coronary artery disease (CAD)

- Pulmonary disease − High risk for CEA:

  ○ Forced expiratory volume and 1 sec (FEV1) <50% predicted
  ○ Severe obstructive pulmonary disease or emphysema

- Systemic diseases − High risk for CEA:

  ○ Dialysis-dependent renal failure
  ○ Liver failure
  ○ Uncontrolled diabetes

- Past medical/surgical history − High risk for CEA:

  ○ Prior neck irradiation/surgery:

    ■ Significant risk of nerve injury during CEA

   ○ Recurrent carotid stenosis after CEA
   ○ Contralateral nerve palsy
   ○ Spinal immobility
   ○ Tracheostomy

- Clinical factors conferring higher risk for CAS:

   ○ Symptomatic patients
   ○ Renal failure − not on dialysis
   ○ Severe contrast allergies
   ○ Extreme aortic arch/carotid artery tortuosity/angulation

Laboratory

- Laboratory analysis similar to that performed in the setting of atherosclerotic disease anywhere:

   ○ Risk-factor evaluation:

      ■ Lipid profile
      ■ Diabetics − blood glucose, hemoglobin A1C
      ■ C reactive protein, homocysteine levels

   ○ Preparation for angiography, contrast administration:

      ■ Serum creatinine and calculated glomerular filtration ratio (GFR)
      ■ Coagulation parameters (PT, PTT, CBC with platelet count) − if clinically necessary:

         • Liver disease
         • Recent history of anticoagulation therapy
         • Other coagulopathies − inherited or acquired

Imaging

- Digital subtraction angiography (DSA) remains the gold standard for the measurement of carotid artery stenosis.
- The NASCET criteria are commonly used for the measurement of percentage stenosis:

   ○ 100 − (narrowest luminal diameter/diameter of the normal distal cervical internal carotid artery).
   ○ DSA provides no information about plaque morphology.

- Ultrasound with color Doppler, spectral analysis, and grayscale imaging is easy to use, relatively inexpensive, and avoids the use of contrast agents and radiation:

○ Can be used for longitudinal follow-up.
○ Disputed role as primary test prior to CEA but can be correlated with angiography at the time of CAS.

- Non-invasive cross-sectional imaging techniques:

○ Contrast-enhanced MRA of the neck correlates well with DSA
○ CTA gives superb anatomic detail but as a sole modality is limited especially in heavily calcified lesions were it can overestimate the degree of stenosis.

- Imaging of the brain prior to CAS is essential. It helps to visualize recent ischemia and hemorrhage. Brain imaging also rules out other lesions such as tumors. In addition, imaging acts as a comparison for post-procedural studies.

Indications for Carotid Artery Stenting

- Who will definitely benefit from CAS?

○ The current role of medical management, CEA, and CAS in relation to carotid artery disease is not always clear. There is no agreed consensus and practices vary widely.
○ The North America Symptomatic Carotid Endarterectomy Trial (NASCET) and the European Carotid Surgery Trial (ECST) showed that patients benefit from surgery as opposed to medical treatment in the setting of symptomatic carotid stenosis greater than 70 and 50%, respectively.

- The indications for CAS have been generally adopted from the surgical trials. CAS is generally performed on

○ Patients at high risk for surgery with a symptomatic carotid stenosis of greater than 70%. Surgical high-risk patients include

■ A prior history of CEA and recurrent stenosis
■ Contra-lateral carotid occlusion
■ Previous radiation therapy
■ Previous radical neck dissection
■ High or low surgically inaccessible lesions
■ Significant medical co-morbidities.

○ High-risk status is not a contraindication to CEA. It depends on the individual surgeon and the skills available. The importance of institutional audit and a multidisciplinary approach when selecting patients for either CAS or CEA is critical.
○ Since most embolic strokes occur in patients with a stenosis less than 70%, is there an indication for stenting such lesions?

■ Ongoing investigation into this area with multiple trials and registries. Currently the role of CAS in symptomatic lesions below 70% is unclear.

- ○ Is there any evidence to support CAS in the setting of asymptomatic carotid artery disease?

    - ■ Little solid evidence exists. However, CAS is infrequently offered to asymptomatic patients with a carotid artery stenosis of greater than 80%.

- ○ Other, less common indications for carotid stent placement:

    - ■ Covered stents have been successfully used for carotid "blowouts" (perforation) from tumor infiltration or traumatic carotid injury.
    - ■ Stents may be used as flow diverters in the setting of post-dissection carotid pseudoaneurysm.

- In the US, the Center for Medicare Services (CMSs) will reimburse CAS only for symtomatic patients with high surgical risk (see above criteria) and carotid stenosis greater than or equal to 70%:

    - ○ Symptomatic patients with 50–70% stenosis or asymptomatic patients with 80% or more stenosis are reimbursed but only for patients enrolled in FDA-approved clinical trials.

- The Society of Vascular Surgery recommends the following treatment guidelines for carotid stenosis:

    - ○ Asymptomatic

        - ■ <60% stenosis – medical management
        - ■ >60% stenosis – CEA
        - ■ >80% stenosis and anatomic risks for CEA – consider CAS

    - ○ Symptomatic

        - ■ <50% stenosis – medical management
        - ■ >50% stenosis – CEA
        - ■ >50% stenosis with high perioperative risks – CAS

Contraindications

- Absolute contraindications: (uncommon):

    - ○ Previous history of anaphylaxis to contrast agents
    - ○ Uncontrolled coagulation problems

- Relative contraindications:

    - ○ Renal impairment:

        - ■ Treat with intravenous hydration and bicarbonate therapy plus oral dosing of *N*-Acetyl cyteine

    - ○ Inability to tolerate anti-platelet therapy

○ Aneurysm or vascular malformation downstream from stented lesion:

  ■ Aneurysms or vascular malformation should be addressed prior to CAS to prevent the increased intracranial flow possibly resulting in hemorrhage.

○ Many physicians consider near total carotid occlusion a relative contraindication, especially in the present of good collateral flow in the Circle of Willis:

  ■ There is an increased risk of peri-procedural stroke with increasing carotid artery stenosis but this risk decreases at near total occlusion.
  ■ A careful consideration of the risks and benefits must be made prior to CAS in the setting of total or near carotid occlusion.

○ Evidence of higher complication rates in octogenarians who undergo CAS suggests that age is a relative contraindication.

  ■ No gender difference has been demonstrated with CAS.

○ Visible luminal clot is also an important consideration (Fig. 3). Crossing such a lesion with a wire or embolic protection device is hazardous and may lead to inadvertent distal embolism:

  ■ CEA with back bleeding of the carotid or a proximal EPD is advantageous.
  ■ Observation and anticoagulation for luminal clot with deferred treatment should also be considered.

○ Severe cognitive impairment:

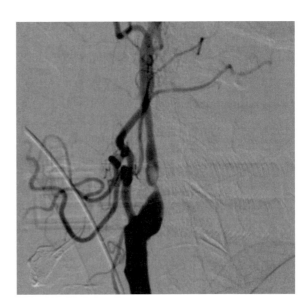

Fig. 3 Lateral digital subtraction angiogram showing visible luminal clot, a relative contraindication to carotid angioplasty and stenting

- There is no evidence of improved quality of life with CAS for the cognitively impaired.

○ Short life expectancy:

- The statistical benefit of CAS is based on a reasonable life expectancy. Surgical experience suggests that patients should have a life expectancy of at least 3 years for symptomatic disease and 5 years for asymptomatic disease to benefit from CAS.

○ Severe tortuosity and heavily calcified lesions:

- CAS can be dangerous with significant risks of iatrogenic vessel rupture or dissection or cerebral emboli.
- Such cases may be better treated by a surgical or medical approach.

Patient Preparation and Selection

- Proper patient selection is mandatory to improve clinical outcomes after CAS. The reliance on measurements of vascular luminal narrowing to predict future ischemic events is somewhat limited. This is certainly an imprecise method:

  ○ There is significant compensatory enlargement of a vessel in response to plaque.
  ○ The majority of culprit lesions causing myocardial infarction in retrospective studies showed luminal narrowing of less than 50%.

- Identification of the "at risk" patient is crucial. Newer imaging techniques will help to more clearly identify patients who will benefit from CAS:

  ○ Hemodynamics – Paired flow studies:

    - Test the ability of the cerebral vessels to increase blood flow in the setting of a vasodilatory stimulus (Fig. 4). If flow does not increase pre-existing vasodilation is inferred.
    - Existing hemodynamic impairment has a strong association with stroke risk and paired flow studies may be used in the future as a means of patient selection for CAS.

  ○ Plaque examination

    - Plaque which contains an extracellular lipid core, active inflammation and a thin fibrous cap is at the highest risk of rupture.
    - Imaging methods to identify high-risk plaque have included

      - Ultrasound, intravascular ultrasound
      - PET/CT.
      - MRI

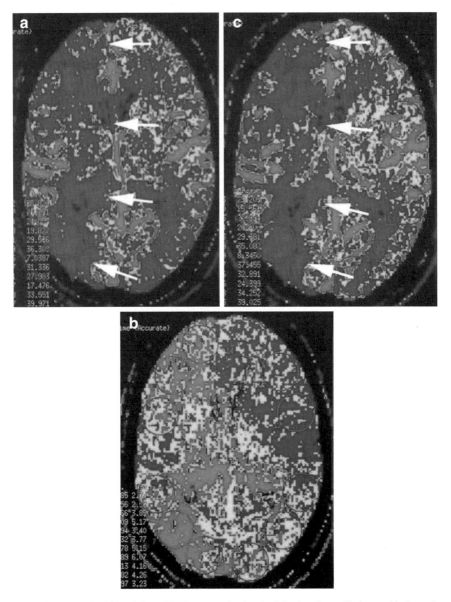

Fig. 4 (**a**) A cerebral blood flow (CBF) map at the level of the basal ganglia in an elderly male with known, high-grade right ICA stenosis reveals significant decrease in the right hemispheric perfusions (*arrows*). (**b**) A mean transit time (MTT) map at the same level also reveals severe elevation of MTT in the entire right hemisphere. Values as high as 11 sec were obtained in some regions of interest in the right MCA territory. (**c**) A CBF map repeated following the administration of acetazolamide fails to reveal any augmentation in the CBF values. In fact, paradoxical response (decreased CBF) was noted in the right MCA territory, suggesting an impaired cerebrovascular reserve

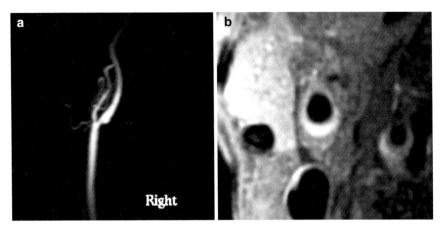

Fig. 5 (**a**) Maximum intensity projection MRA of the carotid bifurcation revealing narrowing of the proximal right internal carotid artery without significant luminal narrowing. (**b**) Post-contrast high resolution, T1-weighted, black blood MR imaging reveals the same lesion. Noted the eccentric posterior lipid core and enhancing cap. Plaque imaging with MR or other techniques may replace our reliance on luminal narrowing to predict future stroke

- T2-weighted images offer good contrast to discriminate plaque components
- Calcification is better identified on T1 imaging.
- Discrimination of the fibrous cap from a lipid core and cap thickness can be accessed with contrast-enhanced MRI.
- These techniques can be used to assess the individual's risk of future cerebral ischemia rather than reliance on luminal narrowing measurements to statically predict stroke risk (Fig. 5).

Relevant Anatomy – Normal and Variant

- Normal aortic arch anatomy is right common carotid originating from first aortic arch branch, the brachiocephalic artery and a separate origin of left common carotid artery from the arch.

  - Frequent variant is left common carotid artery arising off the origin or proximal portion of the brachiocephalic artery (bovine arch)

    - Can be difficult to catheterize due to acute angle of left common carotid artery with the aorta. A Simmons or shephard's-hook catheter is often needed.

- With increasing age, the brachiocephalic and right common carotid arteries may become especially tortuous and/or calcified:

  - Requires stiffer guidewires placed more distal in the carotid circulation (external carotid) in order to successfully catheterize
  - Increased risk of iatrogenic arterial injury or embolic events.

Pre-procedure Medications

- All patients are pre-treated with anti-platelet agents for 5 days prior to the procedure. The use of double anti-platelet therapy commonly using aspirin and clopidogrel is widespread. This practice is derived from coronary artery stenting but lacks evidence in the carotid arteries:
  - The use of various platelet assays to determine the degree of platelet inhibition is also becoming a more common practice.
- Optimal management of blood pressure and blood glucose is critical to a successful outcome:
  - There may be a role for statins in plaque stabilization prior to CAS.

Procedural Considerations

- A full neurological examination should be performed prior to CAS.
- The procedure can be carried out under conscience sedation:
  - Avoids general anesthesia which may be advantageous in the setting of significant medical co-morbidities.
  - Permits neurological examination during the procedure which requires the co-operation of the patient
- Performing the procedure under general anesthesia may be easier on the patient and clinician. Although the ability to perform a neurological examination is lost, intra-procedural angiography with a careful review to assess for missing intracranial branches can be performed.
- With either technique the presence of an anesthesiologist for managing bradycardia and blood pressure instability is invaluable.
- Timing of the procedure is also important:
  - To avoid the risk of hemorrhagic conversion in an infarcted area, wait 4 weeks after an acute ischemic event before performing CAS.
- Detailed review of all imaging is essential for procedural planning. Anatomical considerations, tortuosity, aneurysmal vessels, arch configuration, and heavy calcification can result in a difficult or even dangerous procedure:
  - Access and equipment selection depend on these anatomical factors.
  - Femoral access is commonly used, alternatively brachial or radial access may have advantages for certain lesions.
  - Direct carotid puncture is another option although surgical closure of the puncture is required.
- An arch aortogram will display the anatomy and will often save time by influencing equipment choices:

- ○ Prior to stenting, biplanar views of the intracranial circulation distal to the stenosis are crucial. These angiograms are compared to procedural angiogram to assess for distal emboli.

- Placement of a secure and stable guiding catheter in the common carotid artery is the opening critical step of the procedure. In the setting of challenging anatomy this can be difficult.

  - ○ Cannulation of an external carotid branch and exchange over a stiff wire can be performed.

Intra-procedural Medications and Devices

Embolic Protection Devices

- The use of embolic protection devices (EPDs) is widespread although there is no randomized trial comparing stenting with an EPD and without an EPD.
- EPD rationale:

  - ○ Crossing a tight stenosis or angioplasty and stenting may cause ischemic events by embolization of plaque material or clot into a distal intracranial vessel.
  - ○ Doppler studies confirm emboli occur at the time of CAS.

- EPD may itself cause problems:

  - ○ The distal devices which consist of a filter (Fig. 2) or a balloon that is mounted on a wire still have to cross the stenosis as a first step, there can be incomplete wall apposition, vessel occlusion with debris, vessel spasm or wall damage.
  - ○ There are multiple devices available with a learning curve for each one. Operator inexperience and unfamiliarity can cause significant problems.

- Embolic protection devices are of two main types:

  - ○ Distal-types including occlusive balloons
  - ○ Umbrella-type embolic filters.

- Excessive angulation and heavy calcification can make device deployment hazardous. Crossing profile and capturing efficiency vary with different products.
- Over-sizing of distal filters can ensure luminal adherence and contrast injection will ensure the vessel is patent and not occluded with debris.
- A second type of device is a proximal protection device. These Parodi-type devices avoid the unprotected crossing of a stenosis with a distal filter or balloon:

  - ○ Consists of a large balloon-tipped guiding catheter for aspiration, which occludes the common carotid and a smaller coaxial balloon catheter occluding the external carotid.

○ Reversed flow in the internal carotid artery is induced and the stenosis is crossed for the first time with protection in place. The aspirate is filtered and returned to the femoral vein.

■ Unfortunately not all patients can tolerate reversal of ICA flow.

Intra-procedural Medications

- Atropine 0.5–1.0 mg IV for bradycardia

  ○ Glycopyrrolate IV (alternate) 0.1 mg IV q 2–3 min

- Heparin 5,000 u IV before crossing lesion

  ○ 1,000 u bolus IV every hour
  ○ Maintain ACT near 250

- Heparin alternative is direct thrombin inhibition

  ○ Bivalirudin 0.75 mg/kg IV bolus (about 50 mg)

- GIIbIIIa inhibitors:

  ○ Abciximab 0.25 mg/kg IV bolus, then 0.125 mg/kg/min $\times$ 12 h
  ○ Inhibits platelet accumulation on newly placed stents

- Local preference dictates choice of procedural medications

Crossing a Stenotic Lesion

- The aim is to cross the lesion in a non-traumatic fashion without causing distal embolic events.

  ○ An EPD is carefully advanced
  ○ A micro-catheter and a micro-wire may give better control for crossing a tightly narrowed lesion. Once the lesion is crossed the microwire is then exchanged for an EPD.
  ○ Pre-dilation may be necessary to allow an EPD or stent to pass through the stenosis. In addition, many operators like to perform a definitive angioplasty prior to stent deployment.
  ○ A wide variety of rapid exchange and over the wire systems are available:

    ■ Rapid exchange systems (monorail) allow a single operator to control the wire and advance the device.
    ■ Over the wire devices (OTWs) allow for greater stability and better control.

- Time and care must be spent clearing the dead space of a balloon. Otherwise, balloon rupture may result in air entering the intracranial circulation. Angioplasty balloons are opacified with a half and half mixture of contrast and saline.
- The importance of high-quality equipment and adequately trained staff cannot be overstated:

  ○ The practice of performing angioplasty and stenting with a portable C-arm is hazardous and not in the best interests of the patient.
  ○ An angiographic view, which shows the entire protection device, the stenotic lesion, and the guiding sheath is required.

Stents

- Self-expanding bare mental stents are most commonly used. These deploy in a predictable manner.
- An open-cell design accommodates changing luminal diameter and will adhere to the wall:

  ○ A disadvantage with the open-cell design is the tendency for atheromatous plaque to protrude into the vessel lumen.

- A closed-cell design does not accommodate rapid changes in diameter and may not adhere as well to the wall:

  ○ Tapered stents somewhat overcome incomplete wall adherence
  ○ Closed-cell stents are less tractable and may not be suitable in cases of excessive angulation or tortuosity.

- Balloon mounted stents are also more rigid and are often difficult to navigate into a correct position:

  ○ Used when greater radial force and more precise deployment is needed.
  ○ Primarily used for common carotid origin lesions or at the skull base.

- Oversizing a stent by 1–2 mm helps avoid dead space between the stent and the vessel wall. In addition, the use of a longer stent negates the need for absolute perfect placement and will avoid the need for overlapping stents.
- Covered stents have a role in carotid blowout and tumor infiltration. There is little long-term data in relation to patency to support their use in atherosclerotic disease.
- Drug-eluting stents

  ○ Sirolimus- and paclitaxel-eluting stents are in common use in the coronary arteries. These stents act by the local delivery of drug, which prevents smooth muscle proliferation and intima hyperplasia. These stents have reduced restenosis rates as compared to bare metal stents.

○ Re-endothelialization is significantly delayed in comparison to bare mental stents and so these stents require prolonged use of anti-platelet agents.
○ There is currently no evidence to support their use in carotid artery stenting.
○ There are two important differences between the carotid and coronary arteries which significantly affect intimal hyperplasia and stent restenosis:

   ■ The carotid is a much larger vessel
   ■ The carotid artery has continuous forward flow unlike the coronary.

• Post-stenting angioplasty.
• Nitinol stents will continue to open post-deployment.
• Although angioplasty post-stent deployment may be necessary to correct incomplete stent wall apposition, it is important to avoid aggressive angioplasty as it may induce intimal injury and resultant hyperplasia.

   ○ A functional result with no hemodynamic obstruction is preferred and not a perfect angiographic result.

• Careful examination of pre-procedural and post-procedural angiograms for missing intracranial branches (evidence of emboli) should be done prior to sheath removal.

Immediate Post-procedural Issues

• Patients need to be monitored in a unit with frequent neurological examination and quick access to CT scanning.
• Many centers continue anticoagulation in the immediate post stenting period for 12-24 hours. The role of pre-procedural anti-platelet therapy is likely more critical to prevent acute stent thrombosis.
• Blood pressure monitoring is critical for CAS. All patient should have continuous intra-arterial pressure monitor during and immediately after to help avoid hyperperfusion syndromes.

   ○ Intravenous use of agents such as labetalol and nicardipine are commonly used for blood pressure control.

Follow-Up

• Dual anti-platelet therapy is commonly continued for 3–6 months and then a single agent is used. The higher flow and resultant increased sheer stress seen in the carotid may suggest a role for more prolonged anti-platelet therapy.
• After CAS, risk factor management is desirable:

   ○ Blood pressure control
   ○ Cholesterol management

- ○ Glucose management
- ○ Smoking cessation
- ○ Carotid artery disease is a marker for atherosclerosis and assessment of the coronary arteries may be appropriate.

Results

- Technical success of the procedure lies in the upper 90% range with a low complication rate. In-stent restenosis has been reported in the 6% range at 2years follow-up.
- A recent meta-analysis of CAS and CEA suggested no significant difference in term of stroke, death, and myocardial infarction.
- Other studies have suggested CAS has a higher stroke and mortality rate than CEA in symptomatic patients (EVA-3S trial) although there are problems with patient selection and operator experience in these studies.

Alternative Therapies

- Optimal medical management for carotid occlusive disease has improved dramatically and is recommended for asymptomatic patients with non-critical stenosis or elderly patients with difficult anatomy and high surgical risks.

- ○ Platelet inhibition – aspirin and/or clopidogrel
- ○ Cholesterol and LDL management

  - ■ Statin therapy, others

- ○ Risk factor management

Complications

- CAS can cause the very thing that it aims to prevent, that being transient ischemia or stroke.
- Brain injury will depend on the depth and duration of ischemia:

  - ○ Minor strokes relate to small emboli occluding distal branches.
  - ○ Large clot formation or acute stent thrombosis can lead to devastating clinical outcomes:

    - ■ The risk of stroke depends on patient selection and operator experience.
    - ■ A 30-day stroke rate of 5.8% for CAS was reported in high-risk patients.
    - ■ As complication rates increase, the risk-benefit ratio of the procedure is markedly elevated
    - ■ Centers should aim for stroke rates of 3% or less.

- Angioplasty can result in stretching of the carotid body and resultant hypotension and bradycardia:

  ○ Many centers employ the prophylactic use of atropine.
  ○ Procedural bradycardia and hypotension will often respond to fluid bolus and intravenous atropine.

    ■ Rarely temporary cardiac pacing may be required.

- Post-stenting hyperperfusion syndromes can occur in both the acute and subacute periods. They are caused by impaired cerebral auto-regulation:
  ○ A hyperperfusion hemorrhage typically presents with headache, seizure, or a focal neurological deficit.
  ○ The risk of developing a hyper-perfusion syndrome post CAS is reported at 1%.
  ○ Aggressive management of blood pressure in the post-stenting period is key to preventing such a complication.
- Considering atherosclerosis is a systemic disease, there is often concominant coronary artery disease. Myocardial infarction although rare is reported but at rates lower than following CEA

Key Points

- CAS is used for the treatment of atherosclerotic carotid disease to prevent or reduce the risk of future stroke.
- CAS offers a minimally invasive alternative to CEA with clear advantages in terms of lack of a surgical incision, hospital stay, and avoidance of general anesthesia.
- CAS has a high technical success rate with a low complication rate.
- CAS is commonly performed in symptomatic surgically high-risk patients with a greater than 70% stenosis of the carotid artery.
- CAS is not performed until 4 weeks after an acute ischemic event.
- A consensus-derived multidisciplinary approach is necessary to ensure best practice and good patient outcomes when deciding the role of medical management, CAS, and CEA for carotid artery disease. Adequate training, high-quality equipment, and appropriate patient selection are essential when performing CAS

Suggested Reading

1. Adou-Chebl A, Yadav JS, Reginelli JP, et al. Intracranial hemorrhage and hyperperfusion syndrome following carotid artery stenting: risk factors, prevention and treatment. J Am Coll Cardiol 2004; 43:1591–1601

2. Ambrose JA. Coronary arteriographic analysis and angiographic analysis and angiographic morphology. J Am Coll Cardiol 1989; 13:1492–4

3. Anderson PG, Bajaj RK, Baxley WA, et al. Vascular pathology of balloon-expandable flexible coil stents in humans. J Am Coll Cardiol 1992; 19:372–81

4. Buhk JH, Wellmer A, Knauth M. Late in-stent thrombosis following carotid angioplasty and stenting. Neurology 2006; 66:1594–6.

5. Chaer RA, Makaroun MS. Evolution of carotid stenting: Indications. Semin Vasc Surg 2008; 21:59–63.

6. CMS website http://www.cms.hhs.gov/MLNMattersArticles/downloads/MM5667.pdf regarding carotid stenting reimbursement for medicare patients. Accessed 2/1/2009.

7. Coward LJ, Featherstone RL, Brown MM. Safety and efficacy of endovascular treatment of carotid stenosis compared with carotid endarterectomy; a Cochrane systematic review of the randomized evidence. Stroke 2005; 36(4):905–1

8. Falk E, Shah PK, Fuster V. Coronary plaque disruption. Circulation 1995; 92:657–71.

9. Glagov S, Weisenberg E, Zarins CK, et al. Compensatory enlargement of human atherosclerotic coronary arteries. N Engl J Med 1987; 316:1371–5

10. Glagov S, Zarins C, Giddens DP, et al. Hemodynamics and atherosclerosis. Insights and perspectives gained from studies of human arteries. Arch Pathol Lab Med 1988; 112:1018–31

11. Gorelick PB. Distribution of atherosclerotic cerebrovascular lesions. Effects of age, race, and sex. Stroke 1993; 24(12 Suppl):I16–9

12. Grant EG, Benson CB, Moneta GL, et al. Carotid artery stenosis: Gray-scale and Doppler US diagosis-Society of Radiologists in Ultrasound Consenus Conference. Radiology 2003; 229(2):340–6.

13. Grubb RL Jr, Derdeyn CP, Fritsch SM, et al. Importance of hemodynamic factors in the prognosis of symptomatic carotid occlusion. JAMA 1998; 280(12):1055–60.

14. Hirai T, Korogi Y, Ono K, et al. Prospective evaluation of suspected stenoocclusive disease of the intracranial artery: combined MR angiography and CT angiography compared with digital subtraction angiography. AJNR Am J Neuroradiol 2002; 23(1):93–101

15. Hobson RW, Howard VJ, Roubin GS, et al. Carotid artery stenting is associated with increased complications in octogenarians: 30-day stroke and death rates in the CREST lead-in phase. J Vasc Surg 2004; 40(6):1106–11

16. Hobson RW, Mackey WC, Ascher E, et al. Management of atherosclerotic carotid artery disease: Clinical practice guidelines of the Society for Vascular Surgery. J Vasc Surg 2008; 48:480–86.

17. Joner M, Finn AV, Farb A, et al. Pathology of drug-eluting stents in humans: delayed healing and late thrombotic risk. J Am Coll Cardiol 2006; 48:193–202.

18. Jordan WD Jr, Voellinger DC, Doblar DD, et al. Microemboli detected by transcranial Doppler monitoring in patients during carotid angioplasty versus carotid endarterectomy. Cardiovasc Surg 1999; 7:33–8.

19. Kadkhodayan Y, Derdeyn CP, Cross DT III, et al. Procedural complications of carotid angioplasty and stent placement without cerebral protection device. Neurosurg Focus 2005; 18(1):E1–7.

20. Kolodgie F, Nakazawa G, Sangiorgi G et al. Pathology of Atherosclerosis and Stenting Neuroimag Clin N Am 2007; 17:285–301

21. Mas J-L, Chatellier G, Beyssen B, et al. Endartectomy versus stenting in patients wth symptomatic severe carotid stenosis. N Engl J Med 2006; 355(16):1660–7

22. McKinsey JF. Symptomatic carotid stenosis: Endarterectomy, stenting or best medical management? Semin Vasc Surg 2008; 21:108–114.

23. Mintz GS, Popma JJ, Pichard AD et al. Arterial remodeling after coronary angioplasty: a serial intravascular ultrasound study. Circulation 1996; 94:35–43

24. Mohr JP, Gautier J. Internal Carotid Artery Disease Stroke: Pathophysiology, Diagnosis and Management. Philadelphia: Churchill Livingstone; 1998, 355–400

25. Moses JW, Leon MB, Popma JJ, et al. Sirolimus-eluting stents versus standard stents in patients with stenosis in a native coronary artery. N Engl J Med 2003; 349:1315–23

26. Murad MH, Flynn DN, Elamin MB, et al. Endarterectomy vs. carotid artery stenosis: A systematic review and meta-analysis. J Vasc Surg 2008; 48:487–93.

27. North American Symptomatic Carotid Endarterectomy Trial Collaborators. Beneficial effect of carotid endarterectomy in symptomatic patients with high-grade carotid stenosis. N Engl J Med 1991; 325:445–3

28. Randomised trial of endarterectomy for recently symptomatic carotid stenosis. Final results of the MRC European Carotid Surgery Trial. Lancet 1998; 351:1379–87.

29. Remonda L, Senn P, Barth A, et al. Contrast-enhanced 3D MR angiography of the carotid artery: Comparison with conventional digital subtraction angiography. AJNR Am J Neuroradiol 2002; 23(2):213–9.

30. Rosamond W, Flegal K, Friday G, et al. Heart disease and stroke statistics-2007 update: A report from the America Heart Association Statistics Committee and Stroke Statistics Subcommittee. Circulation 2007; 115:e65–171

31. Thorvaldsen P, Kuulasmaa K, Rajakangas AM, et al. Stroke trends in the WHO MONICA project. Stroke 1997;28:500–506

32. Wasserman BA, Smith WI, Trout 3rd HH, et al. Carotid artery atherosclerosis: in vivo morphologic characterization with gadolinium-enhanced double-oblique MR imaging initial results. Radiology 2002; 223:566–73.

33. Wholey MH, Al Mubarek N, Whley MH. Update review of the global artery stent registry. Catheter Cardiovasc Interv 2003; 60:259–66.

34. Wholey MH, Wholey M, Mathias K, et al. Global experience in cervical carotid artery stent placement. Catheter Cardiovasc Interv 2000; 50:160–7

35. Yadav JS, Wholey MH Kuntz RE, et al. Protected carotid-artery stenting versus endarterectomy in high-risk patients. N Engl J Med 2004; 351:1305–501

Intracranial and Vertebral Artery Angioplasty and Stenting

Jitendra Sharma, J. Mocco, Adnan H. Siddiqui and Elad I. Levy

Introduction

- Intracranial atherosclerosis accounts for 8–12% of all ischemic strokes.
- Diabetes mellitus, hypertension, dyslipidemia, cigarette smoking, and ethnicity increase the risk of intracranial atherosclerosis.
- Patients with severe (>70%) and moderate (50–69%) intracranial stenosis carry a high annual risk of ischemic stroke (17 and 7–8%, respectively), despite aspirin or warfarin therapy.
- Intracranial angioplasty and stenting is an emerging investigational technique for use in patients with clinically significant *or* critical *or* severe stenosis refractory to medical therapy.

Clinical Features and Patient Selection

- Patients with intracranial stenosis most commonly present with an acute stroke or a transient ischemic attack.
- Intracranial angioplasty and stenting can play a significant role in patients with frequent transient ischemic attacks who have moderate to severe stenosis that is refractory to medical therapy.
- Intracranial angioplasty and stenting can be considered on an emergent basis in patients who have fresh thrombus or severe intracranial stenosis with fluctuating symptoms in acute stroke settings in conjunction with intravenous or intra-arterial thrombolytic therapy.
- Patients who present with stroke in evolution with stable symptoms can be treated electively in 4–6 weeks to reduce the risk of hemorrhagic transformation.

R.A. Morgan, E. Walser (eds.), *Handbook of Angioplasty and Stenting Procedures*, Techniques in Interventional Radiology, DOI 10.1007/978-1-84800-399-6_15, © Springer-Verlag London Limited 2010

Diagnostic Evaluation

Clinical

- Stroke scale score
- Duration of symptoms
- Assuming the patient will need further imaging:
  - Allergies to contrast agents
  - Is a pacemaker in use? Are there other metallic foreign bodies ineligible for MR imaging?
  - Renal function evaluation − serum creatinine

Imaging

- Initial diagnostic evaluation can be done by using either magnetic resonance imaging (MRI) of the brain along with magnetic resonance angiography (MRA) or computed tomography angiography (CTA) of the head and neck along with CT of the head with perfusion imaging.
- We prefer CTA and CT of the head with perfusion imaging for the initial evaluation of symptomatic patients, because it provides information regarding vascular anatomy and degree of stenosis, as well as insight into the patient's physiology.
- MRI with MRA can provide useful information regarding posterior fossa lesions, as well as identify small cortical and subcortical lesions.
- We recommend a catheter angiogram in all cases as it is the most sensitive and specific in confirming the diagnosis and estimating the severity of stenosis.

Laboratory

- Basic blood tests (including complete blood count, comprehensive metabolic panel, and coagulation profile) are obtained in conjunction with the initial evaluation.

Indications

- Primary therapy in symptomatic severe vertebral or intracranial stenoses
- Secondary therapy in moderate stenoses that have failed medical management

Contraindications

- Large (hemispheric) stroke, hemorrhage, or early stroke in evolution with stable symptoms
  - Risk of intracranial hemorrhage

- Old stroke with chronic intracranial arterial occlusion/stenosis
- Multiple stenoses from known vasculitis.

Patient Preparation

Pre-procedure and Peri-procedure Medications

- To prevent thrombosis, patients receive antithrombotic and anticoagulant medications before the procedure.
- Aspirin (325 mg daily) and clopidogrel (75 mg daily) are initiated at least 3 days before the procedure; in emergent cases, clopidogrel (600-mg loading dose), and aspirin (650 mg orally) are given 4 h before the procedure.
- When intraprocedural events require use of angioplasty/stenting, a glycoprotein IIb−IIIa inhibitor may be substituted for antiplatelet therapy.

  ○ The three commercially available glycoprotein IIb−IIIa inhibitors are abciximab, eptifibatide, and tirofiban. The use of glycoprotein IIb−IIIa inhibitors is an *off-label indication*. The caveat in the use of these agents is that their effect cannot be reversed and, ideally, a CT scan is obtained prior to their administration to exclude the presence of an intracranial hemorrhage.

- After the placement of an arterial sheath or a guide catheter, the patient is started on a heparin drip. An intravenous bolus of 50 U/kg of heparin is administered, and the baseline activated coagulation time (ACT) is obtained.
- An ACT of between 250 and 300 sec is maintained during the procedure.
- The catheter should be frequently flushed with heparinized saline before and after each wire exchange to prevent the formation of thrombus.

Anesthesia

- To allow regular neurologic assessment of patients throughout the procedure, we use conscious sedation rather than general anesthesia.
- We prefer to use a combination of fentanyl and midazolam administered in short intravenous pushes (of 50 and 1 mg, respectively) until light sedation is achieved.
- Occasionally, in pediatric patients or uncooperative adults, the use of general anesthesia is required. In such cases, neurophysiologic monitoring is recommended.

Procedure

Percutaneous Vascular Access

- Selection of the puncture site is based on the individual patient anatomy. The common femoral artery is the most typical site for vascular access. The femoral artery should be palpated and punctured approximately 2–3 cm below the level of the inguinal ligament.

- An entry site that is too low increases the risk of the development of an arteriovenous fistula or pseudoaneurysm, whereas one that is too high may lead to retroperitoneal bleeding.
- Fluoroscopy should be used to locate the femoral artery if anatomical landmarks are difficult to assess, e.g., in obese patients.
- Femoral access is relatively contraindicated in cases of severe peripheral vascular disease, aortic aneurysm or dissection, and morbid obesity.
- We use the radial artery approach for better access to the vertebral artery origin in certain patients. Before using the radial artery as an access site, an Allen test should be performed to confirm that the palmar arch is patent.
- We rarely use the brachial artery; however, we may if the femoral artery is not accessible for intervention and the patient fails the Allen test. The brachial artery approach is associated with a high risk of neurologic complication and hand ischemia as the brachial artery is an end artery with little collateral blood supply.
- The carotid artery is extremely rarely used as an access site when other access sites are impossible to use.

Angiography

- A baseline angiogram is performed to estimate the length and geometry of the lesion and to assess the collateral blood supply.
- This study also provides a baseline roadmap for the procedure and documents the severity and location of the stenosis and the caliber of the adjacent normal vessel.

Angioplasty

- A 6 French (F) guide catheter or a 6F long sheath is placed in the selected access vessel. A microcatheter and a 0.014-inch microwire are used to cross the lesion, and the wire and catheter advanced to a sufficient distance beyond the portion of artery that needs to be dilated. The microwire is then removed and a stiffer 300-cm, 0.014-inch exchange wire is placed through the microcatheter which is then withdrawn.
- The balloon is then advanced over the 0.014-inch guidewire to the intracranial artery of interest and inflated to 6–12 atmospheres of pressure at the site of stenosis. The balloon is undersized, with a diameter ranging between 80 and 100% of the normal adjacent vessel, to reduce the risk of arterial damage or rupture.
- Primary complications associated with PTA are distal embolization, vessel dissection, vasospasm, and acute stenosis. The higher complication rate seen with PTA of intracranial versus coronary and peripheral vessels is thought to be secondary to decreased adventitia and structural support around intracranial vessels, as well as the critical nature of cerebral tissue.

Angioplasty Versus Stent-Assisted Angioplasty

- To potentially avoid restenosis, lesion recoil, or vessel dissection, PTA may be combined with stent placement (PTAS). The benefits of intracranial PTAS over PTA alone are less immediate post-procedural stenosis and low risk of target vessel dissection.
- For stent placement, a 6F guide catheter or a 6F long sheath is placed in the intracranial vessel of interest. A microcatheter and a 0.014-inch microwire are used to cross the lesion and the wire is advanced to a sufficient distance beyond the portion of artery that needs to be stented. The microwire is then removed and a stiffer 300-cm, 0.014-inch exchange wire is placed through the microcatheter and advanced across the lesion. Subsequently, the microcatheter is exchanged out and the stent is deployed across the stenotic region.
- Staged stent-assisted angioplasty is our technique of choice, in an attempt to reduce the peri-procedure and post-procedure complication rates. In this approach, the stent is placed several weeks after angioplasty. Our rationale behind the use of staged PTAS is that it allows time for healing post-angioplasty, resulting in intimal proliferation and scar formation that can work as a protective shield during stent deployment. The limitation of PTAS is late luminal loss secondary to in-stent restenosis.

Guiding Catheter and Sheath

- We prefer firm guiding catheters or sheaths with a flexible soft tip.
- We use the common carotid artery as the most common location to exchange the guiding catheter in order to prevent vasospasm in the internal carotid artery.
- We place the arterial sheath either all the way into the parent artery or in the femoral artery during initial access. If the sheath is placed in the femoral artery, it is essential to use the appropriate sheath size to allow passage of the chosen guide catheter.
- The guiding catheter is then advanced over a hydrophilic wire by using a road map into the internal carotid artery; care is taken not to advance the catheter into the petrous segment of the internal carotid artery in order to avoid dissection of the vessel.
- Sometimes, owing to severe atherosclerotic disease of the internal carotid artery or a sharp angle relative to the common carotid artery, the guiding catheter can be left in the distal common carotid artery.
- The guiding wire for a posterior circulation intervention is chosen on the basis of the anatomy and caliber of vertebral and basilar artery. To obtain firm support, the catheter is advanced as high as possible in the vertebral artery but with care taken not to advance the catheter above the horizontal turn of the vertebral artery at C2 in order to avoid vasospasm and dissection of the vessel.

- Most guiding catheter are 6F, but 5F catheters are preferred for vertebral or basilar artery angioplasty. The 6F catheter can be used for a large diameter vertebral artery.
- Once the position of the guidewire is confirmed, contrast agent is administered to check for vasospasm in the internal carotid or vertebral artery. Should the contrast agent show significant vasospasm, the guidewire is withdrawn slightly and the procedure is halted while an intra-arterial vasodilators, such as verapamil, is administered. Once the spasm has resolved, the procedure is resumed.

Guidewire Selection

- The choice of the wire is highly personal and also depends on whether the balloon and/or stent were brought up primarily or via an exchange maneuver. In either case, the wire should have a tip that is both steerable and flexible enough to navigate the tortuous cerebral vasculature. Additionally, the shaft of the wire should be firm enough that the dilation device can track easily.

Stent Selection

- We use bare metal, self-expanding, or drug-eluting stents (DESs) for intracranial PTAS. The selection of stent is based on patient profile, degree of stenosis, and anatomy of the vessels.
- The self-expanding Wingspan stent (Boston Scientific, Natick, MA) provides several advantages over balloon-mounted stents, as delivery can be achieved with less aggressive guiding catheter positions, resulting in less iatrogenic parent vessel spasm and dissection or distortion of the vessel.
- Occasionally, sirolimus or paclitaxel DES are chosen for their antiproliferative, anti-inflammatory, and immunosuppressive properties in a bid to reduce the occurrence of in-stent restenosis. However, DES require a longer time for endothelialization; and as a result, prolonged antiplatelet therapy is necessary to avoid late in-stent thrombosis.

Follow-Up Evaluation and Postprocedure Management

- An immediate post-procedure angiogram is performed and compared with the baseline angiogram to determine the degree of post-procedure stenosis. It is also critical to assess for post-procedure complications such as dissection flap, vessel damage, or distal artery embolus.
- The heparin drip is usually discontinued post-procedure, but it can be continued for a longer period of time if a thrombus is present or in the case of a severe lumen irregularity that can predispose to thrombus formation.

- Combination antiplatelet therapy (aspirin and clopidogrel) should be continued after the procedure for a duration of 30 days to 1 year. Aspirin is continued permanently in patients after angioplasty or stenting. Clopidogrel should be continued in conjunction with aspirin for 30 days in post-angioplasty patients, for 90 days after bare-metal stent placement, and for 1 year after DES placement.
- We perform repeat angiography 3–6 months after the procedure to evaluate for subacute to late stenosis or in-stent restenosis, or if symptoms occur.

Complications

- The major complications associated with intracranial PTA and stenting are distal embolization, vessel dissection, vasospasm, and acute stenosis.
- In the case of vessel dissection, if the flow through the vessel is normal with no residual stenosis, thrombus formation, or flow delay and the patient is clinically stable, we continue the heparin drip overnight. On the next day, we perform angiography to evaluate the status of the dissection. If the dissection looks stable and improving, we discontinue the heparin drip and continue to maintain the patient on antiplatelet medications.
- However, if the dissection is affecting the flow through the vessel, treatment is undertaken by deploying a bare metal or self-expanding stent across the stenosis and the dissection.
- If a thrombus has already formed around the area of dissection, leading to decreased flow through the vessel, we use intravenous abciximab or intra-arterial fibrinolytic therapy to lyse the clot.
- Distal embolus is another complication that is seen post intervention. If distal embolus is affecting the blood flow through the vessel and leading to cerebral infarction begin intravenous abciximab or fibrinolytic intra-arterial therapy. Minor emboli with normal blood flow and good collateral supply needs no further intervention.
- A serious but rare complication is arterial rupture leading to intracranial hemorrhage. Intracranial hemorrhage should be suspected with rapid rise in blood pressure and decline in pulse associated with worsening clinical status. In this case, the heparin therapy should be actively reversed by administering protamine.
- If bleeding still continues, gentle inflation of a balloon *proximal* to the site of bleeding should be done to temporarily occlude the flow through the vessel. The patient should be clinically monitored with serial CT head scans in a critical care unit. An external ventricular drain should be placed if the patient's mental status does not allow quality serial examinations.

Key Points

- Pay close attention to antithrombotic and anticoagulation medications before, during, and after the procedure. Frequently check ACT values.

- Familiarity with the approaches for vascular access and the indications and contraindications for each is crucial.
- Always obtain baseline and immediate post-procedure angiograms.
- Frequent monitoring of the patient's vital signs, clinical status, ACT, and position of devices throughout the procedure is crucial.
- Undersize the balloon during angioplasty to reduce the risk of arterial damage or rupture.
- Use the common carotid artery for guiding catheter exchange to prevent vasospasm in the internal carotid artery.
- Check for vasospasm in the internal carotid or vertebral artery by injecting contrast material after the guidewire is in position.

Suggested Readings

1. Chimowitz MI, Lynn MJ, Howlett-Smith H, Stern BJ, Hertzberg VS, Frankel MR, Levine SR, Chaturvedi S, Kasner SE, Benesch CG, Sila CA, Jovin TG, Romano JG: Warfarin-Aspirin Symptomatic Intracranial Disease Trial Investigators. Comparison of warfarin and aspirin for symptomatic intracranial arterial stenosis. N Engl J Med 352:1305–1316, 2005.
2. Cross DT, 3rd, Moran CJ, Derdeyn CP: Technique for intracranial balloon and stent-assisted angioplasty for atherosclerotic stenosis. Neuroimaging Clin N Am 17:365–380, ix, 2007.
3. Fiorella D, Levy EI, Turk AS, Albuquerque FC, Niemann DB, Aagaard-Kienitz B, Hanel RA, Woo H, Rasmussen PA, Hopkins LN, Masaryk TJ, McDougall CG: US multicenter experience with the Wingspan stent system for the treatment of intracranial atheromatous disease: periprocedural results. Stroke 38:881–887, 2007.
4. Hanel RA, Levy EI, Guterman LR, Hopkins LN: Advances in stent-assisted management of intracranial occlusive disease and cerebral aneurysms. Tech Vasc Interv Radiol 7:202–209, 2004.
5. Ingall TJ, Homer D, Baker HL, Jr, Kottke BA, O'Fallon WM, Whisnant JP: Predictors of intracranial carotid artery atherosclerosis. Duration of cigarette smoking and hypertension are more powerful than serum lipid levels. Arch Neurol 48:687–691, 1991.
6. Levy EI, Hanel RA, Bendok BR, Boulos AS, Hartney ML, Guterman LR, Qureshi AI, Hopkins LN: Staged stent-assisted angioplasty for symptomatic intracranial vertebrobasilar artery stenosis. J Neurosurg 97:1294–1301, 2002.
7. Morris PP: Practical Neuroangiography, 2nd ed. Baltimore MD, Lippincott Williams & Wilkins/Wolters Kluwer, 2007, pp. 40–42.
8. Osborn AG: Diagnostic Cerebral Angiography, 2nd ed. Baltimore MD, Lippincott Williams & Wilkins, 1999, pp. 424–431.
9. Sacco RL, Adams R, Albers G, Alberts MJ, Benavente O, Furie K, Goldstein LB, Gorelick P, Halperin J, Harbaugh R, Johnston SC, Katzan I, Kelly-Hayes M, Kenton EJ, Marks M, Schwamm LH, Tomsick T: Guidelines for prevention of stroke in patients with ischemic stroke or transient ischemic attack: a statement for healthcare professionals from the American Heart Association/American Stroke Association Council on Stroke: co-sponsored by the Council on Cardiovascular Radiology and Intervention: the American Academy of Neurology affirms the value of this guideline. Circulation 113:e409–e449, 2006.
10. Sacco RL, Kargman DE, Gu Q, Zamanillo MC: Race-ethnicity and determinants of intracranial atherosclerotic cerebral infarction. The Northern Manhattan Stroke Study. Stroke 26:14–20, 1995.
11. Schneider PA: Endovascular Skills: Guidewire and Catheter Skills for Endovascular Surgery 2nd ed. New York, NY, Informal Healthcare, 2003, pp. 6–29.

Angioplasty/Stenting of the Subclavian and Axillary Arteries

Trevor John Cleveland

Clinical Features

- Clinically significant upper limb vascular disease is much less common than lower limb vascular disease.
- The most likely pathology causing subclavian and axillary artery stenoses and occlusions is atheroma. However, lesions may occur as a result of fibromuscular dysplasia (FMD), irradiation, inflammatory arteritis, and arterial spasm.
- Symptoms may result from either a reduction in blood flow or as a result of the formation of emboli.
- If subclavian or axillary artery disease causes a significant reduction in blood flow, the patient will present with intermittent claudication of the arm on exercise.

  - If the occlusive lesion is proximal to the vertebral artery, arm exercise may result in a "steal" of blood down the vertebral artery from the cerebral circulation. In such circumstances, arm exercise will result in cerebral symptoms such as dizziness.
  - If an occlusive lesion lies proximal to the internal mammary artery that has been used as a conduit for coronary artery bypass, arm activity may "steal" blood from the coronary circulation resulting in return of the patients symptoms of angina.

- If an atheromatous plaque in the subclavian or axillary artery becomes unstable and thrombogenic, it may become a nidus for the formation of blood clot and subsequently embolize. Some emboli may be large and may become lodged in large arteries, causing acute limb ischemia; smaller emboli may cause digital infarcts ("blue finger syndrome").
- Subclavian and axillary artery stenoses of lesser severity, if symptomatic, tend to present with embolic symptoms. More severe stenoses or occlusion are more likely to produce flow-related symptoms.
- The left subclavian artery is the most common site for disease.

R.A. Morgan, E. Walser (eds.), *Handbook of Angioplasty and Stenting Procedures*,
Techniques in Interventional Radiology, DOI 10.1007/978-1-84800-399-6_16,
© Springer-Verlag London Limited 2010

Diagnostic Evaluation

Clinical Assessment

- Patients with upper limb vascular disease should undergo a full general vascular examination, including lower limb pulse evaluation, cardiac assessment, and abdominal palpation to exclude an abdominal aortic aneurysm.
- More focused assessment of the upper limbs should include a clinical history to assess the timescale over which symptoms have developed and the details of the symptomatology. Particular attention should be paid to symptoms of upper limb claudication, steal, or embolic events.
- Pulses should be palpated, including the supraclavicular, axillary, brachial, radial, and ulna pulses, to make an assessment of the level of the obstruction. The Allen test may be useful to assess the presence and patency of the radial and ulna arteries.
- The presence of bruits should be sought, particularly in the supraclavicular fossa.
- The brachial artery blood pressure should be measured in both arms. A lower blood pressure in one arm suggests a significant proximal lesion. Care should be taken in the interpretation of this sign, as there may be bilateral disease and embologenic foci may not cause a hemodynamic effect.
- As the main treatment options lie between endovascular and open surgical techniques, an assessment should be made regarding the patients' suitability for anesthesia.
- An endovascular option is highly likely to be dependent on access from the femoral approach, so particular attention should be paid to the presence and quality of the femoral pulses when making a more general vascular assessment.

Laboratory Investigations

- Renal function should be checked because of the necessity to use contrast medium during angioplasty and stenting.
- The blood coagulation should be checked – platelet count and I.N.R.

Imaging

- Imaging strategies are dependent to some extent on local expertise and availability. Imaging is required to identify the location of disease, the degree of disease and the local anatomy affecting the treatment options. The strategy will involve a combination of Duplex ultrasound, CT angiography (CTA), and MR angiography (MRA).

- If axillary artery disease is suspected, Duplex ultrasound can directly assess this segment and provide information regarding the degree of stenosis and the lesion location. If the disease lies more proximally, direct insonation of the lesion may not be possible. Pulse wave analysis will indicate the presence or otherwise of disease.
- MRA (3D Gadolinium enhanced) is preferable to CTA due to the lack of ionizing radiation. Both CTA and MRA have the ability to provide excellent images of the aortic arch and the supra-aortic vessels, and to make an assessment of the carotid and vertebral artery circulations, which may be relevant. Both techniques (also Duplex) may be confounded by heavy calcification and MRA is particularly susceptible to motion artifact at the aortic arch.
- MRA and CTA give excellent anatomical maps of the subclavian and axillary arteries, which enable the identification of anatomical variants (see below), and the planning of therapy. Moreover, vessel diameters and lesion lengths can be accurately measured, so that the appropriate endovascular equipment is available at the time of the intervention.

Indications for Treatment

- Symptomatic vascular disease of atheromatous origin
- Fibromuscular dysplasia
- Post radiotherapy

Contraindications

- Asymptomatic vascular disease
- Active infection in the region of the access site
- Active vasculitis
- Disease in a location, which will require stent placement across the origin of significant side branches (such as the vertebral or internal mammary arteries) is a relative contraindication.

Patient Preparation

- All patients should have informed consent obtained and baseline blood tests performed as detailed above.
- Leg and arm pulses should be palpated to assess available access points.
- The majority of subclavian and axillary artery procedures can be performed under local anesthesia, without any need for sedation. Such patients do not need to be starved prior to their procedure and they should be encouraged to maintain good

Fig. 3 This reconstructed CT
angiogram shows four
branches from the aortic arch.
The third branch from the left
(*arrow*) is the left vertebral
artery arising directly from
the aortic arch

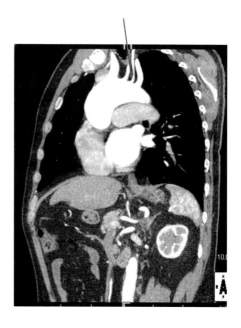

Equipment Specific to This Scenario

- Ultrasound guidance for access is often vital for the success of these procedures, particularly for brachial artery access, as the brachial pulse is often faint
  or impalpable.
- Long sheaths (70 cm or longer) or guiding catheters are needed for the introduction of balloons and stents from the femoral approach. Such devices can usually
  be inserted through 6F sheaths or 8F guiding catheters.
- Embolic protection devices (such as those used for carotid and coronary artery
  stenting) may be useful in these procedures (see below).

Pre-procedure Medications

All patients should already be prescribed before the procedure:

- A statin
- An antiplatelet agent (such as aspirin or Clopidogrel)
- Antihypertensive medication, as indicated by blood pressure measurements

Procedure

Arterial Access

- Subclavian and axillary artery lesions may be approached from either the brachial or the femoral approach, or a combination of the two.
- Femoral artery access is performed in a standard fashion.
- In the presence of a subclavian or axillary artery stenosis or occlusion, the brachial pulse downstream to the lesion is likely to be either weak or impalpable. Therefore, ultrasound should be used as guidance to puncture the artery. In the past, when most delivery systems for stents were greater than 6F, a formal cut-down was used for brachial access. This is no longer necessary, but may be used if ultrasound guidance is either unsuccessful or not available.

Angiography

- Diagnostic angiographic images can be obtained using conventional catheter techniques, MRA or CTA.
- Prior to intervention, catheter angiography should be performed, using a pigtail catheter, placed in the aortic arch.

   Assessment should be made of the following:

- Whether the lesion is an occlusion or a stenosis
- The relationship of the lesion to important side branches (most notably the vertebral artery and the internal mammary artery)
- The lesion morphology
- The hemodynamics of the lesion, particularly if there is reverse flow in the vertebral arteries.

Intra-procedural Medications

- All patients should already be taking the medications described previously, e.g., Statin, antiplatelet medication, and antihypertensive medication (as required).
- Patients should receive intra-procedural doses of short-acting anticoagulant drugs (such as heparin) to ensure that they remain anticoagulated for the duration of the procedure to prevent pericatheter thrombosis and thrombosis of arterial segments which have stasis of flow during balloon inflation.

Assessing the Lesion

Morphology

- Stenoses are technically easier to treat than occlusions.
- During angioplasty and stenting, atheromatous material may be dislodged along the wall of the artery, thus close proximity of side branches may result in compromise of those side branches.
- Heavily calcified lesions, particularly occlusions may be very resistant to endovascular treatment, both in terms of the ability to cross the lesion with a guidewire and resistance to expansion by balloons and stents.

Location

- Lesions located at the origin of the subclavian or brachiocephalic arteries may be very difficult to engage from a femoral approach, reducing the chances of successful recanalization.
- Close proximity of the lesion to the vertebral artery may result in vertebral artery compromise during angioplasty or stent placement.
- Lesions which have a segment of subclavian or axillary artery either proximally or distally are generally easier to engage with guidewires.

Pressure Measurements

- Pressure measurements are generally of little use for these procedures as the intention of primary angioplasty (PTA) may not be for flow-limiting disease (in the context of embolic symptoms). When stents are placed they are sized to match the arterial diameter outside the lesion and so full expansion is the desired outcome.
- There are no data to support any prognostic value in measuring intra-arterial pressures for such procedures.

Choosing a Balloon or Stent

- If balloon angioplasty is the planned procedure, the balloon should be sized to match the artery just distal to the lesion. Such measurements can be obtained from a number of sources:

  o Diagnostic CTA or MRA
  o Duplex
  o Calibrated catheter angiography

- If the primary intention is to place a stent, or a stent is used for a failed PTA, then the intended stent diameter should match the adjacent artery. For a balloon-mounted stent, these diameters should be the same. For a self-expanding stent, the unconstrained diameter should be 1–2 mm larger than the index artery.

- If the arterial segment is not likely to be subject to compressive forces, and accurate placement is needed, then balloon-mounted stents are generally favored. If recovery from compressive forces is likely to be important, then a self-expanding stent must be used.

Performing the Procedure

Crossing the Lesion

- Stenoses are technically less challenging than occlusions.
- Stenoses may be approached from either the brachial or the femoral approach.

  - Generally, they are easier to traverse if they are approached from a smaller diameter artery, i.e., from the brachial approach.
  - In addition, the crossing of such lesions may be less likely to cause any associated thrombus to be dislodged if approached from a brachial access. This is of particular importance when treating lesions in the brachiocephalic artery, where any emboli produced will potentially travel to the cerebral circulation and cause a stroke. In such circumstances, the use of cerebral protection devices may be advantageous.

- Subclavian and axillary artery occlusions usually arise from the formation of chronic plaque which is both well organized and often calcified. As a result they are very resistant to traverse with a guidewire.

  - To achieve success, these lesions may need to be approached from both the brachial and femoral approach (Fig. 4). The intimal lining of the occluded artery is destroyed by the disease process and the guidewire is likely to pass in a plane within the media of the arterial wall.

- If the lesion lies close to the origin of an important branch artery, consideration should be paid to protection of this vessel, by passing a wire or balloon into this artery during treatment of the primary lesion.

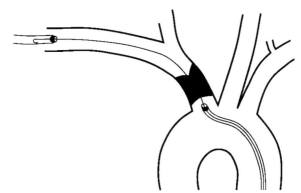

Fig. 4 A diagrammatic representation of a combined approach to a brachiocephalic occlusion from both a femoral and brachial approach

Deploying the Balloon/Stent

- Balloons and stents should be selected to obtain the desired diameter of the target artery and should be of sufficient length to cover the lesion.
- If the selected stent is not long enough to cover the lesion, additional stents should be available to adequately cover the lesion. Additional stents should be placed with an overlap of at least 1 cm.
- It is important to have the facility to perform angiograms before and after PTA or stent insertion. This is generally achieved by the placement of a pigtail catheter in the aortic arch, usually from a femoral approach.

Endpoint

- If the original symptoms were of embolic origin, the primary intention is to perform PTA and to stimulate the arterial lining to heal with a smooth neointima. Thus the aim of the procedure is not for a perfect hemodynamic result, although the flow through the segment must be sufficient to prevent a significant risk of acute thrombosis. Once PTA has been performed the arterial wall must be allowed sufficient time to heal.
- If the original symptoms were the result of poor blood flow, then the primary intention is to remove the hemodynamic lesion. This may be achieved by PTA or stent placement. For stenotic lesions, either strategy is reasonable, as there is no definite difference in outcomes between PTA and stents. However, for occlusions, the results of primary stenting are better than PTA. Therefore, the lesion should be stented with the intention of achieving as small a residual stenosis as possible.

Immediate Post-procedural Care

- The access points should be closed.

  - In the ante cubital fossa, this should be achieved by application of digital pressure.
  - A closure device may be used to seal a femoral artery puncture.

- The access points should be observed for bleeding or hematoma, and the patient's vital signs should be monitored.
- Stroke may occur both during these procedures and in the immediate post-operative period. Routine neurological observations should be undertaken.
- There is no need to continue heparin after completion of the procedure, but antiplatelet medication should not be interrupted.

Follow-Up and Post-procedure Medications

- These procedures may be performed on a day case basis, provided that patients are observed for at least 4 h after their procedure, and are discharged to a safe environment (responsible company, telephone availability, information sheet

regarding complications to be aware of, a point of contact at the treating hospital available 24 h a day).
- Statins, anti-hypertensives, and antiplatelet agents should be continued indefinitely.

Results

- There are few series of significant size in the literature and no randomized trials.
- The success at crossing complete occlusions is variable ranging from 30 to 94%.
- The patency results for treated stenoses are generally better than those for occlusions and stent series report higher patency than PTA series. However, the vast majority of series contain a wide range of lesion and treatment types, making it difficult to draw definite conclusions regarding the efficacy of PTA versus stents.
- Primary patency of 80% at 6 and 16 months are described along with patency of 75% at 8 years. Other series describe less durable results.

Alternative Therapies

- Conservative therapy with best medical management should be considered for relatively minor symptoms.
- Open surgery (bypass, transposition, or endarterectomy) are alternatives.

Complications

- Complications include
  - ○ Acute stent/PTA thrombosis
  - ○ Stroke
  - ○ Arm emboli
  - ○ Access site hematoma

How to Treat

- Acute stent/PTA thrombosis may be treated by thrombectomy, thrombolysis, or surgical bypass.
- Stroke may be hemorrhagic or embolic and should be investigated by CT or MRI.
  - ○ Thrombolysis may be considered in the hyperacute phase of embolic stroke.
  - ○ Reversal of anticoagulation.
  - ○ Cessation of antiplatelet agents in the case of hemorrhagic stroke.
- Distal embolization to the arm is often asymptomatic. If patients are symptomatic, they may be treated by aspiration or Fogarty embolectomy.

How to Avoid

- Avoidance is largely dependent upon good technique, drug therapy, effective planning, and not treating morphology poorly suited to PTA/stenting.

Key Points

- Review symptoms and ensure that the procedure is indicated.
- Ensure that the pre-procedural imaging is adequate, take time to plan the procedure, and check that all the appropriate equipment is available.
- Know how to use all of the equipment.
- Ensure that the patient is taking appropriate drug therapy.
- Limit manipulation of the lesion to a minimum by use of the brachial approach.
- Consider cerebral protection if embolization to the brain is a possibility.
- Have a low threshold for seeking the advice/help of someone with a large experience of the treatment of these lesions.

Suggested Reading

1. Kessel D, Robertson I. Interventional Radiology: A Survival Guide – 2nd Edition. Elsevier.
2. Przewlocki T, Kablak-Ziembicka A, Pieniazek P, et al. Determinants of immediate and long-term results of subclavian and innominate artery angioplasty. Catheter Cardiovasc Interv 2006; 67: 519–526.
3. Rutherford RB (Ed) Rutherford Vascular Surgery – 6th Edition. Elsevier 2008, Chapter 90.
4. The Royal College of Radiologists (2005). Standards For Iodinated Intravascular Contrast Agent Administration To Adult Patients. Royal College of Radiologists, London. http://www.rcr.ac.uk
5. Woo EY, Fairman RM, Velazquez OC, et al. Endovascular Therapy of Symptomatic Innominate-subclavian Arterial Occlusive Lesions. Vasc Endovasc Surg 2006; 40: 27–33.

Stent-Grafting of the Thoracic Aorta

Jean-Paul Beregi and Marco Midulla

Clinical Features

Thoracic endovascular repair is often known by the acronyms TEVAR or TEVR.

The technique was introduced in the early 1990s and has become increasingly used worldwide to treat a variety of aortic pathologies.

Types of the Pathology Treated by TEVR

- Thoracic aortic aneurysm (TAA): These include atherosclerotic aneurysms, post-traumatic false aneurysms, anastomotic pseudoaneurysms post-aortic surgery, mycotic aneurysms, and pseudoaneurysms post-coarctation repair.
- Acute Aortic Syndromes (AAS): Aortic dissection, Intramural Hematoma (IMH), and penetrating aortic ulcer (PU).

The term AAS was introduced in 2001 to describe acute chest pain related to three acute aortic pathologies:

- Chronic aortic dissection
- Acute Traumatic Aortic Rupture (ATAR)
- Aortobronchial fistula

Diagnostic Evaluation

Clinical

Most aortic pathology is silent until there is evidence of rupture or impending rupture:

- The majority of aortic lesions are discovered by chance as a result of chest radiography, MRI or CT examinations performed for other clinical indications.

R.A. Morgan, E. Walser (eds.), *Handbook of Angioplasty and Stenting Procedures*,
Techniques in Interventional Radiology, DOI 10.1007/978-1-84800-399-6_17,
© Springer-Verlag London Limited 2010

- Chest pain in the presence of a known aortic lesion suggests impending or established rupture.
- Established rupture is usually accompanied by severe chest pain, hypotension, or death.

Laboratory

Clearly aortic rupture is usually accompanied by a fall in the serum hemoglobin.

- In acute dissection or IMH, involvement of the renal and other visceral branches may be accompanied by deterioration in renal function and serological signs of intestinal ischemia such as an increase in lactate dehydrogenase.

Pre-interventional Imaging

It is essential to review the preoperative imaging to

- Identify the nature of the aortic pathology
- Assess the indications, if any, for treatment
- Decide a plan for therapy

The main non-invasive modalities used for the evaluation of the thoracic aorta are chest radiography, CT, and MR imaging.

Chest Radiography

Assess chest radiographs performed for other indications for signs of aortic pathology.

- Observe for enlargement of the thoracic aorta and signs of rupture: mediastinal widening, left pleural effusion.

CT and CTA

The main imaging method used for the assessment of the thoracic aorta.

- The scan should cover the entire aorta commencing above the aortic arch and extending inferiorly to include the abdominal aorta and the iliac arteries as far as the inguinal ligament.

- Use multiplanar reconstructions (MPRs) and view the maximum intensity projection (MIP) images on the CT workstation to assess:

  ○ Location and extent of the aortic lesion
  ○ For the presence of proximal and distal landing zones for an endograft(s)
  ○ The configuration of the aorta and iliac vessels with regard to tortuosity and kinking which might cause problems in delivery of the endograft to the required site
  ○ The access site and iliac arteries for their diameter, amount of calcification, and the presence of aneurysms

- Diameter measurements of the aorta should always be made orthogonal to the vessel. This is most easily done using the reformatted images. If only axial images are available, the diameter of the short axis of the vessel should be measured.
- The following diameter measurements should be obtained:

  ○ The maximum diameter of the aorta.
  ○ The diameter of potential landing zones for an endograft proximal and distal to the aortic lesion.
  ○ The diameter of the access vessels — i.e., the iliac and common femoral arteries.

- Length measurements are best made using oblique sagittal or curved reformatted images.
- The following length measurements should be obtained:

  ○ The length of the aneurysm if present
  ○ The length of normal diameter aorta proximal and distal to the aortic lesion (landing zones)

MRI and MRA

Less commonly used than CT for pre-procedural imaging for TEVR:

○ A combination of MRI and MRA is best.
○ Gated scans improve image quality.
○ Axial coverage from the aortic arch to the iliac arteries is not possible.

The necessary measurements required when planning TEVR are summarized in Table 1 and Fig. 1.

Table 1 Preoperative measurements required when planning for TEVR

D1 a	Aortic diameter proximal to the lesion	2 cm proximal to the lesion
D1 b		Immediately proximal to the lesion
D2	The diameter of the aortic lesion	
D3 a	Aortic diameter distal to the lesion	Immediately distal to the lesion
D 3 b		2 cm distal to the lesion
L1	Proximal neck length (proximal landing zone)	Distance of lesion-LSCA; or distance of lesion-LCA; or distance of lesion−innominate artery or distance of lesion−aortic sinotubular junction
L2	Length of the lesion	
L3	Length of the distal neck (distal landing zone)	Usually distance from lesion−coeliac trunk
D4	Iliac artery diameters	Right and left

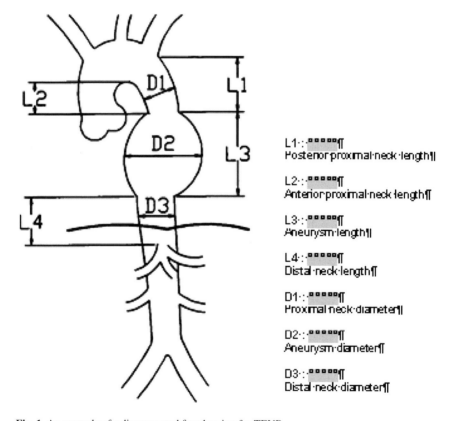

L1·:· ▪▪▪▪▪¶
Posterior proximal neck length¶|

L2·:· ▪▪▪▪▪¶
Anterior proximal neck length¶

L3·:· ▪▪▪▪▪¶
Aneurysm length¶|

L4·:· ▪▪▪▪▪¶
Distal neck length¶

D1·:· ▪▪▪▪▪¶
Proximal neck diameter¶|

D2·:· ▪▪▪▪▪¶
Aneurysm diameter¶

D3·:· ▪▪▪▪▪¶
Distal neck diameter¶

Fig. 1 An example of a diagram used for planning for TEVR

Indications

Urgent Indications

- Aortic rupture:
  - Aneurysm
  - Aortic trauma
  - Aortic dissection, intramural hematoma, and PAU
- Non-ruptured symptomatic atherosclerotic aneurysms
- Non-ruptured traumatic aortic pseudoaneurysms
- Visceral ischemia due to true lumen collapse (dynamic compression) in aortic dissections
- Persistent thoracic pain in the presence of acute type B dissection or intramural hematoma
- Enlarging aorta on consecutive CT scans in acute aortic syndrome

Elective Indications

- Atherosclerotic aneurysm larger than 5.5 cm.
  - 5 cm in women or small adults
- Aortic dissection with an aortic diameter greater than 5.5 cm.
- Chronic traumatic pseudoaneurysm greater than 5.5 cm

Extended Indications

The technique can be extended to treat lesions involving the aortic arch and thoracoabdominal pathology by the following techniques:

- Hybrid procedures – these involve elective bypass of the supra-aortic or abdominal visceral vessels followed by the insertion of endografts.
- The use of branched or fenestrated endografts.

These complex procedures are outside the scope of this chapter.

Contraindications

The following are relative and not absolute.

- Marfan syndrome or other connective tissue diseases
- Systemic infection
- Unfavourable anatomy

Patient Preparation

- Procedures are either performed under general or regional anesthesia. Therefore, patients are prepared in the standard manner for the type of anesthesia they require.
- Imaging of the carotid and vertebral arteries is sensible if the stent-grafts have to be deployed close to these vessels, or if the supra-aortic vessels require elective bypass to extend the proximal landing zones.

Relevant Anatomy

The key anatomical inclusion criteria for TEVR are

- The presence of landing zones of normal aorta proximal and distal to the lesion to provide a seal between the endograft and the aortic wall and prevent leakage into the aneurysm or false lumen.
- Adequate caliber access vessels.

Proximal Landing Zone

Diameter:

- The maximum diameter landing zone is decided by the maximum available endograft diameter – currently 46 mm (Valiant, Medtronic, Santa Rosa, CA).
- Endografts should be oversized by 10–20% to achieve an adequate seal.
- Therefore, the maximum diameter of the landing zone is 42 mm.

Length:

- 20 mm between the lesion and the left subclavian artery is optimal for straight-forward procedures.
- If the lesion is more proximal and close to the aortic arch and supra-aortic vessels, one or more of these vessels can be covered after pre-procedural elective bypass of the relevant supra-aortic vessels.
- Coverage of the left subclavian artery *without* bypass was previously performed, but this practice is now known to be associated with increased stroke and paraplegia risk.

Distal Landing zone

Diameter:

- Similar dimensions to the proximal landing zone.

Length:

- Optimally, there should be 2 cm between the distal aspect of the lesion and the celiac artery.
- The distal landing zone can be extended inferiorly by elective bypass of the celiac and/or the other visceral vessels.

Access Vessels

The iliac and common femoral arteries should be of adequate caliber to enable passage of the endograft delivery system.

- In practical terms, the access vessels should be at least 7 mm in diameter to allow passage of the smaller caliber endografts.
- Wider iliac arteries are required for the widest endografts.

Equipment

Endografts

Flexibility, conformability, ease of deployment, accuracy of deployment, durability, availability in a wide range of diameters and lengths, and low-profile delivery systems are desirable attributes for the ideal endograft.

Several types of endograft are currently commercially available.

These include

- Talent (Medtronic)
- Valiant (Medtronic)
- Zenith TX2 (Cook, Bloomington, IN)
- Gore TAG (W.L. Gore & Associates, Flagstaff, AZ)
- Relay (Bolton Medical, Sunrise, FL)
- Evita (Jotec, Hechingen, Germany)
- Endofit (Endomed Phoenix, AZ)

The technical features of the most commonly used devices are presented in Table 2.

Endograft Selection

The following are true about the current devices:

- No device is perfect.

Table 2 Technical features of some commercially available devices (author's personal assessments)

Device	Introducing sheath	Introducing system size (F)	Available diameter size (mm)	Available lengths(mm)	Bare proximal portion	Delayed deployment of more proximal stent	Radial force	Flexibility	MRI compatibility (images artifacting)	Delivery System
TAG (GORE)	Y	20–24	26–40	20	N	N	+	++	Y	Pull- knob
Talent (MEDTRONIC)	N	22–27	22–46	100	Y	N	++	+	Y	Pull-back
Valiant (MEDTRONIC)	N	20–24	22–46	100–220 150-	Y	N	+++	++	Y	Pull-back xcelerant system
Zenith TX2 (COOK)	Y	20–22	22–42	100–216 150-	Y	Y	++	+	N	Pull-back
Relay (BOLTON)	N	22–26	22–46		Y	Y	++	+	Y	Pull-back

- There is no good quality scientific evidence that any one device is better than the others.
- The majority of devices are chosen on the basis of personal preference and experience.
- The nitinol stent-grafts are MR compatible so that the risk of irradiation can be reduced for the follow up examinations.
- In general devices are oversized by 10–20% for aneurysms and slightly less for acute dissection (e.g., 5–10%).
- When selecting a device diameter for use in dissections, the caliber of the aorta just proximal to the dissection should be used. This will generally be the diameter of the mid-aortic arch.
- In acute dissections, a device length should be chosen to cover the main entry tear.
- In chronic dissection, devices should extend from just proximal to the entry tear to the diaphragm.

Other Equipment Required for TEVR

Other equipment required for standard TEVR includes

- Vascular Sheaths: 6–24F

  - A 6F sheath is useful for the diagnostic catheter.
  - A 16–18F sheath is required for passage of a balloon for dilatation of the endografts.
  - Some endografts, e.g., Gore TAG require placement through a sheath.

- Diagnostic catheter – 90–100 cm long pigtail/flush catheter.
- Guidewires: 260-cm long Lunderquist guidewire (Cook), or similar
- Balloons to mold the endografts after deployment, e.g., Coda (Cook), Reliant (Medtronic).

Pre-procedure Medications

- No specific medications are required before the procedure.

Procedure

Arterial Access

Endograft Insertion

Most procedures involve device insertion through standard surgical femoral arteriotomies:

- The procedure can be performed totally percutaneously with certain closure devices (e.g., Prostar XL, Abbott Vasc), although this technique is subject to quite a steep learning curve with the risk of severe hemorrhage and damage to the access arteries.
- Patients with poor access vessels may not be suitable for TEVR. However, other access routes may be used. For example, endograft deployment via a surgical conduit or cut-down on to the common iliac artery, the abdominal aorta, the axillary artery, the subclavian artery and the common carotid artery have all been reported.
- The exposed artery is punctured with an arterial needle. A conventional guidewire and catheter is advanced to the aortic arch. The conventional guidewire is exchanged for a Lunderquist exchange guidewire which is looped in the ascending aorta.
- The endograft delivery system is advanced to the site of the lesion over the Lunderquist guidewire under constant fluoroscopic observation.
- It is better to advance the tip of the endograft to a centimeter or so proximal to the lesion before deployment. The device can be pulled back if required, but cannot be advanced.
- If the patient has a dissection, care must be taken to advance the delivery catheter up the aortic true lumen and not the false lumen.

Diagnostic Catheter

A diagnostic flush catheter is required to guide accurate placement of the endograft:

- This is most commonly placed from the contralateral femoral artery through a percutaneous 6F sheath.
- An alternative access is the ipsilateral femoral artery (by a separate puncture) or via an upper extremity access (usually the low brachial artery).

Angiography

- If patients have a dissection, angiography should be performed in the upper abdomen to ensure that the catheter is in the true and not the false lumen.
- In patients with aneurysms, procedural angiography is first performed with the endograft delivery system placed at the approximate location for deployment. Performing aortography before this stage is unnecessary, involves unnecessary irradiation to patient and interventionalists, and is a waste of contrast medium.
- If the lesion is close to the aortic arch, it is important to see the supra-aortic vessels in profile. Therefore aortography should be performed in the appropriate oblique projection. Usually LAO ranges from 30 to 75°.
- Standard precautions should be observed with regard to flushing catheters placed in the aortic arch or ascending aorta to avoid cerebral air or thromboemboli.
- Aortography should be performed using 20–30 mL contrast medium at 15–20 mL/sec.

Intra-procedural Medications

- Heparin: 5,000 IU administered intra-arterially, unless there is evidence of aortic rupture.
- Broad-spectrum intravenous antibiotics are usually given to prevent endograft sepsis.
- Drugs are administered by the anesthesiologist to reduce the blood pressure to 100 mmHg peak systolic pressure immediately prior to endograft deployment.

Deploying the Endograft

Each endograft has a different method of deployment. A description of the methods for the different endograft types is outside the scope of this chapter.

The following points are generic for all endografts:

- Be sure to familiarize yourself with the method of deployment for the endograft you are using before the procedure starts. Reading the instructions at the time of deployment with the device in the aorta is poor clinical practice and increases complications.
- If you have never used an endograft before, it is wise to see other practitioners deploy the endograft first. This may involve visits to other hospitals.
- For your first or second deployments, it is sensible to ask an expert with the device to attend the procedure to help you.
- For most endograft designs, check aortograms should be performed after partial release of the endograft to ensure that the graft is being released in the desired position.
- If more than one endograft is required to cover the length of the lesion, make sure that there is adequate overlap between the adjacent devices to prevent future device separation.
- Molding of the endografts is usually performed after deployment to ensure full expansion of the endograft and to enhance the seal between adjacent devices and between the endografts and the landing zones.
- When placing endografts in true lumens in patients with dissection, balloon molding is generally not performed because of a risk of rupture of the dissection flap.

Endpoint

Before completion angiography can be performed, the pigtail catheter, which is "trapped" between the endograft and the aortic wall, must be withdrawn to a level below the endografts and readvanced through the endograft lumen again, to a level proximal to the endografts. This procedure is performed over a standard guidewire to prevent dislocation of the endograft by the pigtail.

Technical success is defined by a completion angiogram which

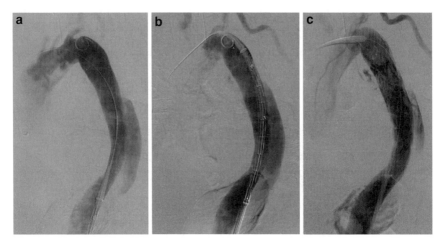

Fig. 2 (a, b, and **c)** Treatment of an acute dissection with a Valiant endograft. Figure (a) shows a dissection of the descending thoracic aorta. The main communication between the true and the false lumen is in the upper descending aorta. After insertion and deployment of a single Valiant endograft, the main fenestration has now been covered. A follow-up CT scan performed a week later showed no residual false lumen perfusion in the thorax

- Shows a patent endograft (or endografts)
- Exclusion of the aneurysm sac with no endoleak
- Closure of the main thoracic fenestration between the true and the false lumen in patients with dissection
- Patency of the supra-aortic vessels and/or the celiac artery if these vessels are close to the lesion

Examples of TEVR in a patient with acute type B dissection and in another patient with a ruptured aneurysm of the descending thoracic aorta are presented in Figs. 2 and 3.

Immediate Post-procedural Care

This consists of standard recovery procedure after general or regional anesthesia. Specific points after TEVR include

- Patients should be monitored for stroke or paraplegia.
- If there is evidence of paraplegia, a percutanous spinal drain should be placed to reduce the pressure of the cerebrospinal fluid. This is performed by anesthesiologists.
- There is no evidence to support routine prophylactic preoperative spinal drainage for all TEVR procedures.

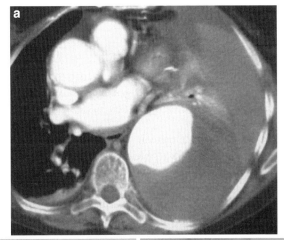

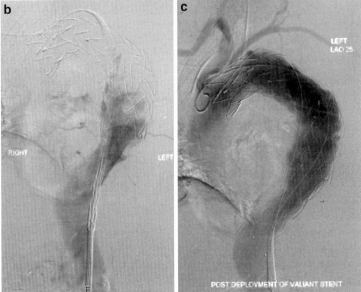

Fig. 3 (**a, b,** and **c**) Treatment of a patient with a contained rupture of an aneurysm of the descending thoracic aorta. Figure (a) shows the aneurysm and a hemothorax. The patient was treated by the emergent insertion of two overlapping Valiant endografts. The procedure was successful and the patient was discharged 14 days later

- Some interventionalists place preoperative spinal drains in patients who have previously undergone abdominal aortic surgery or in patients in whom it is planned to cover a long length of thoracic and abdominal aorta with endografts.

Follow-Up and Post-procedure Medications

Follow-Up

- Regular follow-up by CT or MR is mandatory to monitor for complications.
- Regular plain radiographs of the endografts are also necessary to monitor for continued integrity of the devices, i.e., disconnection and metallic strut fracture.
- Follow-up protocols vary. Our patients undergo CT scans pre-discharge, at 3 months, at 1 year, and at annual intervals thereafter. Plain radiographs are performed before discharge and at annual intervals.
- Specific features to look for on follow-up imaging include endoleaks, change in aneurysm sac size, endograft disconnection, persistent perfusion or thrombosis of the false lumen, and any new relevant findings involving the aorta or other viscera.

Post-procedure Medications

There are no specific medications to be taken after TEVR:

- Most patients take antiplatelet therapy in the form of aspirin.
- Routine antibiotics or clopidogrel are not required

Results

The technical success of TEVR is very high and is reported as constantly above 90% for all indications.

Apart from technical success, the outcome data tend to vary slightly with indication.

Aneurysms

- For descending thoracic aneurysm, the EUROSTAR collaborators reported data in 249 patients with 30-day mortality for elective TEVR of 5.3% and paraplegia of 4%.
- Similarly, the European Talent Registry reported technical success of 98%, in-hospital mortality in 5%, paraplegia in 1.7%, and stroke in 3.7%. Similar outcomes have been reported for the newest generation of endografts, despite the fact that patients in these later series had more challenging anatomy compared with earlier series.

Dissection and Acute Aortic Syndrome

- For acute type B dissections, the results of TEVR are better than surgery.
- Most series report mortality rates below 10% with paraplegia rates of less than 3%.
- Most vascular centers would now regard endovascular therapy to be the first-line treatment for acute complicated type B dissections.
- Indications for repair of chronic dissections have usually been limited to the onset of complications and an aortic diameter exceeding 5.5–6.0 cm.
- The availability of data regarding the outcomes of EVR for chronic dissections is very poor. In the series to date, the mortality rates have been acceptable but the long-term success in preventing aortic expansion is unclear.

Traumatic Aortic Injury

- Although TEVR seems to have become the gold standard for TAI, there are relatively limited data on outcomes. However, the procedural mortality is less than 10% throughout and the reported risk of paraplegia is negligible
- However, there remain concerns with the poor suitability and durability of the available devices for this predominantly young population.

Complications

Stent Related

Maldeployment

- Failure to land the endograft in the correct location usually requires placement of an additional device, either an additional endograft or a cuff. A supply of these should be available for use if required to prevent procedural failure.
- Maldeployment is avoided by

    ○ Avoid hurrying during deployment
    ○ Perform check angiograms during deployment
    ○ Perform check angiograms in the appropriate obliquity

Endoleak

Similar to abdominal EVAR, these may be type 1, 2, or 3. Type 1 is the most frequent followed by type 3 and finally type 2.

- Endoleaks are avoided by

    ○ Accurate pre-procedural planning and correct device selection
    ○ Accurate deployment of the endografts

- Type 1 and type 3 endoleaks generally require treatment.
- Treatment of endoleaks may involve repeat balloon dilatation. However, insertion of additional endografts is usually required.
- Type 2 leaks may be due to retrograde filling from the left subclavian artery if this artery has been covered without bypass, or bypassed but not tied off at its origin. Embolization of type 2 leaks from the left subclavian artery is usually performed, if necessary, using Amplatz plugs or coils.

Related to Vascular Access

This may consist of iliac artery rupture because of trauma caused by the large endograft delivery system.

- This is best treated by insertion of a covered stent. A supply of these should always be kept in stock.

General Complications

- **Stroke**
  - Increased by excessive manipulations in the aortic arch
  - Increased by covering the left subclavian artery without bypass
  - Increased in the presence of atheroma in the aortic arch
- **Paraplegia**
  - Increased by endografting long lengths of aorta
  - Increased by previous abdominal aortic repair
  - Treat by spinal drainage
- **Fever**: It may occur as a result of thrombosis of aneurysmal sac or the false lumen.

Key Points

- TEVAR should be considered for the treatment of aortic pathology involving the descending thoracic aorta.
- The diameter threshold for intervention on the descending aorta is 5.5 cm.
- In most cases, insertion of these devices is straightforward and does not involve a long procedure time.
- A femoral arteriotomy is usually required, although percutaneous insertion using closure devices is feasible.
- The technical success rates are very high and approach 100% in most series.
- The conversion rate to open surgery is negligible.

- The paraplegia rate is around 2% and the stroke rate is approximately 4% in most series.
- The most common complication is a type 1 endoleak. This requires reintervention and usually involves the insertion of additional endografts.
- The technique is relatively new and follow-up by imaging should be lifelong.

Suggested Reading

1. Rousseau H, Verhoye JP, Heautot JF eds. Thoracic Aortic Diseases. Springer-Verlag, Heidelberg, Berlin, 2006.
   A recent comprehensive text book collecting the experiences of the worldwide best known people who devoted their activity to thoracic aortic issues
2. Vilacosta I, Román JA. Acute aortic syndrome. Heart. 2001 Apr; 85(4):365–8. No abstract available.
   The introduction of the term "Acute Aortic Syndromes" with the description of the relative anatomo-pathological entities
3. Gaxotte V, Thony F, Rousseau H, Lions C, Otal P, Willoteaux S, Rodiere M, Negaiwi Z, Joffre F, Beregi JP. Midterm results of aortic diameter outcomes after thoracic stent-graft implantation for aortic dissection: a multicenter study. J Endovasc Ther 2006 Apr; 13(2):127–38.
4. www.ctsnet.org
   A thematic e-site dedicated to the cardiothoracic surgery with on-line books available for consultations

Elective Endovascular Aneurysm Repair (EVAR) of Abdominal Aortic Aneurysms (AAA)

Johannes Lammer and Maria Schoder

Clinical Features

- The incidence of AAA is 4% in the adult population and 11% in males older than 65 years.
- Men are 4–8 times more affected by AAA than women.
- Between 1993 and 2003 the overall rates of treated unruptured and ruptured AAAs in the US remained stable (unruptured 12–15/100,000; ruptured 1–3/100,000).
- Aneurysms should be treated when they are 5.5 cm or larger, symptomatic or increase in size by 5 mm per year.

Diagnostic Evaluation

Clinical

- May present with a palpable non-tender abdominal mass.
- May present with a palpable tender abdominal mass.
- May present with abdominal or back pain.
- May present with symptoms related to distal embolization.
- May present with pain and hypotension because of rupture.

Ultrasound

- Ultrasonography is the basic tool for the diagnosis of AAA.
- Ultrasound is used for the screening of patients at risk for AAA.

CT Angiography (CTA)

- The main method used for the assessment of patients with a known AAA.
- CTA protocol (e.g., 64 row multislice CT).

R.A. Morgan, E. Walser (eds.), *Handbook of Angioplasty and Stenting Procedures*, 225
Techniques in Interventional Radiology, DOI 10.1007/978-1-84800-399-6_18,
© Springer-Verlag London Limited 2010

- ○ Coverage from the superior mesenteric artery to the groin.
- ○ 80–100 cc contrast medium (300–400 mg J/mL).
- ○ 160–300 mAs, 120 kV, 64 × 0.625 mm, 0.75 sec rotation, pitch 1.2, trigger level 150 HU, 8-sec delay post trigger.
- ○ Cross-sectional image reconstruction – 3 mm slice, reconstruction index (RI) 2 mm, soft kernel, W 900/C 250.
- ○ 3D reconstruction − 1 mm slice, RI 0.5 mm, soft kernel (B-filter), W 900/ C 250, thin maximum intensity projection (MIP), MIP every 15° in z-axis.

Contrast-Enhanced Magnetic Resonance Angiography (MRA)

- Less commonly used than CT.
- Useful for patients with abnormal renal function or allergy to iodinated contrast medium.
- Protocol: Localizer, T1 weighted FFE axial, T2 weighted GRE axial, bolus tracking.
- Contrast medium: 0.2 mmol/kg body weight, Gd-chelate (Omniscan, Dotarem, Gadovist, MultiHance), saline solution flush, contrast-enhanced 3D-GRE (TFE, FLASH) coronal, short TR (<3 ms), small flip angle (<30°).
- 3D reconstruction – MIP every 15° in z-axis.

Catheter Angiography

- Has largely been replaced by CTA and MRA.
- Used mainly as a problem solver:

  - ○ To assess borderline neck.
  - ○ To assess borderline iliac arteries.

- Method:

  - ○ Performed with a calibrated flush catheter (pigtail, straight) with 1-cm lead markers.
  - ○ 20–35cc contrast medium (300 mg J/mL).
  - ○ Injected at 10–15 cc/sec.
  - ○ Image abdominal aorta and pelvic arteries, oblique views if required.

Information Required from Imaging Studies

- Superior mesenteric artery (SMA) – this must be patent because the inferior mesenteric artery (IMA) will be occluded after endograft placement.
- Renal arteries and accessory renal arteries.

- Length, diameter, kinking, thrombus, and calcification of the aneurysm neck (aorta between the renal arteries and the AAA), which forms the proximal landing zone for the endograft.
- Length, diameter, kinking, thrombus, and calcification of the iliac arteries (which form the distal landing zone and the access arteries).
- Diameter and calcification of the common femoral artery.

Indications for EVAR

- AAA with a diameter of 5.5 cm or larger.
- Symptomatic aneurysms (pain, tenderness, distal embolization). These should be treated even if they are smaller than 5.5 cm diameter.
- Documented growth of more than 0.5 cm per year.

Contraindications

Because EVAR can be performed under local and spinal anesthesia, anatomic factors are the dominant contraindications:

- Short infrarenal neck <10–15 mm.
- Wide infrarenal neck – >33 mm.
- Excessive neck angulation >65°.
- Excessive thrombus or calcification in the neck is relative contraindication.
- A very conical neck.
- Small access vessels – <7 mm.
- Excessive iliac artery tortuosity and calcification.

Patient Preparation

- Chest X-ray.
- ECG.
- In symptomatic patients, exercise ECG, Thallium scanning, coronary CTA, or cardiac MRI may be required.
- Laboratory parameters:

  o Coagulation tests.
  o Renal and liver function tests.
  o Blood cell count, hematocrit.
  o Cross-match four units of blood.

- Informed consent.
- Urinary catheter.

Relevant Anatomy

- There should be proximal and distal landing (or sealing) zones of adequate dimension.
- With increasing experience, the absolute values of diameter, length, and angulation may change.
- Standard inclusion criteria for EVAR:

  - Neck diameter 33 mm or less.
  - Neck length 15 mm or longer.
  - Angulation of <65°.
  - Thrombus and severe calcification <50% circumference of neck.
  - CIA diameter 22 mm or less.
  - CIA length >35 mm.
  - Absence of excessive tortuosity and calcification.
  - The access vessels, i.e., femoral and external iliac arteries should be of adequate caliber to accept the endograft delivery system, i.e., >7 mm diameter.

Equipment Required for EVAR

Stent-Grafts

- Types – Bifurcated, Aortouniiliac, or fenestrated:

  - Bifurcated – the most common type used for the majority of patients with standard anatomy.
  - Aortouniiliac devices – used in patients with unilateral iliac artery disease or in emergency aneurysm repair.
  - Fenestrated – used in patients with aneurysms unsuitable for conventional stent-grafts (usually short and/or angulated necks).

- Examples of devices – Zenith (W. Cook, Europe), Endurant, Talent (Medtronic, Santa Rosa, CA), Excluder (W. Gore, Flagstaff, AZ).
- Stent structure – stainless steel or nitinol.
- Graft fabric – polyester or ePTFE.
- Proximal fixation – infrarenal with hooks, suprarenal with or without hooks.
- Bifurcated design – modular or unibody.
- Delivery system 18–22F.

Catheters

- Pigtail catheter for aortography.
- A selection of selective catheters for manipulations in the iliac arteries and aorta, and for cannulation of the contralateral limb:

- ○ Cobra.
- ○ Multipurpose.
- ○ Vertebral or Berenstein.
- ○ Simmons 1 or Sos Omni catheters.
- Balloon catheters:
  - ○ Compliant balloon up to 36 mm in diameter for balloon molding the attachment sites, and anastomoses between the components.
  - ○ Angioplasty balloon for dilating iliac stenoses.

Guidewires

- Standard guidewires.
- Exchange length very stiff guidewires to support the endograft delivery system:
  - ○ Lunderquist (W. Cook).
  - ○ Meier (Boston Scientific Corp.).
- Hydrophilic guidewires.

Additional Tools

- Introducer sheaths of different sizes − 6–18F.
- Palmaz stent – in case of a proximal type Ia endoleak.
- Self-expanding stents – in case of stenosis or kinking of stentgraft limbs.
- Wire loop snare – to aid retrograde cannulation of the contralateral limb if the ipsilateral route is unsuccessful.
- Closure device if a surgical femoral arteriotomy is not used.

Technique of EVAR

Anesthesia

- The procedure is usually performed under general anesthesia.
- Spinal and local anesthesia are also options.

Arterial Access

Femoral access:

- Unilateral or bilateral surgical femoral arteriotomy
- Percutaneous femoral artery access using closure devices

- Conduit to the common iliac artery:
  - Used if the patient has small, narrowed, or even occluded external iliac arteries, which are unsuitable for passage of the large stent-graft delivery system.
  - A vascular surgeon sutures a bypass graft to the common iliac artery.
  - The stent-graft can be inserted through the bypass graft. At the end of the procedure, either the bypass can be closed or it can be used as an iliofemoral graft.

Intra-procedural Medications

These are administered before insertion of the stent-graft:

- Heparin 5000 IU.
- Broad spectrum antibiotics.

Procedure

Before Stent-Graft Deployment

- The contralateral femoral artery is catheterized and a 6F sheath is inserted.
- A diagnostic pigtail catheter is inserted via this access into the aorta to the level of T12/L1.
- The ipsilateral femoral artery is catheterized.
- A standard guidewire and selective catheter (e.g., cobra) are advanced into the upper thoracic aorta.
- The standard guidewire is exchanged for a very stiff guidewire (260-cm long Lunderquist), which is placed with the tip in the ascending aorta.
- The stent-graft is inserted under fluoroscopic guidance.
- Care should be taken if there is resistance during passage of the stent-graft through the iliac arteries to avoid dissections or rupture.
- The stent-graft should be advanced to the level of L1.

Deployment of the Stent-Graft

- Catheter angiography is performed to define the level of the renal arteries (Fig. 1a):
- The stent-graft is deployed so that the graft material is located immediately below the renal arteries.
- After deployment of the main body of the device, the pigtail catheter is withdrawn over a standard guidewire.
- The contralateral limb is cannulated from the contralateral groin with a selective catheter and a hydrophilic guidewire.

Fig. 1 (**a**) Angiogram of AAA before EVAR. (**b**) Angiogram after stentgraft placement

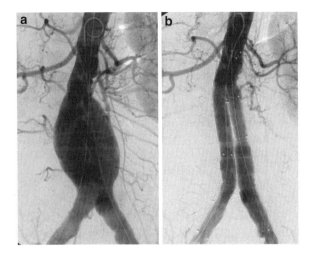

- After cannulation of the contralateral limb opening, the position of the guidewire within, rather than without, the body of the graft should be confirmed either by the injection of contrast through a catheter, or by the rotation of a pigtail catheter.
- If retrograde cannulation of the limb is difficult, contralateral limb cannulation can be achieved using a cross-over technique:
  - A sidewinder (Simmons 1) or Sos Omni catheter is placed across the flow divider of the stent-graft main body.
  - A hydrophilic guidewire (curved, 260 cm) is advanced to the contralateral iliac artery and snared.
- After inserting a second Lunderquist guidewire through the contralateral limb opening into the aorta above the stent-graft, the contralateral limb is inserted.
- Balloon angioplasty should be performed at the proximal landing zone, the distal landing zone and at the device connections to enhance the seal.
- If there is an aneurysmal common iliac artery (>23 mm diameter) as well as an aortic aneurysm, it will be necessary to land the endograft limb in the external iliac artery.
- Before this is performed, it is necessary to embolize the internal iliac artery before insertion of the stent-graft to prevent retrograde flow into the aneurysmal common iliac artery and aortic aneurysm sac.
- This is achieved by coils or an Amplatzer plug usually before the procedure.

Endpoint

- This is decided by good quality catheter angiography.
- The procedure is completed when angiography shows a patent stent-graft, patent endograft limbs, and absence of flow into the aneurysm sac (endoleak) (Fig. 1b).

Insertion of an Aortouniiliac Stent-Graft

- Aortouniiliac (AUI) stent-grafts are chosen if

  ○ One iliac artery is diffusely narrowed and is not suitable for a contralateral limb.
  ○ One iliac artery is occluded.
  ○ Severe tortuosity of one iliac artery prevents insertion of the contralateral limb.
  ○ If there is rupture of the aneurysm, rapid exclusion of the aneurysm is required, and there is insufficient time to place a bifurcated device.

- The AUI device is available as either a single or two-piece device.
- The opposite common iliac artery must be occluded to prevent retrograde filling of the aneurysm sac. This is usually achieved with an occluder of appropriate size.
- The procedure is completed by a femorofemoral cross-over graft.

Immediate Post-procedure Care

- Recovery after EVAR is much quicker than after open surgery.
- A period of time on the ITU or HDU is not usual; patients may spend 24 h or so, if they have severe comorbidity, which manadates this.
- Most patients are mobilized early and are discharged 3–5 days post EVAR.

Follow-Up and Post-procedure Medications

- Follow-up is by a planned schedule of CT scans, and/or ultrasound, and plain radiography.
- A typical CT protocol is

  ○ Predischarge or 6 weeks.
  ○ 3 months.
  ○ 12 months.
  ○ Annually thereafter.

- Annual plain radiographs.
- Many centers are replacing CT scans with ultrasound, which, in combination with plain abdominal radiographs, does not seem to affect the detection of important complications.
- Follow-up medication consists in most cases of once daily aspirin, and in some centers, a statin, e.g., Simvastatin.

Results

- Technical success is very high occurring in over 98% of procedures.
- Conversion to open surgery is rare occurring in 0.6% of patients.
- Transfusion requirements are significantly lower in EVAR compared with surgery.
- In-hospital stay is lower after EVAR compared with open surgery.
- In hospital mortality from registry data is low occurring in 3.3%.
- In two randomized multicenter trials, the EVAR I trial and the DREAM trial, the 30-day mortality rates were 1.7 and 1.2%, respectively. The mortality rates of open surgery in the two randomized trials were 4.7 and 4.6%, respectively, which was significantly higher than the mortality rate of EVAR. However, while the difference between the two treatments was maintained at 3 years, all cause mortality was similar after EVAR and open surgery.
- Reinterventions are required in 15% of patients.
- Cost-effectiveness analyses show that EVAR is more expensive than open surgery. This is largely due to the costs of the devices, the cost of reinterventions, and the costs of follow-up, especially CT scans.
- Efforts to reduce the costs of EVAR by addressing the factors above are ongoing.

Complications

- Complications occur in up to 35% of procedures.
- Most complications can be avoided by meticulous pre-procedural planning, procedural technique, and the correction of any problems before the procedure is completed.
- Complications include

  - Endoleaks
  - Limb occlusion
  - Limb or external iliac artery stenosis
  - Iliac artery rupture
  - Renal artery occlusion
  - Partial or complete renal infarction
  - Renal impairment due to contrast
  - Modular disconnection
  - Device migration

- Rupture:

  - The incidence of late rupture was reported to be 1.6% in the EUROSTAR registry, 1.2% in the Talent registry, 0.5% in the Zenith US trial and 0% in the Excluder US trial.
  - Type I and type III endoleaks are significant risk factors for rupture

Endoleaks

- The most common complications are endoleaks.
- Endoleaks are classified as follows
    - Type I – Leak at attachment sites: Ia – proximal, or Ib – distal
    - Type II – Leak due to side branch reperfusion (from lumbar arteries, IMA, renal arteries)
    - Type III – Modular disconnection or a fabric tear
    - Type IV – Graft fabric porosity
    - Type V – Endotension, i.e., increasing sac size without a visible leak.
- Type I and III leaks are risk factors for rupture and should be treated when diagnosed.
- Type II leaks are not a definite risk factor for rupture, and the majority resolve spontaneously.
- There is controversy as to whether Type II leaks ever require treatment, even if the aneurysm sac increases in size.

Management of Endoleaks

- **Type Ia endoleaks:**
    - Type Ia endoleaks are due to poor apposition between the endograft and the wall of the aneurysm neck.
    - If the stent-graft has been inadvertently placed too low, a cuff should be placed so that the graft material extends to the renal arteries.
    - If the stent-graft extends correctly to the renal arteries, contact between the graft material and the wall of the aorta should be improved by placement of a Palmaz stent.

        - Equipment required: Palmaz P4054 stent (Johnson & Johnson NJ), 30 or 35 mm non-compliant balloon, pressure inflation device, 18F sheath.
        - The stent is mounted on the balloon, advanced through the sheath, and deployed inside the aortic endograft at the level of the neck.
        - The balloon is inflated until the pressure reaches 2 atm (Fig. 2).

- **Type Ib endoleaks**
    - These may be due to poor apposition between the endograft limb and the iliac artery or due to inadequate extension into the iliac artery.
    - Management is by repeat balloon dilation or insertion of further endograft limbs.

- **Type II endoleaks**
    - These are generally only treated if there is evidence of sac enlargement and no other cause.

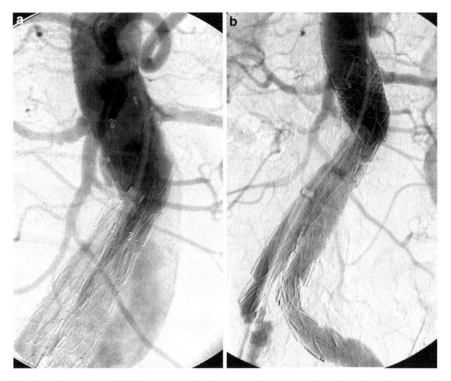

Fig. 2 (**a**) Type Ia endoleak after stent-graft placement. (**b**) Closure of endoleak after placement of Palmaz stent

- Embolization of the vessels (e.g., IMA, lumbar arteries) involved in the endoleak is required.
- This can be achieved by transarterial embolization or percutaneous puncture of the sac followed by embolization.
- Transarterial embolization requires superselective cannulation of the lumbar artery or the inferior mesenteric artery with a microcatheter. The catheter tip should be placed as close as possible to the aneurysm sac. Embolization can be performed with microcoils or glue.

- **Type III endoleaks**

  - Modular disconnection requires the insertion of additional bridging endografts.
  - A fabric tear is hard to diagnose and is effectively a diagnosis of exclusion after all other causes of endoleaks have been discounted.
  - Treatment of fabric tears requires either relining with an additional aortic endograft, usually an AUI device, or surgical conversion.

Management of Other Complications

- Iliac artery occlusion:

  - Commonly occurs in unsupported graft limbs.
  - Occurs due to limb kinking.
  - Occurs due to impingement of the end of the endograft limb on the side of the iliac artery wall.
  - Avoid by prevention at the time of completion angiography.
  - Perform completion angiography without stiff guidewires in situ, which might conceal any potential kinks or stenoses.
  - Prevent by placement of uncovered stents in potential problem areas.
  - Treat limb occlusion by either Fogarty balloon embolectomy and correction of underlying problem, or a femorofemoral cross-over.

- Limb stenoses discovered at follow-up should be treated by uncovered stents.
- Iliac artery rupture should be treated by balloon tamponade, followed by insertion of an endograft.
- Renal artery occlusion:

  - If the stentgraft is placed too high and a main renal artery is occluded, an attempt can be made to pull the stent-graft down. However, if the stent-graft has hooks or barbs, severe damage to the aortic wall is possible.
  - If renal artery occlusion is due to the displacement of mural thrombus or atheroma across the renal artery ostium, it may be possible to recanalize the renal artery with a sidewinder catheter and hydrophilic guidewire, followed by subsequent stent placement.

- Migration:

  - Acute migration may occur in patients with severely angulated or conical necks.
  - Late migration is a major independent risk factor for rupture and occurs in up to 2% of endografts.
  - Treatment of migration is by a cuff or an additional aortic stent-graft.

Key Points

- Perform meticulous pre-procedural planning to optimize patient and endo-graft selection.
- Early in your experience adhere to the standard anatomic criteria for EVAR.
- Remember to evaluate the access arteries for suitability for passage of an endograft and for use as the distal landing zones.
- Use the optimal angiographic facilites available.
- Take care not to cover the renal arteries.

- Treat Type I and III endoleaks before the procedure is regarded as complete.
- Predict and treat potential kinks or stenoses of the iliac limbs or arteries.
- Maintain careful follow-up by CT or by ultrasound and by plain abdominal radiographs.

Suggested Reading

1. Curci JA for the Excluder Bifurcated Endoprosthesis Investigators. Clinical trial results of a modified gore excluder endograft: comparison with open repair and original device design. Ann Vasc Surg 2007 May; 21(3):328–38.
2. Greenberg RK et al. for the Zenith Investigators. Zenith AAA endovascular graft: intermediate-term results of the US multicenter trial. J Vasc Surg 2004;39:1209–18.
3. Greenhalgh R for the EVAR trial participants.Endovascular aneurysm repair and outcome in patients unfit for open repair of abdominal aortic aneurysm (EVAR trial 2): randomised controlled trial. Lancet. 2005 Jun 25–Jul 1; 365(9478):2187–92.
4. Matsumura JS et al. A multicenter controlled clinical trial of open versus endovascular treatment of abdominal aortic aneurysm. J Vasc Surg 2003; 37:262–71.
5. Prinssen M et al. A randomized trial comparing conventional and endovascular repair of abdominal aortic aneurysms. N Engl J Med 2004; 351:1607–18.
6. Torsello G for the Talent AAA Retrospective Longterm Study Group. Long-term outcome after Talent endograft implantation for aneurysms of the abdominal aorta: a multicenter retrospective study. J Vasc Surg 2006; 43:277–84.
7. van Marrewijk CJ et al. for EUROSTAR. Risk of rupture due to type II endoleak. J Vasc Surg 2002; 30:461–73.

Endovascular Management of Ruptured Abdominal Aortic Aneurysm

William C. Loan and Chee Voon Soong

Clinical Features

- Ruptured abdominal aortic aneurysms (rAAAs) remain a significant source of morbidity and mortality. The use of endovascular repair (eEVAR) for their management may offer a valuable alternative to open surgery.
- Presentation: >50 years; four times more common in men, abdominal and/or back pain, hypotension.
- Endovascular treatment of rAAA can offer rapid control of the leaking vessel and, potentially, recovery from the condition.
- The object of endovascular management of ruptured aneurysms is to achieve hemostasis and to allow recovery from the acute condition. Long-term management may include reintervention or elective conversion to open repair.
- Case selection is the key to success and the implications of poor selection are likely to be serious.

Diagnostic Evaluation

Laboratory

- Baseline full blood count
- Group and cross-matched for minimum of 6 units of packed cells
- U&E
- Coagulation screen

Imaging

Computed Tomography (CT) remains the basis for preoperative assessment.

Angiography has been successfully used as the primary imaging modality for unstable patients.

R.A. Morgan, E. Walser (eds.), *Handbook of Angioplasty and Stenting Procedures*,
Techniques in Interventional Radiology, DOI 10.1007/978-1-84800-399-6_19,
© Springer-Verlag London Limited 2010

Use contrast enhanced CT to

- Confirm the diagnosis
- Demonstrate the anatomy of the aneurysm neck: length, shape, calcification, and thrombus
- Assess access vessels: Tortuosity, diameter, calcification, and length
- Plan management of iliac aneurysms if they are present
- Measure for graft selection
- Should the anatomy be unsuitable for eEVAR:

  ○ Note the position of renal veins relative to aortic neck
  ○ Note the relation of the aneurysm neck to the renal arteries to inform choice of clamp position during open repair
  ○ Note any iliac aneurysm which may not be appreciated at open operation
  ○ Assess for any pathology which might affect the likely outcome or life expectancy

N.B. During the assessment and the imaging phase, all equipment for open and endovascular repair should be made ready.
  Continuing stability must not be assumed.
  Percutaneous equipment for balloon aortic occlusion should be available.

Indications

Inclusion criteria for Eevar:

- Neck diameter <34 mm.
- Neck length – at least 5 mm, preferably longer (longer if there are any other negative features present such as calcification, thrombus, angulation, or conical shape).
- Minimum access vessel diameter ≥ 7 mm (6.5 mm if the vessels are non-calcified and minimally tortuous).
- Suitable device available.
- Appropriate staff available.

Contraindications

Absolute

- Contraindications must be weighed against the extreme nature of the condition, and significantly increased risk may be acceptable in the clinical context.
- Juxtarenal or suprarenal AAA.
- Small iliac arteries <6 mm.
- Neck diameter >34 mm.

Relative

- Neck length <5 mm, unless sacrifice of the renal arteries is acceptable
- A patient who is determined to be at low risk for open repair, particularly with less than optimal anatomy for eEVAR.
- Access vessels <7-mm diameter.
- Complex anatomy with iliac aneurysms.

Anatomy

This is the key to planning of the procedure.

Desired Normal Anatomy

- The mesenteric vessels arise 1–1.5 cm above the renal arteries.
- The dominant renal arteries arise at approximately the same level.
- The aneurysm usually extends to the aortic bifurcation.

Aberrant Anatomy

- Multiple renal arteries, often with low origins from the sac or iliac artery
- Superior mesenteric artery arising at the level of the renal arteries
- Ectopic or transplanted kidneys
- Superior mesenteric artery and celiac trunk disease making the inferior mesenteric artery crucial for bowel perfusion
- Normal or a small diameter distal aorta with the potential for constricting a bifurcated endograft
- Lumbar artery hypertrophy should raise suspicion of occult iliac stenosis

Equipment

Emergency Access Trolley

A basic percutaneous trolley should be set up as soon as a rupture is diagnosed.

- This can be used to insert an occlusion balloon should the patient deteriorate.
- It is possible to insert an occlusion balloon from a brachial artery access without fluoroscopy guidance.
- Achieving aortic occlusion from the femoral or brachial approach should be relatively straightforward under fluoroscopic control.

Stent Grafts

- Either aortouniiliac or bifurcated systems can be used.
- An adequate stock with a comprehensive variety of sizes of stent components should be available to cover as wide a range of anatomy as possible.
- An AUI two-part system with a top (or proximal) diameter between 24 and 36 mm, and a bottom (or distal) diameter of 12–24 mm will cover most anatomical combinations (Fig. 1a, b). An occluder for the contralateral limb is required for an AUI system.
- Stock management is critical to have correct equipment available.

Catheters/Balloons

- **Non-selective catheters:** Pigtail or straight multi-hole catheter for aortography
- **Selective catheters:** Cobra, hockey stick, multipurpose, range of rear facing (sidewinder) shapes to negotiate tortuous iliac arteries and aneurysm neck
- A 16F 45 cm sheath to support an occlusion balloon inserted from a femoral access

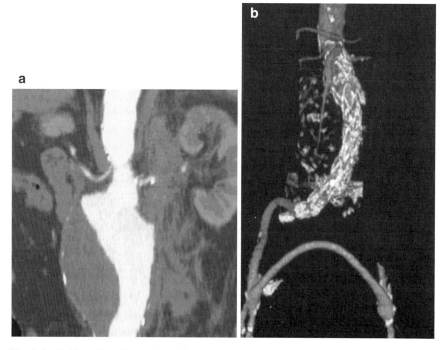

Fig. 1 (**a, b**) Short, irregular neck, confirmed rupture. Treated with an AUI device and fem–fem cross-over graft

- A 12F $\geq$45 cm sheath to support an occlusion balloon inserted from a brachial access
- A molding balloon (can be used for aortic occlusion)
- A range of angioplasty balloons and stents to deal with access vessel stenoses
- A giant balloon expandable stent for proximal aneurysm neck, e.g., Palmaz stent (Johnson & Johnson)
- 25 and 30-mm diameter balloon for insertion of the giant balloon-expandable stent into the proximal aneurysm neck

Guidewires

- Standard guidewires for access
- Stiff guidewires – e.g., Lunderquist 260 cm or Back up Meier guidewire 260 cm
- Hydrophilic/selective wires for cannulation of the contralateral limb opening and for negotiating tortuous iliac arteries

Procedure

Resuscitation/Anesthesia

- Hypotensive resuscitation: Fluid administration should be kept to the minimum required to maintain cerebral perfusion as indicated by the level of consciousness and systolic BP $\geq$60 mmHg.
- Only once the aneurysm is excluded, should volume replacement begin.
- An early request for fresh frozen plasma or other coagulation factor replacement should be considered.
- The procedure should preferably be started under local anesthesia; some sedation may be required. The entire procedure can frequently be performed under local anesthesia, including femorofemoral cross-over grafting.
- General anesthesia should be avoided until the aneurysm is excluded to prevent precipitous hemodynamic decompensation during muscle relaxation.
- It should be emphasized that the volume of concealed blood in the retroperitoneum or peritoneal cavity, which cannot be seen, must still be replaced.

Access

- Percutaneous access is attractive for bifurcated systems, and in less stable patients.
- Surgical exposure of the femoral arteries can assist delivery system insertion in diseased access vessels, and will be required for AUI systems, as a fem–fem cross-over graft.

- In a grossly unstable patient an occlusion balloon can be inserted percutaneously from femoral access. Inflating the balloon at the top of a 16F sheath, and using a stiff/super stiff guidewire will allow balloon position to be maintained. (Fig. 2a, b) An assistant should be tasked with maintaining balloon position, which must be checked frequently.
- It is possible for operators to gain access simultaneously on both sides, requiring two sets of puncture needles/wires to be available on the trolley.

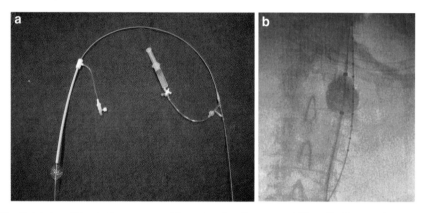

Fig. 2 (a) A molding balloon supported by a sheath to improve stability of balloon during occlusion. **(b)** Balloon system as seen in (a), balloon inflated in the sac and advanced into the aneurysm neck, allowing aortic occlusion without causing mesenteric and renal ischemia. Note the conical upper surface of the balloon as it is held against the aneurysm neck from below. The calibrated catheter alongside the balloon allows imaging and measurement during balloon occlusion

Initial Angiography

Following Pre-operative CT

- There should be no need for angiography prior to insertion of the stent-graft delivery system.
- The first digital subtraction run can be delayed until the system is placed at the approximate level of the renal arteries.
- High-quality imaging is critical to enable rapid, accurate deployment of devices in emergency cases.
- A significant proportion of patients with ruptured AAA are obese. This may limit image quality and increase radiation exposure to the patient and staff.

Primary Imaging with Angiography

- Calibrated angiography allows sufficiently accurate evaluation of the anatomy and measurement.

- Should the patient deteriorate, the aorta can be occluded, and both angiography and graft insertion can be carried out with an occlusion balloon in place.

Clinical Scenarios

The specific procedure plan is dependent upon the clinical setting.

A "Stable" Patient

- Avoid aortic occlusion.
- The endograft insertion procedure similar to elective cases.
- Avoid general anesthesia.
- Regional anesthesia can be time consuming; local anesthesia is sufficient at least until the aneurysm is excluded.

Continuing stability cannot be assumed, decompensation can be extremely rapid.

An Unstable Patient

- Rapid exclusion of the aneurysm is the priority.
- Aortouniiliac devices allow more reliable, rapid aneurysm exclusion.
- Balloon occlusion can be maintained in an infra-renal position, with rapid movement to a supra-celiac position and reinflation possible if required. The stent-graft can be deployed alongside the sheath supporting the balloon. The balloon can then be removed through the sheath, which will slide out alongside the graft.
- The duration of balloon occlusion, particularly in the supra-renal position should be kept to a minimum.

Management of Iliac Aneurysms

- Rupture of isolated iliac aneurysms is rare.
- Aortoiliac aneurysms are relatively common, requiring graft extension into the external iliac artery, with embolization of the internal iliac artery.
- Internal iliac embolization can be time consuming. A vascular occlusion plug (Amplatzer) can reduce the time to aneurysm exclusion.
- Avoid excessive over-sizing of the graft to be implanted into the external iliac artery. Plan to leave the distal end of the device in as straight a segment of external iliac artery as possible.
- Completion angiography must be carried out after stiff wires have been removed, to visualized any kinking, particularly of the external iliac arteries.
- Insertion of uncovered stents may be necessary to overcome kinking at distal landing zones.

Detection of Procedural Endoleaks

Patient Stable

- Perform careful angiography of the proximal anastomosis first.

    o Use a high rate of injection.
    o Use a fast frame rate acquisition.
    o Image in two planes.

- Pull down the catheter into the body of the graft. Perform angiography with a reduced injection rate of approximately 7 mL/s to ensure contrast does not reflux above the top of graft.

    o If the leak is still present, it is not a proximal type 1 endoleak.

- Repeat angiography with balloons inflated in both iliac arteries to occlude flow.

    o Inject contrast from below via the balloon catheters.
    o Use a rapid frame rate.
    o Contrast will "spill" out of the leak when it reaches the level of the leak.

- Minor leaks (type 4 or 2) can be left, if hemodynamic stability is maintained.

Patient Unstable: Requiring Significant Fluid Volumes to Maintain Consciousness and Systolic ≥ 60 mmHg

- The occlusion balloon can be inflated initially in the supra-renal position and angiography performed beneath the balloon.
- Should the proximal seal appear intact, the balloon can be repositioned in the juxta- or infrarenal position. The balloon must be supported with a large sheath to prevent the water hammer effect dislodging the balloon and possibly also the graft.

Management of Procedural Endoleaks

- Type 1 leaks: Proximal or distal. If there is room, extend the endograft coverage with a cuff for a proximal leak, a limb extension for a distal leak, or a Palmaz stent to increase radial force.
- Type 2 leaks: These can generally be left as long as the patient is maintaining hemodynamic stability.
- Type 3 leak: Repeat balloon dilation of the junctions between device components; if this fails bridge the junction with a further stent-graft.
- Type 4 leaks: These do not appear to cause significant problems, at least in the short or medium term.

Aftercare

- Immediate post-operative imaging is generally not necessary unless there is evidence of continued or recurrent bleeding.
- Adequate blood transfusion and fluid replacement is difficult to gauge, as visible and recordable intra-operative blood loss will not reflect the true loss of blood volume.
- Intensive care is frequently, but not universally necessary. The average ICU stay post-operatively is on average, around 1 day.
- High ventilation pressures and abdominal distension with poor urine output suggest abdominal compartment syndrome. Intra-abdominal pressure can be monitored via the urinary catheter. Early decompression may be necessary.
- Prolonged restriction of oral intake may be necessary. This may be related to delayed gastric emptying, perhaps due to retroperitoneal hematoma impinging upon the duodenum.

Follow-Up

- These patients have worse anatomy and often more advanced disease than elective patients. The follow-up therefore needs to be at least as intensive as for elective patients.
- CT is the mainstay of follow-up imaging. However, contrast-enhanced ultrasound and MRI can aid endoleak detection and characterization.
- Plain X-rays of abdomen should be performed to identify wire fracture and impending or established separation of components.

Results

- The published data are limited.
- The mortality of open repair for ruptured aneurysms is around 41%, despite improvements in surgical techniques, anesthesia and intensive care support.
- The outcomes of eEVAR vary greatly from center to center and reflect reporting bias and differences in patient selection.
- A recent metaanalysis of the worldwide experience from 48 centers involving 442 patients demonstrated an average mortality of 18%.
- A randomized trial comparing eEVAR with open repair, failed to demonstrate any difference between the two groups, although the findings have been the subject of great controversy.
- There is as yet no strong evidence that eEVAR is better than surgery, especially in unstable patients.

Alternative Therapies

- Open surgical repair
- Palliative care

Complications

Early

- Thrombosis/Coagulopathy

  ○ These patients are not routinely heparinized and thrombosis of the graft is not uncommon. With the common femoral arteries exposed, balloon thrombectomy is usually straightforward. Beware not to dislodge the proximal end of the graft.
  ○ Thromboembolic events in the legs are common. These should be treated by balloon thromboembolectomy.
  ○ Despite the lack of visible blood loss, clotting factors are diminished and coagulopathy should be suspected if hemodynamic control proves difficult to achieve. Early replacement of lost factors should be considered.

- Failure to seal with continued hemorrhage.
- Injury to access vessels: dissection/perforation/avulsion of iliac arteries.
- Impairment of the various organs: renal failure, respiratory failure, cardiac failure, and intestinal ileus.
- Intestinal ischemia.
- Abdominal compartment syndrome.
- Gastric outlet obstruction by hematoma.
- Deep vein thrombosis.

Late

- Late complications of eEVAR are similar to those of elective EVAR. However, probably due to less favorable anatomy, or more advanced aneurysmal disease, they seem to be more common.
- The presence of uncovered stents at the proximal neck of the graft can complicate the management of migration and proximal endoleaks (Fig. 3).
- Graft infection is probably more common than in elective series.
- Conversion to open repair as an elective procedure to manage late complications may be necessary. However endovascular management of most complications is possible, and in general, is associated with a low morbidity.

Fig. 3 Follow-up CT of an AUI graft inserted for rupture showing kinking of the graft body and distal migration. This occurred despite a large self-expanding stent which was inserted for a type 1 endoleak intra-operatively, and has been left behind by migration of the stent-graft. Treatment by a proximal extension is made more difficult by the presence of the balloon-expandable stent

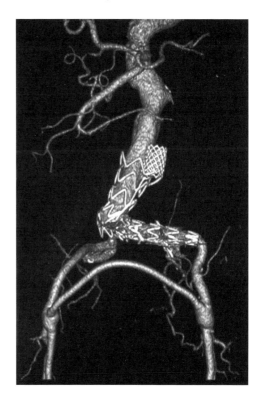

Key Points

- Agree a management protocol with a multidisciplinary team in advance.
- Assessment of CT/Angiogram for suitability must be carried out by specialists with extensive experience in planning elective cases.
- Not every case is suitable. Each must be assessed realistically.
- It is impossible to predict future stability of a patient with a ruptured aneurysm.
- Do not waste time and have a plan for managing the unstable patient.

Suggested Reading

1. Badger SA, O'donnell ME, Makar RR, Loan W, Lee B, Soong CV. Aortic necks of ruptured abdominal aneurysms dilate more than asymptomatic aneurysms after endovascular repair. J Vasc Surg 2006 Aug; 44(2):244–9.

2. Frank J. Veith, Takao Ohki, Evan C. Lipsitz, William D. Suggs, Jacob Cynamon Treatment of ruptured abdominal aneurysms with stent grafts: a new gold standard? Seminars Vasc Surg 2003 June; 16(2):171–5.
3. Malina M, Veith F, Ivancev K, Sonesson B. Balloon occlusion of the aorta during endovascular repair of ruptured abdominal aortic aneurysm. J Endovasc Ther 2005 Oct; 12(5):556–9.
4. Matsuda H, Tanaka Y, Hino Y, Matsukawa R, Ozaki N, Okada K, Tsukube T, Tsuji Y, Okita Y. Transbrachial arterial insertion of aortic occlusion balloon catheter in patients with shock from ruptured abdominal aortic aneurysm. J Vasc Surg 2003 Dec; 38(6):1293–6.
5. Rose DF, Davidson IR, Hinchliffe RJ, Whitaker SC, Gregson RH, MacSweeney ST, Hopkinson BR. Anatomical suitability of ruptured abdominal aortic aneurysms for endovascular repair. J Endovasc Ther 2003 Jun; 10(3):453–7.

Angioplasty/Stenting/Lysis/Thrombectomy of Hemodialysis Access

Himanshu Shah and Gordon McLennan

Clinical Features

- Chronic kidney disease (CKD) affects approximately one in nine people in the United States with over 300,000 patients on hemodialysis.
- Hemodialysis access failure is a major cause of morbidity, cost, and hospitalization for patients with end-stage renal disease.
- Access stenosis is a major cause of dialysis access (graft, fistula) failure.
- Screening combined with prophylactic angioplasty lowers the rate of dialysis access thrombosis.
- The National Kidney Foundation's Kidney Disease Outcomes Quality Initiative (K/DOQI) provides evidence-based clinical practice guidelines for the placement and management of hemodialysis access.

Diagnostic Evaluation

Clinical

- Access dysfunction is screened at the dialysis center and patients are referred for intervention when an abnormal screening parameter is identified.
- K/DOQI guidelines recommend at least monthly screening with physical exam as well as surveillance by measuring access flow (e.g., Transonic device), venous pressures, recirculation, or by duplex ultrasound.
- Patients with an abnormal screening parameter are sent for a fistulogram and intervention.
- Access stenosis is the most common cause of dialysis graft failure. It results in an increase in intra-access pressure, decrease in flow rate, and ultimately leads to thrombosis.

Imaging

- Neointimal hyperplasia is the most common cause of access stenosis in the outflow veins. A less common cause is valve hypertrophy (Fig. 1).

R.A. Morgan, E. Walser (eds.), *Handbook of Angioplasty and Stenting Procedures*,
Techniques in Interventional Radiology, DOI 10.1007/978-1-84800-399-6_20,
© Springer-Verlag London Limited 2010

Fig. 1 (**a**) Dialysis fistulogram shows a hypertrophied valve in the outflow forearm cephalic vein resulting in significant stenosis as evidenced by jetting of contrast. (**b**) Significant stenosis is also evident by the "waist" on the angioplasty balloon during balloon inflation

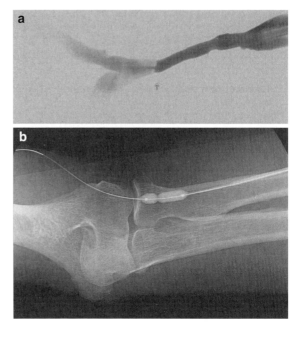

- Concentrated needle sticks can result in stenosis or dilatation/aneurysm formation (Fig. 2).
- Central venous stenosis and occlusion is often secondary to prior central venous catheters (especially subclavian vein catheters) but may also be secondary to prior trauma, surgery, or pacemakers (Fig. 3).
- The classic location of stenoses in native dialysis fistulae is in the juxta-anastomotic outflow vein. In dialysis grafts the classic location is at the venous anastomosis (Fig. 4).
- Stenosis can occur anywhere along the dialysis access circuit including the inflow artery, intragraft, at the arteriovenous anastomosis, at the arterial or venous anastomoses, in the outflow vein, or in the central veins.

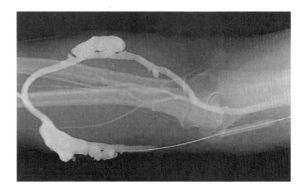

Fig. 2 Forearm dialysis graft with large arterial limb and venous limb pseudoaneurysms

Fig. 3 Left subclavian pacemaker with central venous stenosis/occlusion

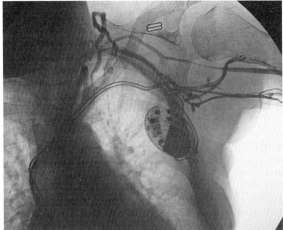

Fig. 4 (**a**) Left wrist fistula with focal juxta-anastomotic cephalic vein stenosis. (**b**) Left forearm graft with venous anastomotic stenosis

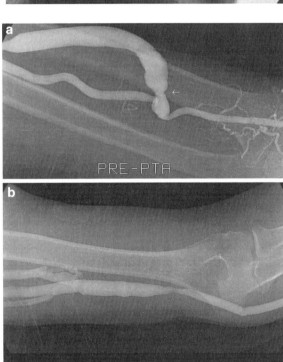

Indications

- Angioplasty of dialysis grafts and fistulae is indicated when there is greater than 50% diameter stenosis and an abnormal clinical/physiologic indicator of dysfunction:

- Low flows – less than 600 mL/min or less than 1,000 mL/min with greater than 25% decrease in flow over 3–4 month period
- Elevated dynamic or static venous pressures
- Elevated urea recirculation (more useful in fistulae than grafts)
- Arm swelling – central venous stenosis
- Abnormal physical exam – poor thrill, pulsatile
- Poor maturation of fistula
- "Pulling Clots" – arterial inflow stenosis

- Extremity edema caused by central venous stenosis should be treated by angioplasty. Stent placement is recommended for elastic recoil (>50%) after angioplasty or for restenosis within 3 months following angioplasty.
- Stent placement in the peripheral veins is indicated for failed angioplasty (>2 angioplasties needed within 3 months) in a surgically inaccessible lesion or other surgical contraindication as well as for angioplasty-induced rupture.
- It is critical to determine whether the stented segment will impact the viability of a functional fistula in the future prior to placing a stent in the periphery. It may be better to surgically revise an access than stent it if the surgeon can create a viable fistula.
- Thrombectomy is indicated for occluded grafts and fistulae and should be performed as early as possible.

Contraindications

- Prophylactic angioplasty of a stenosis in the *absence* of a clinical indicator of access failure (low flows, high venous pressures, elevated recirculation, etc.) is discouraged.
- Uncorrectable severe coagulopathy is a relative contraindication.
- Thrombosed grafts and fistulae which are suspected of being infected should not undergo percutaneous thrombectomy due to the risk of sepsis and septic emboli.

  - Be aware that a reactive phlebitis can occur in the region of the clotted outflow vein and less commonly over the clotted graft resulting in local erythema and tenderness that can mimic an infection.

- Severe allergy to iodinated contrast agents is a relative contraindication. Options include pre-medication or use of alternate contrast agents (carbon dioxide gas, gadolinium-based agents).

  - Limit the use of gadolinium-based agents in an effort to reduce the risk of nephrogenic systemic fibrosis.

- Percutaneous intervention on a newly placed (less than 2–4 week old) graft is a relative contraindication.

Patient Preparation

- Patient NPO for at least 6 h – for moderate sedation
- Labs – coagulation studies (INR, PTT), platelet count, electrolytes
- If potassium elevated consider management options:
  - Check EKG for spiked T waves
  - Give calcium gluconate
  - Consider temporary catheter and urgent dialysis and then treat the patient the following day

Anatomy: Grafts and Fistulae

- Upper extremity fistulae are the preferred access for hemodialysis patients. These include wrist (radiocephalic), elbow (brachiocephalic), or transposed brachial basilic arteriovenous fistulae (Fig. 5).

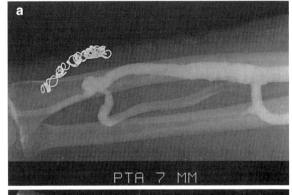

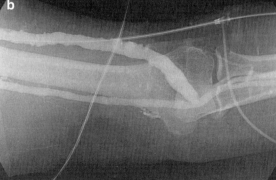

Fig. 5 (**a**) Right wrist radiocephalic fistula. Note the metallic coils from prior embolization of a "competing" side branch of the cephalic outflow vein. (**b**) Left elbow brachiocephalic fistula

- Each extremity can support nine different fistula configurations

    - Radiocephalic
    - Brachiocephalic
    - Transposed brachiobasilic
    - Transposed radioulnar
    - Graz variation
    - Transposed brachiobrachial
    - Transposed radiointerosseous
    - Transposed femoral vein to brachial artery
    - Transposed femoral vein to radial artery

- Understanding the surgery that was performed is critical to understanding the potential access sites and interventions needed
- Forearm or upper arm grafts are acceptable for access if a fistula cannot be placed (Fig. 6)
- Lower extremity fistulae or grafts are acceptable if upper arm sites are exhausted (Fig. 7)
- Tunneled catheters are the least preferred type of chronic access for hemodialysis patients.

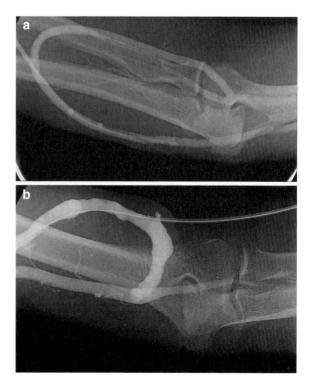

Fig. 6 (**a**) Right forearm loop graft. (**b**) Left upper arm bovine graft

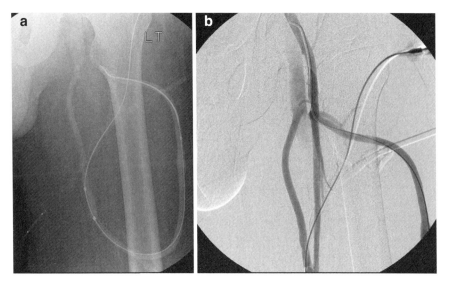

Fig. 7 (**a**) Lower extremity loop graft. (**b**) Closeup of the arterial and venous anastamoses to the femoral artery and vein

Equipment

- Needles

    ○ 18 or 19G single or double-wall that accept 0.035" guidewires
    ○ 21G needle in micropuncture set
    ○ Sheathed needles such as the Amplatz needle

- Wires

    ○ 0.018" wire in micropuncture set
    ○ 0.035" guidewires for most angioplasty and stent interventions
    ○ Hydrophilic, non-hydrophilic
    ○ Steerable, non-steerable
    ○ 0.014" wires for "coronary" type angioplasty balloons
    ○ 0.018" wires for other low-profile angioplasty balloons

- Catheters

    ○ Micropuncture catheter with 3F inner cannulas and 4 or 5F outer catheter
    ○ 4 or 5F diagnostic catheters

- Sheaths

    ○ Most commonly used are 5–7Fr sizes. Depends on type of intervention planned.

- ○ 4F can be used for arterial interventions with coronary or other low-profile angioplasty balloons.
- ○ 5–6F can be used for most peripheral angioplasties, mechanical thrombectomy, and peripheral stents
- ○ High-flow sheaths often useful in mechanical thrombectomy cases.
- ○ 7F usually needed for central angioplasties and stents

- Angioplasty balloons

  - ○ Generally, high-pressure non-compliant balloons are used.
  - ○ 5–8 mm diameter sizes are commonly used for peripheral venous stenoses
  - ○ 10–12 mm and larger diameter sizes usually needed for central venous stenoses.
  - ○ 3–6 mm diameter sizes often required for arterial inflow stenoses with smaller sizes for wrist fistulae and larger for elbow fistulae and upper and lower extremity grafts.
  - ○ Semicompliant "coronary" type balloons are often useful in wrist fistulae with radial artery inflow stenosis as they allow a range of balloon diameter size depending on the inflation pressure applied.
  - ○ Cutting balloons not routinely used but have a niche role in resistant stenoses or when high-pressure angioplasty may not be desired due to potential barotrauma or rupture risk such as at the arteriovenous anastomosis of fistulae. The microsurgical blades of the cutting balloon allow for complete balloon waist effacement at low pressures.

- Pressure inflators – commonly used especially for high-pressure inflation or when using coronary type balloons.
- Stents

  - ○ Self-expanding stents most commonly used due to their flexibility.
  - ○ Balloon-expandable stents are contraindicated in areas which are potentially compressible such as the peripheral veins and across joints.
  - ○ Bare stents typically used but covered stents may be needed for large ruptures.
  - ○ No current evidence to support use of drug-eluting stents
  - ○ Some evidence suggests lower restensosis rate of covered stents versus angioplasty in venous stenosis associated with dialysis grafts (Impra Trial)

- Guiding catheters in 5–8F sizes may be useful for thromboaspiration
- Embolectomy catheters (Fogarty-type)

  - ○ 4–6F
  - ○ Over-the-wire and not-over-the-wire available
  - ○ Most commonly used for thrombectomy cases and disrupting the arterial plug at the anastomosis

- Adherent clot catheters

    ○ Useful for removing resistant adherent clot/pseudointimal hyperplasia in grafts.
    ○ Do not use in native vessels

- Pulse spray catheters – 4 or 5F commonly used with a variety of infusion side hole lengths (5–50 cm)
- Mechanical thrombectomy devices

    ○ Wide variety available
    ○ Over-the-wire and not over the wire devices
    ○ Wall contact versus non-wall contact devices
    ○ Limited run-time for some devices due to hemolysis
    ○ Adenosine release from mechanical disruption may lead to bradycardia/dysrythmias

Pre-procedure Medications

- Sedation and analgesia

    ○ A local anesthetic (e.g., Lidocaine) is used for the access puncture site
    ○ Moderate sedation and analgesia with agents such as Fentanyl (Sublimaze) and Versed (Midazolam) enhances patient comfort

- Antibiotics

    ○ Recommended that an antibiotic be used for thrombectomy cases to cover skin organisms (e.g., Cefazolin).
    ○ Optional use for other interventions.

- Antispasmodic agents

    ○ Venospasm at the venous puncture site may be severe, especially in outflow veins of immature fistulas. An antispasmodic skin cream (e.g., Nitropaste, papaverine cream) applied to the anticipated puncture site prior to the procedure may be helpful for prophylaxis against spasm but is not routinely or widely used.

Procedure

Physical Exam

- A normal access will have a nice thrill throughout the venous outflow.
- Pulsatility, except near the arterial anastomosis of a graft, signifies an outflow stenosis.

- There should be no abrupt transition in the thrill along the graft or outflow vein.
- In the case of a single outflow stenosis, the access will be pulsatile from the arterial anastomosis to the site of stenosis and then have a weak thrill and poor turgor of the outflow vein beyond the stenosis.
- A cord may be palpable at the site of the stenotic lesion.
- An arterial inflow stenosis will demonstrate a weak thrill or pulse with collapsed ("flat") graft or outflow vein.
- A thrombosed access will have no thrill or pulse beyond the arterial anastomosis.
- A central venous stenosis will manifest as extremity swelling/edema with possible visible chest wall collaterals.
- Evaluate the peripheral pulses, especially if performing a thrombectomy because of the risk of arterial emboli from the procedure.
- Also, evaluate the hand for ischemia as treatment of a venous outflow stenosis will aggravate steal syndrome if present (Fig. 8).
- Limited ultrasound exam in the interventional suite can be a useful adjunct to the physical exam and is especially helpful when evaluating non-mature or dysfunctional fistulae. It can evaluate the site(s) of stenosis, identify non-palpable outflow vein(s), and evaluate the extent of thrombosis.

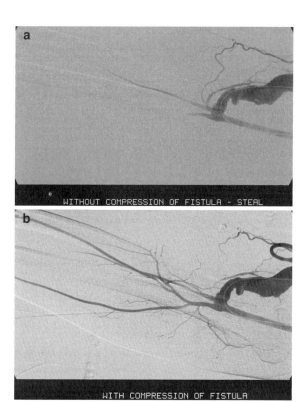

Fig. 8 (**a**) Right brachicephalic elbow fistula with diminished flow to the distal forearm arteries. (**b**) Marked improvement in flow to the radial and ulnar arteries with compression of the outflow cephalic vein in this patient with steal syndrome

Arterial/Venous Access

- Access the graft or fistulae based on the clinical scenario, physical exam findings, and findings on prior exams.
- More than one access may be required, especially for treating thrombosed grafts and fistulae and also if there are multiple stenoses located in different areas (e.g., central stenosis with additional stenosis near the arterial anastomosis) that cannot be treated with a single access site.
- In patients with loop grafts, a perpendicular access into the graft apex can allow access into both the arterial and venous limbs without requiring an additional puncture site.
- For wrist (radiocephalic) fistulae, a single retrograde access near the elbow/antecubital fossa allows access to most non-central lesions.
- For wrist and elbow fistula, a single antegrade access just central to the arteriovenous anastomosis allows access to most lesions except for arterial inflow, anastomotic or immediate juxta-anastomotic lesions. Hemostasis following the procedure may be more difficult, however, given the higher pressures near the anastomosis as opposed to further central in the venous outflow.
- Brachial artery access may be required for evaluation of non-maturing dialysis fistulae when the outflow vein is non-palpable, non-visible, or diminutive in size.
- The inner catheter of a micro-puncture set is suitable for this purpose and its small size (3F) minimizes complications such as access site thrombosis, hematoma, or pseudoaneurysm (Fig. 9) .
- Ultrasound is often useful especially when treating dialysis fistulae. It can help decide where to access, and allow access into non-palpable, non-visible outflow veins.
- A number of access needles can be used for initial access into the graft or fistula including angiocatheters, 18/19G thin-wall needles, micropuncture type set, and sheathed needles.
- A vascular sheath is typically required for performing angioplasty, stent placement, or mechanical thrombectomy.

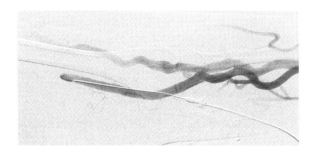

Fig. 9 Immature left antecubital fistula with fistulogram performed by retrograde brachial artery access using the 3F inner cannula of a micropuncture set

Fistulography

- The entire access needs to be evaluated including the inflow artery, anastomosis, graft (if present), outflow vein(s), and central veins.
- If there is a contraindication to iodinated contrast then consider using carbon dioxide gas and/or gadolinium contrast agents. Try to avoid refluxing the arterial anastomosis with carbon dioxide gas because of the risk of stroke but carbon dioxide can be injected directly into the artery above the anastomosis via retrograde catheter or microcatheter in the brachial artery. This avoids reflux. Also carbon dioxide tends to overestimate the degree of stenosis, as it tends to "float" in the blood as opposed to admixing with the blood. Minimize the volume of gadolinium agents used in order to reduce the risk of nephrogenic systemic fibrosis.
- The arterial anastomosis of grafts can be imaged using several techniques:

    ○ Extrinsic compression of the outflow vein or graft central to the puncture site
    ○ Balloon occlusion (i.e., Fogarty, angioplasty balloon) of the outflow vein/graft
    ○ Retrograde puncture into the graft with advancement of a diagnostic catheter (typically 4 or 5F) across the arterial anastomosis into the inflow artery.

- Visualization of the arteriovenous anastomosis of fistulae can be difficult. In addition to the techniques described above for grafts, the following can be performed:

    ○ For wrist fistulae, inflation of a blood pressure cuff in the upper arm to suprasystolic pressure will aid in refluxing the anastomosis.
    ○ 3F catheter (inner cannula of micropuncture set) access into the inflow artery.

- Perform multiple views, especially at the site(s) of suspected stenosis, when the angiographic findings are discordant with the clinical or physical exam findings (Fig. 10).
- Perform the fistulogram with the arm in different positions (abduction, adduction, internal/external rotation) if there is a narrowing of the axillary or subclavian veins or cephalic vein in the region of the humeral head to ensure that it does not represent positional extrinsic compression.
- Identify all the sites of significant stenosis. Determine if a new or additional site of access will be required to treat all lesions.
- For thrombosed accesses, typically a "pull-back" venogram is performed prior to declotting the graft/fistula to identify outflow stenoses and delineate the extent of thrombus. This is then followed by a complete fistulogram once flow is restored.

Intra-procedural Medications

- Sedation and analgesia as needed for patient comfort.
- Heparin

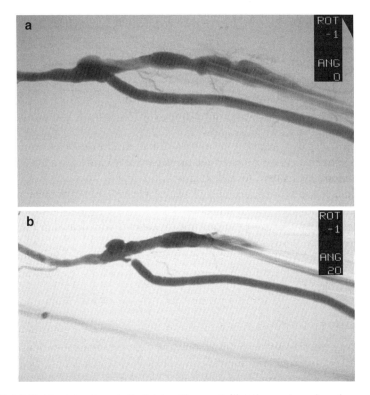

Fig. 10 (**a**) Right wrist radiocephalic fistula with poor thrill at the anastomosis and poor distention of the outflow cephalic vein reveals no obvious significant stenosis. (**b**) Repeat imaging with craniocaudal angulation reveals severe juxta-anastomotic inflow radial artery stenosis

- ○ Recommended when treating clotted grafts and fistulae but is optional for angioplasty and stent procedures.
- ○ Typical doses are 3,000–5,000 units IV.
- ○ Consider its use when treating complex lesions or when prolonged angioplasty balloon inflation time is anticipated or needed.
- ○ No data to support or refute its routine use.
- ○ May result in difficulties with hemostasis once the sheath is removed.

  - ■ If given, consider checking an activated clotting time (ACT) prior to pulling the sheath. If ACT is greater than 200 sec, then consider delaying sheath removal or using an adjunctive method of hemostasis (see Section "Immediate Post-procedure Care") in addition to or in place of manual compression.

- • Nitroglycerin

  - ○ Use as needed to treat arterial or venous spasm.
  - ○ Typical dose is 100 μg intravenous/intra-arterial infused at the site of spasm. Repeat dosing as needed, but monitor for hypotension.

- ○ Especially useful when treating poorly maturing fistulae which are prone to spasm.
- Thrombolytics (tPA, Urokinase, etc.)
  - ○ Can be used alone or in conjunction with mechanical thrombectomy devices.
  - ○ Typical doses of tPA vary between 2 and 20 mg.
  - ○ 1 mg tPA is approximately equivalent to 100,000 units of Urokinase.
- Antibiotic
  - ○ Give when treating thrombosed accesses due to concern over subclinical infection in the clot.
  - ○ Typically use second-generation cephalosporin to cover typical gram positive bacteria and other typical skin flora.
  - ○ May use Quinolones as a second line for patients with penicillin allergy.
  - ○ No evidence to support routine use of antibiotics.

Assessing the Lesion

- Morphology/Complexity
  - ○ Rarely calcified although this is sometimes seen in intragraft lesions.
  - ○ May exhibit recoil and respond only to high-pressure balloon angioplasty.
  - ○ Severe venous stenoses may look long and diffuse or even like a complete occlusion but this is often an artifact of imaging with very poor contrast opacification downstream from a severe, but focal stenosis.
- Location
  - ○ Most all venous (85%)
  - ○ 10–15% arterial
- Pressure measurements are typically not needed for assessment of stenosis.
- Choosing a balloon or stent
  - ○ Oversized balloons are commonly used with typical oversizing of 10–15% for arterial stenoses and 20–30% (or at least 1-mm oversizing) or greater for venous stenoses (Fig. 11). Progressive oversizing of balloons during subsequent interventions of recurrent stenosis of the same lesion may result in increased patency.
  - ○ When treating arterial inflow lesions, especially of small caliber arteries such as the radial artery in wrist fistulas, small profile (coronary type) balloons advanced over 0.014" guidewires may be useful (Fig. 12).
  - ○ Typically, self-expanding stents are used because of their flexibility.
    - ■ Balloon-expandable stents, if used, should not be placed at potentially compressible sites such as the peripheral veins or across joints but are acceptable in central locations deep in the thorax.

Fig. 11 (**a**) 6mm forearm loop graft with long segment stenosis extending from the venous anastamosis into the basilic outflow vein. (**b**) 8 mm diameter x 10 cm length angioplasty balloon chosen. (**c**) No significant residual stenosis following angioplasty

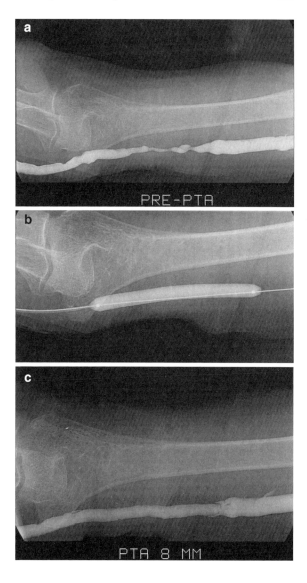

Performing the Procedure

- Crossing the lesion

  - Is usually straightforward.
  - For difficult lesions or occlusions, angled catheters (e.g., Berenstein) and/or steerable hydrophilic guidewires (Glidewire, Roadrunner, etc.) are useful (Fig. 13).

Fig. 12 (**a**) Left wrist radiocephalic fistula with juxta-anastomotic radial artery inflow and cephalic vein outflow stenoses. (**b**) Angioplasty via cephalic vein access using a 3.75 mm "coronary" balloon. (**c**) Post angioplasty of radial artery and cephalic vein stenoses

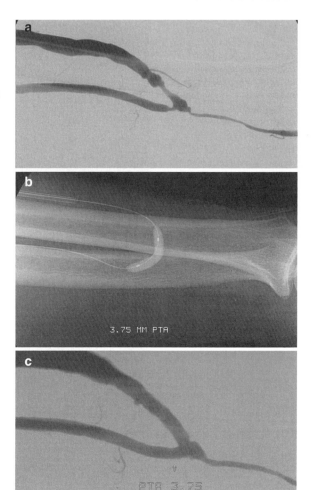

- ○ If there is difficulty passing wires, catheters, or devices beyond areas of severe tortuosity or pseudoaneurysm then extrinsic compression or manipulation may be a useful adjunct.

- • Deploying the balloon/stent

  - ○ High-pressure non-compliant angioplasty balloons advanced over 0.035″ guidewires are commonly used. It is not unusual for venous stenotic lesions to require in excess of 20 atm pressure in order to completely efface the balloon waist (Fig. 14). Pressure inflators are often needed.
  - ○ Most angioplasty balloons can be inflated beyond the rated burst pressure, often up to 25–50% over the rated burst pressure.

Fig. 13 (**a**) Tortuous antecubital outflow vein with focal stenosis which may represent a hypertrophied valve. (**b**) Lesion crossed and treated using hydrophilic catheter and guidewire and low profile angioplasty balloon

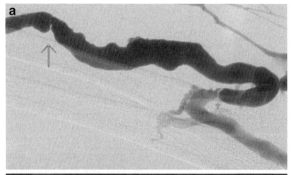

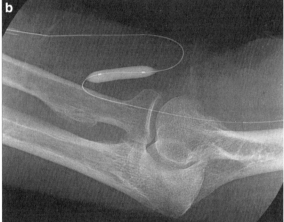

- ○ Typical balloon inflation times range from 1 to 3 min. Prolonged balloon inflation times of greater than 3–5 min may be useful for central or elastic stenoses.
- ○ Cutting balloons may be used if the high-pressure balloon waist can not be effaced (resistant stenosis) or if there is concern about "barotrauma" when using a very high-pressure angioplasty balloon.
- ○ Stents should not be placed for resistant stenoses (Fig. 15).

  - ■ Stents may be placed for elastic stenoses, ruptures, and failed peripheral angioplasty when there is no good surgical option and for failed angioplasty in central venous stenoses.

- • Treatment of clotted graft or fistulae

  - ○ Mechanical Methods (Figs. 16 and 17):

    - ■ Access the graft or fistula directed toward the venous outflow.
    - ■ Pull-back venogram is performed to demonstrate the most central extent of thrombus and to evaluate the central veins for stenosis.

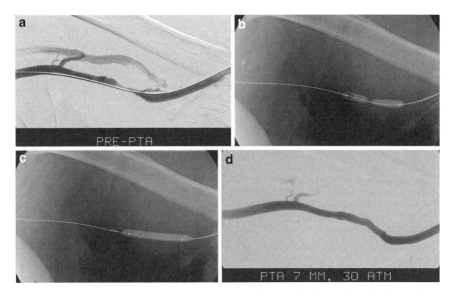

Fig. 14 (**a**) Left upper arm graft with venous anastomotic stenosis. (**b**) Persistent balloon waist at 15 atmospheres pressure. (**c**) Complete balloon waist effacement at 30 atmospheres pressure. (**d**) Post angioplasty fistulogram shows no residual stenosis

- Administer adjunctive drugs: Heparin and antibiotics.
- Use the device to clear the venous end of the clot. Aspirate the access after using the device.
- Puncture the access directed toward the arterial inflow.
- Use the device to clear to the mid portion of the arterial end of the access without crossing the anastomosis. The goal is to remove as much clot as possible prior to re-establishing flow.
- Use the thrombectomy device or fogarty-type balloon catheter across the anastamosis to pull the arterial plug and re-establish flow.
- Examine the access and assess for pulsatility and patency.
- If the access feels like it is patent and there is forward flow, then slowly inject a small amount of contrast to determine if there is forward flow. If not, then continue to use the device to clear the clot until antegrade flow is established.
- Once flow is established, then perform a complete fistulogram.
- Identify the underlying stenoses and treat with angioplasty and other measures as appropriate.

- Lyse and Wait Technique:

  - In the holding room, access the thrombosed access with an angiocather.
  - Compress the anastomosis to prevent peripheral arterial emboli and inject 2–4 mg of tPA with 3,000–5,000 units heparin into the access.
  - Wait for 30–90 min prior to placing patient in the angiography suite.

Fig. 15 (**a**) Severe rupture of basilic outflow vein following balloon angioplasty. (**b**) Treated by placing a long self-expanding uncovered stent

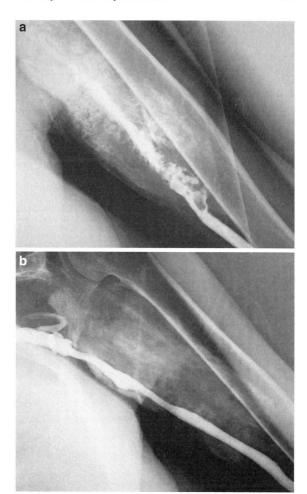

- When patient is in the suite, access the graft and assess whether there has been partial or complete thrombolysis. Treat any residual clot with a fogarty balloon catheter.
- Once clot is removed and flow is re-established, perform a complete fistulogram and treat underlying stenoses as appropriate.

Endpoint

- The typical endpoint is restoration of a normal thrill to the graft or fistula.
- A successful angioplasty will have complete effacement of the balloon waist and result in 0–30% residual narrowing. In addition, the previously abnormal clinical indicator should return to normal.

Fig. 16 (**a**) Clotted upper arm graft with clot extending into the outflow graft. (**b**) Fistulogram following successful mechanical thrombectomy and angioplasty of severe venous anastomotic stenosis

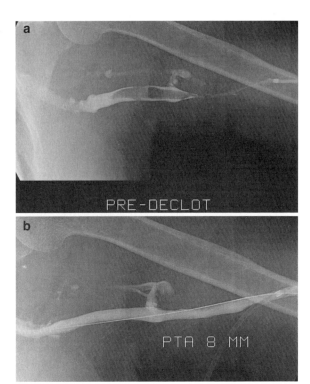

- If the angiographic result is equivocal, pressure measurements can be obtained. Pull-back pressures as well as static venous pressure measurement can be performed.

  ○ For grafts, the pressure in the venous limb should be less than 30% of systolic systemic arterial pressure to signify that there is no significant residual venous outflow stenosis remaining.
  ○ Also, flow measurement devices are available for use in the interventional suite and may be used to document increases in access flow pre- and post-intervention.

Immediate Post-procedure Care

- The access sheaths are removed and hemostasis is obtained by manual compression.
- Typically 5–10 min of light compression is required for hemostasis. If the outflow stenosis could not be adequately treated with significant residual stenosis or if heparin was given during the procedure and the activated clotting time (ACT) is

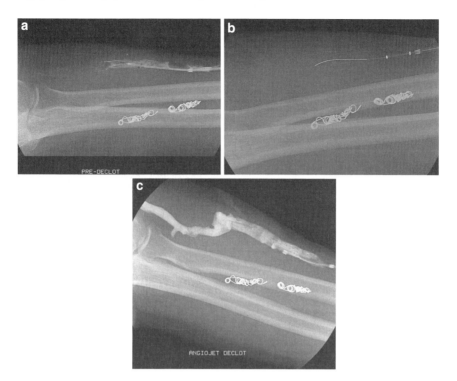

Fig. 17 (**a**) Clotted left wrist radiocephalic fistula with sheath directed towards venous outflow and clot in forearm cephalic vein. (**b**) Mechanical thrombectomy device (Angiojet). (**c**) Successful mechanical thrombectomy

above 200 sec, then hemostasis may take longer due to elevated pressures in the graft or fistula or residual anticoagulation effect.
• Other options for hemostasis include use of gelfoam, hemostatic pad, purse-string suture, or compression device.

Follow-Up and Post-procedure Medications

• No specific follow-up is required. If a purse-string suture was used for hemostasis, then this should be removed either prior to discharge from the department or at a follow-up visit the next day or the dialysis center should be instructed to remove the suture.
• The treated dialysis graft or fistula may typically be used for dialysis immediately following the procedure, except for immature fistulae which will likely require a few additional weeks to mature prior to use. The dialysis center should continue their dialysis access surveillance program and ensure that the previously abnormal clinical parameter (low flows, high venous pressures, elevated recirculation, etc.) has returned to normal following the intervention.

- No specific medications are required.
- Plavix may be considered following small vessel (e.g., arterial inflow) angio-plasty.

Results – Per K/DOQI Guidelines

- Angioplasty is expected to have at least a 50% primary patency rate at 6 months.
- Thrombectomy is expected to have a 40% primary patency rate at 3 months.
- An immediate patency rate of at least 85% is expected for graft thrombectomy.
- Clinical outcome goals are to have a fistula thrombosis rate of less than 0.25 episodes per patient-year and graft thrombosis rate of less than 0.5 episodes per patient year at risk. This can be accomplished by access screening combined with prophylactic angioplasty.

Alternative Therapies – Surgical Intervention

- Surgical therapy for dialysis access dysfunction should be thought of as comple-mentary and not competitive to percutaneous intervention.
- Due to the expense, invasiveness and potential depletion of veins as compared to percutaneous intervention, surgery is held to a higher standard with an expected 50% primary patency at 1 year (compared to 50% at 6 months for angioplasty).
- Surgical revision is indicated for angioplasty failures (two failures within 3 months).
- Surgical revision is also suggested for percutaneous thrombectomy failures (two failures within 1–2 months).
- Surgical therapy is the treatment of choice for suspected infected grafts.

Complications and Treatment

- Complications include vessel dissection, rupture, arterial emboli, and thrombosis.
- Dissections do not typically require treatment if they are not flow limiting.

  ○ Flow-limiting dissections can be managed by prolonged balloon inflation. If unsuccessful a stent can be placed.

- Venous rupture is expected to occur in about 5% of cases, especially if the balloons are being appropriately oversized.

  ○ Treatment can include prolonged balloon inflation +/– manual compression over the rupture site to "seal" the rupture.
  ○ Bare stents and/or covered stents can be used if prolonged balloon inflation is unsuccessful.

Fig. 18 (**a**) Occlusive ulnar artery embolus following mechanical thrombectomy of left forearm loop graft. (**b**) Successful treatment using the "backbleed" technique

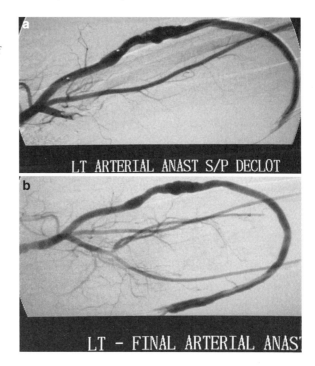

- Arterial emboli may occur during graft and fistulae thrombectomy procedures (Fig. 18).

  ○ Symptomatic emboli should be treated by thromboaspiration, fogarty, or mechanical thrombectomy, thrombolysis, "backbleeding" technique, or surgery if other measures are unsuccessful.
  ○ Asymptomatic emboli may be left alone especially if they cannot be treated using relatively simple techniques.

- Focal thrombosis typically results from dissection or rupture or from prolonged balloon inflation time (typically greater than 3–5 min) especially if anticoagulants were not given.

  ○ Treatment can include lytics, thromboaspiration, and mechanical thrombectomy.

Key Points

- Remain up to date with the knowledge and skills necessary to take care of these patients.

- Be familiar with and follow evidence-based guidelines related to dialysis access intervention (K/DOQI Vascular Access Guidelines)
- A proper workup will allow the most appropriate and successful intervention to be performed. Take into consideration the patient's medical history, current clinical indicator(s) of access failure, physical exam findings, prior imaging findings, and prior surgical and percutaneous interventions performed.
- Perform meticulous fistulography with additional views as needed, especially if the clinical findings of access failure and findings (or lack thereof) at fistulography are discrepant.
- Be familiar with and stock an adequate inventory of equipment including catheters, guidewires, angioplasty balloons, stents, and thrombectomy devices.
- Ultrasound can be a very useful adjunct in the interventional suite when evaluating and treating dysfunctional dialysis fistulae.

Suggested Reading

1. Aruny JE, Lewis CA, Cole PE, et al. Quality improvement guidelines for percutaneous management of the thrombosed or dysfunctional dialysis access. J Vasc Interv Radiol 1999; 10:491–498.
2. Gray RJ, Sacks D, Martin LG, et al. Reporting standards for percutaneous interventions in hemodialysis access. J Vasc Interv Radiol 1999; 10:1405–1415.
3. National Kidney Foundation. K/DOQI Clinical practice guidelines for vascular access. American Journal of Kidney Diseases July 2006; 48(suppl):S248-S273.
4. Patel AA, Tuite SM, Trerotola SO. Mechanical thrombectomy of hemodialysis fistulae and grafts. Cardiovasc Intervent Radiol 2005; 28:704–713.
5. Trerotola SO, Johnson MS, Shah H, et al. Backbleeding technique for treatment of arterial emboli resulting from dialysis graft thrombolysis. J Vasc Interv Radiol 1998; 9:141–143.
6. Trerotola SO, Stavropoulos SW, Shlansky-Goldberg R, et al. Hemodialysis-related venous stenosis: treatment with ultrahigh-pressure angioplasty balloons. Radiology 2004; 231:259–262.
7. Vesely TM, Siegel JB. Use of the peripheral cutting balloon to treat hemodialysis-related stenoses. J Vasc Interv Radiol 2005; 16:1593–1603.
8. www.kidney.org – Official website of the National Kidney Foundation, Inc.

Thrombolysis for Acute Lower Limb Ischemia

Thomas O. McNamara and Susie J. Muir

Introduction to Acute Lower Limb Ischemia (ALLI)

- Most acute vascular occlusions occur without the patient noting either sudden pain, or altered appearance of the limb. They can remain clinically silent or manifest as new onset or worsening of claudication.
- ALLI is a small subset of acute occlusions that is dramatically different:

  - The onset is painfully obvious to the patient.
  - The appearance of the limb is frightening to the patient (and doctor).
  - The patient intuitively fears for the survival of his/her limb.

- The negative features of this condition are

  - The residual slow-flow state can result in progressive thrombosis (clot propagation), and obliteration of the entire vascular bed which can cause tissue death/amputation.
  - Emergency surgical treatment (thromboembolectomy) has been associated with a surprisingly high mortality (10–20%) which is higher than that associated with revascularization for claudication (chronic occlusions). Death usually due to acute myocardial infarction (AMI).
  - Historically, the amputation rate in the survivors of emergency surgical revascularization is also frustratingly high (10–20%).

- The positive features of this condition are

  - Occluding clot is always "fresh"
  - Collateral flow can preserve resting tissue for many hours.
  - Therefore, ideally suited to treatment with thrombolysis (lysis and/or mechanical devices).
  - Once the long occlusion is cleared the cause is usually found such as an arterial stenosis which can be treated with angioplasty/stent, obviating the need for bypass surgery
  - Following lysis the patient can be discharged the next day

R.A. Morgan, E. Walser (eds.), *Handbook of Angioplasty and Stenting Procedures*, Techniques in Interventional Radiology, DOI 10.1007/978-1-84800-399-6_21, © Springer-Verlag London Limited 2010

Diagnostic Evaluation of Acute Lower Limb Ischemia (ALLI)

Clinical

- Symptoms: Sudden onset of foot pain, coldness, numbness, and/or paresthesias which can progress to anesthesia and paraysis.
- Signs: Foot pallor, coolness, and absence of pulse, which can progress to absence of capillary refill, fixed skin mottling, bullae, and necrosis.
- Pathophysiology: Collateral flow is inadequate for resting tissue.

  ○ In contrast, a claudicant has adequate tissue perfusion at rest and only has symptoms during exercise.

- The clinical categories of ischemia are Viable, Threatened, and Irreversible.

  ○ Terminology is based on the expectations of tissue loss in the absence of restoration of flow.
  ○ Categorized by sensorimotor exam, skin perfusion, pedal Doppler, and angiographic pattern.

Laboratory

- Chemistry panel, coagulation screen (INR, aPTT, platelets, fibrinogen), and CBC.
- Type and screen for possible need for transfusion

Imaging

- CXR if pulmonary edema suspected
- Possibly CT head if neurologic indications and/or cancer history
- Consider vascular ultrasound examination of bypass graft or vein to clarify the extent and severity of thrombosis

Indications for Thrombolysis of ALLI

- Symptomatic acute arterial occlusion (<10–14 days)

Contraindications for Thrombolysis of ALLI

- Most are relative:

  ○ Hemorrhagic diabetic retinopathy
  ○ History of gastrointestinal blood loss

- ○ Recent abdominal surgery (1 month)
- ○ Recent neurological surgery or stroke (6 months)

- Absolute contraindications

  - ○ Non-viable extremity
  - ○ Active bleeding

Patient Preparation and Monitoring for Thrombolytic Infusion in ICU

- Foley catheter
- Air mattress to prevent/reduce back pain during lysis
- Lambs-wool and cradle to foot of bed to protect foot
- Adequate venous access: central line or PICC
- Morphine IV or PCA pump for pain
- CBC, electrolytes, creatinine every morning
- Fibrinogen each morning

  - ○ Consider reducing lytic dose as fibrinogen falls below 150 mcg/dL

- Monitoring during lysis: During lysis we routinely monitor patients with either Viable or Threatened ALLI on a ward for vascular disease. However, we would strongly consider admission to an intensive care unit when treating the patient with Irreversible/Profound Ischemia.
- Occult Bleeding:

  - ○ BP, Pulse q 2 h. Call if systolic is <100, or $P > 90$.
  - ○ Daily Hct. 3% drop is common, >6% is significant.
  - ○ CT of abdomen and pelvis if retroperitoneal bleed suspected.

- Access Site Bleeding:

  - ○ Observe q 2 h. Mark limits and call if diameter >10 cm.

Procedure

- Heparinize to prevent worsening of ischemia due to clot propagation/extension:

  - ○ Heparinization alone is associated with improvement in color and comfort.
  - ○ Clot propagation/extension is not common, but it would be hazardous.

    - ■ Converts a non-emergent problem to an emergent one
    - ■ Significantly increases the risk of the compartment syndrome following revascularization
    - ■ Worsened ischemia can be followed by post-ischemic neuropathy

- Initiate clot clearing promptly, but not necessarily emergently

  - Emergent cases performed when limb is severely threatened

- Access from contralateral femoral artery.

  - Introduce contralateral sheath that terminates in common femoral artery of affected limb
  - Occlusions should all be soft and easily traversable with a regular guidewire (gw)

- Traversal with a non-hydrophilic gw confirms the clinical impression that the occlusion is due to new clot

  - Caveat: The proximal few millimeter may be firm due to compaction

- New clot (0–14 days) will promptly clear with lytic therapy and/or can be largely aspirated with devices

  - The exception is when there is no place for the blood to go due to the occlusion having extended into the pedal vessels
  - Infuse via multi-side hole infusion catheter that extends across most of the clot
  - Currently prefer to use infusion catheter that combines multiple side holes plus ultrasound emissions (EKOS, Bothell, Washington).

- **Treat** with low-dose of the lytic of your choice:

  - Urokinase (UK) = 50,000–60,000 units/h
  - Tenecteplase (TNK) = 0.2 mg/h
  - Alteplase (tPA) = 0.5 mg/h
  - Reteplase (rPA) = 0.20–0.24 mg/h
  - Markedly decrease heparin once lysis has begun

    - Exception is that UK appears to be associated with less bleeding, despite concurrent systemic heparinization.

Medications for ALLI

- Editor does not use any heparin (even via sheath) when infusing tPA.
- Usually infuse 150 units/hr of heparin via sheath when infusing TNK or rPA.
- Antibiotics – especially if puncturing surgical graft material
- Drugs for spasm – Nitroglycerin, Diltiazem
- GIIa/IIIb inhibitors – Abciximab

Complications and Treatment

- Bleeding at access site(s)

  - Increase sheath size.
  - Decrease lytic by 50%, stop heparin.

- ○ Try to finish with other interventions (Angiojet, stents).

- Overhydration:

  - ○ Call if intake is greater than output by 1,000 mL in 24 h.

- Nephrotoxicity:

  - ○ Call if urine output is <300 ml q 8 h.

- Intracranial Hemorrhage:

  - ○ Call if systolic BP is >170.
  - ○ Interrupt lysis until BP is <170.
  - ○ Consider labetalol 50 mg IVPB q 15 min up to 400 mg or significant bradycardia.
  - ○ Avoid lysis if known vascular malformation/aneurysm.
  - ○ Avoid lysis if stroke or intracranial surgery within past 6 months (author would be reluctant to treat irrespective of elapsed time since surgery or prior intracranial surgery).

- Hyperkalemia:

  - ○ Electrolytes q 24 h.

- Systemic Revascularization Syndrome: Systemic response to revascularization of dead muscle and other tissues

  - ○ Hypotension,
  - ○ Arrhythmias due to hyperkalemia, lactic acidosis
  - ○ Nephrotoxicity due to myoglobinuria
  - ○ Adult respiratory distress syndrome (ARDS) due to embolization of clots/fibrin-platelet aggregates from the limb
  - ○ Disseminated intravascular coagulopathy (DIC) from the release of procoagulants from the ischemic tissues.

- Local post-revascularization complications consist of the compartment syndrome.

  - ○ Swelling, tenderness of the compartment,
  - ○ Worsening difficulty with either dorsal or plantar flexion.
  - ○ Treatment is surgical fasciotomy.

    - ■ Lack of detection and timely treatment can result in necrosis of muscle with resultant foot drop versus amputation.
    - ■ Timely consultation with either orthopedic or vascular surgery is recommended if the symptoms and signs present following successful revascularization (it is a complication of success).

Clinical Categories, Angiographic Patterns, Treatment(s)

- Appropriate patient and clot selection is critical to the success of interventional therapies to treat acute lower limb ischemia (ALLI). To optimize selection of patients and determination of method(s) of treatment it is considered essential that they be categorized based on the composite of

  - Symptoms
  - Physical findings
  - Pedal Doppler signal
  - Angiographic pattern

- The thrombolytic or mechanical clot-clearing approaches have several advantages

  - Clarification of the location, nature, and extent of the flow-limiting lesion
  - Better treatment planning: Fewer stents versus atherectomy versus laser versus simple balloon angioplasty versus type of bypass
  - Improvement of endovascular alternative success rates
  - Avoidance, or at least postponement, of the need for bypass graft (bpg)

    - In general, surgery should be postponed as long as possible and preservation of the native artery should be a priority.
    - The options available when a graft occludes are fewer than when a native artery either reoccludes or develops a restenosis.
    - Prosthetic grafts do not develop collaterals and therefore reocclusion results in severe ischemia.

- A recanalized native vessel can be associated with the development of collaterals as a restenosis develops resulting in less severe ischemia if occlusion occurs.
- Thus, graft failure is more likely to be associated with a return of ALLI than restenosis or reocclusion of a previously recanalized native artery.

Viable

- This presentation accounts for approximately 10% of ALLI cases

  - Not in immediate danger of limb loss

    - Tissue blood supply adequate for survival if condition does not worsen

  - Heparinization will improve appearance of the limb, diminish symptoms, and stabilize the clotting process to prevent further propagation of clot with worsening of ischemia.

    - Will not enable the limb to return to the pre-occlusive state
    - Subsequent severe claudication expected

○ Urgent restoration of blood flow is recommended, but immediate/emergency restoration not required.

■ Tissue loss not expected if occlusive pattern does not progress.

Clinical/Physical Findings

- History:

  ○ Sudden, unrelenting pain, coldness, and numbness in the affected limb.
  ○ Onset will usually have been within the past 24 h, but may have occurred several days earlier.

- Older and/or post-bpg patients will frequently wait a few days to see if symptoms will clear spontaneously (denial, fear of treatment).
- Rest pain usually clears with time and immobilization, but the coolness and pallor will not clear as the collateral flow is inadequate at rest in the subset of patients with the ALLI syndrome.
- Severe pain in the calf and foot brought on by walking only a few steps.
- Physical examination:

  ○ The affected foot is pale and cool.
  ○ Sensation is intact (even light touch).
  ○ Motor function is intact (toe and ankle movements symmetrical).
  ○ Calf muscle tenderness and swelling would be unusual in this category and indicate a heightened risk of the compartment syndrome following revascularization.
  ○ Capillaries refill rapidly.
  ○ No palpable pedal pulse.

Doppler Findings

- Pulsatile signals audible at ankle
- Ankle pressure >25 mmHg below brachial pressure
- Ankle/brachial index 0.0–0.4

Angiographic Findings (Examples)

- Occlusion of a single arterial segment
- Iliac versus SFA versus popliteal versus one tibial artery (two still widely patent)
- Collateral vessels are patent, but not large, numerous or tortuous

- Occlusion of femoral–popliteal bpg, but patent popliteal artery.

- Embolus to popliteal, but patent normal trifurcation system distally and SFA proximally

- Embolus to common femoral, but patent normal common/external iliac proximally and normal profunda/superficial femoral distally

  ○ Usually more ischemic as flow into both the superficial and profunda femoris arteries is obstructed.

Action

- Heparinization, wire/catheter passage and lytic administration as described above.

Threatened

- This presentation accounts for approximately 75% of ALLI
- Imminent danger of tissue necrosis and further clot propagation

  ○ Collateral flow is inadequate, and threatens survival of tissue at rest

- Heparinization expected to stabilize status and prevent clot propagation

  ○ Not likely to significantly improve either color or temperature of limb.

- Further clot propagation could be very hazardous to survival of limb, survival of patient, and increases risk of post-revascularization complications (local = compartment syndrome, systemic = hyperkalemia, lactic acidosis, arrhythmias, hypotension, adult respiratory distress syndrome, acute tubular necrosis, death)
- Urgent improvement in blood flow advisable
- Thrombolysis/other clot-clearing treatments are effective alternatives to emergency surgery

  ○ Many reports document lower mortality and amputation rates
  ○ Interventional skills and experience are imperative

1. **Clinical/Physical Findings**

- History:
- ALLI; same onset as with viable
- In contrast to VIABLE, the pain does not relent with time and rest, and is more severe

  ○ Pain typically involves both calf and foot
  ○ Unlike viable where typically the foot alone is painful

- Patients usually seek medical help sooner than do those in the viable category
- Examination:

  ○ Signs of coldness and pallor are more advanced than in the viable category
  ○ Sensory Function

    ■ Loss to even light touch qualifies for THREATENED

    ■ Can use readily available Kleenex to test for asymmetry leg to leg
    ■ More serious (worse) if there is loss of sensation to pin prick

      • Unable to differentiate between sharp and dull ends of pin

    ■ More serious (worse) if patient can only sense deep pressure (squeezing of foot)
    ■ More serious (worse) if loss of proprioception (toe position)
    ■ Put in Profound/Irreversible category if anesthetic (only 10% of cases)

  ○ Motor Function

    ■ Weakness of toe dorsiflexion is first motor dysfunction apparent
    ■ Motor impairment lags behind sensory impairment
    ■ Compare bilateral vigorous toe dorsiflexion
    ■ Less rapid and not as extensive on affected side = first sign of motor impairment.
    ■ If no movement, categorize as Profound/Irreversible not Threatened

  ○ Foot examination

    ■ Marked blanching of foot when elevated and very slow capillary filling when returned to horizontal
    ■ Foot becomes ruborous when dependent
    ■ Patient more comfortable when foot dependent, so foot is often edematous if ischemia has been present for a few days
    ■ Gangrene is not present
    ■ Usually only seen with Chronic Critical Limb Ischemia (CLI)
    ■ Tenderness of calf muscles not uncommon (probably due to preference for dependency, and resultant edema +/– lactic acid in the interstitial fluid). Induration (muscle that is firm, but still compressible and can contract) is uncommon, but worrisome as it may be a sign of impending rigor (rock hard, dead muscle tissue)
    ■ Rigor changes the category to irreversible and is probably best treated with amputation
    ■ Induration prompts use of rapid clot-clearing techniques versus surgery
    ■ Careful monitoring during clot clearing is essential to detect evidence of worsening ischemia and need to accelerate clot clearing
    ■ Careful monitoring following clot clearing is essential to detect localized (compartment syndrome) or systemic revascularization syndrome (outlined above)

Doppler Findings

- No audible pulsatile flow in pedal arteries
- No ankle/brachial pressure ratio
- Audible pedal venous flow (with compression of foot)

Angiographic Findings

- Multi-vessel, multi-level occlusion
- Requirement for blood to traverse more than one collateral bed
- Usually in series

  - Occlusion of SFA and popliteal arteries with profunda collaterals to geniculate collaterals to reconstitute flow in major distal vessel = trifurcation
  - Occlusion of common and external iliac arteries or one limb of aortobifemoral bpg with collateral pathway via lumbars to internal iliac branches to common femoral artery

- Occasionally in parallel

  - Origin occlusions of all three trifurcation arteries with collateral flow around each

- Sometimes see a single level of acute occlusion, but obstruction of inflow to collateral bed

Actions for Threatened

- **Heparinize** (initial and maintenance doses dependent on severity of sensorimotor impairment)

  - Bolus of 3,000–5,000 units
  - Try to achieve a PTT of 80–100 sec.
  - Maintenance dose ~1,000 u/h I.V. to keep PTT 80–100 sec prior to lysis

    - Dependent upon degree of ischemia
    - If only hypesthesia→ aPTT of 60 sec probably sufficient

  - Cut back when lysis has been initiated
  - Therapeutic levels of heparin anticoagulation usually not deemed critical during lysis
  - With urokinase aPTT of 60–80 sec is acceptable, but <45 sec with other lytics
  - Usually do not use heparin during tPA infusions and 150 units/h via sheath when infusing either rPA or TNK

- Urgent angiography

○ Probably best-performed ASAP, unless dramatic improvement following heparin

- For Threatened the authors usually begin with continuous low-dose infusion (now supplemented with ultrasound device – EKOS)
- Remember that the spectrum of ischemia within Threatened category extends from minimal to marked sensorimotor impairment – treat accordingly

  ○ For minimal sensorimotor impairment, begin with low dose of lytic and re-exam after overnight infusion.
  ○ Consider short-term high dose (4 h) if either sensory deficit is more than hypesthesia or if there is some motor impairment.
  ○ High dose varies from 2 to 4 times low dose (given under Viable) depending upon severity of ischemia, but prefer duration of <4 h followed by rean-giogram at 4 h with intent to finish by aspirating any residual clot (Possis) or just switch to low dose for overnight infusion if the clinical exam has improved and no easy access to the interventional suite.

- Author prefers beginning with continuous infusion as it can be initiated with a minimum of instrumentation, room time, sedation, and analgesia. Also, less risk of embolization, hypertension, and hemoglobinuria that can follow use of the POSSIS device
- Would use Angiojet to completely clear any residual clot at time of follow-up angiogram as there is less clot which is more hydrated and easier to aspirate, embolization less likely, and less significant.
- For worsening sensorimotor exam, no improvement with heparin, sluggish toe movement, and/or sensation to only firm foot pressure, strongly consider initial use of mechanical devices or other lytic adjuncts:

  ○ Consider Power Pulse Spray (PPS) versus just aspiration

    ■ PPS = loading dose of lytic into clot via Possis and then aspirate
    ■ PPS requires 20-min dwell time of drug in clot before aspiration

  ○ Bolus of abciximab into the clot (slowly deposit 0.25 mg/kg [diluted in 10 mL] as catheter is withdrawn from distal to proximal end of clot)
  ○ If Angiojet does not re-establish flow consider either bolus of abciximab and initiate low-dose lysis versus no abciximab, but use of high-dose lytic × 4 h
  ○ Consider infusions via EKOS catheter

- If ischemia worsens after above attempts (uncommon) consider surgery or repeat effort with Possis.

  ○ Surgery is an excellent, but bigger, more stressful procedure and carries more risk to these patients, who are likely to have associated coronary, carotid, and lung disease.
  ○ Blaisdell's review of the results of the emergency surgical treatment of 3,330 acutely ischemic limbs demonstrated a 27% mortality and a 14% amputation rate

- Our experience in treating these same types of occlusions with continuous-infusion thrombolysis has yielded a 2% mortality and 5% amputation rate
- The additions of the potential accelerating effect of GP IIb/IIIa (abciximab, others) and the AngioJet would be expected to at least maintain those improved results
- The incidence of post-revascularization complications is less following lysis

  ○ Localized = compartment syndrome
  ○ Systemic syndrome = hypotension, arrhythmia, ARDS, ATN, death.

Irreversible/Profound Ischemia

- The clotting process is so extensive, collateral flow so reduced, and ischemic changes so advanced that major amputation will be necessary if revascularization is unsuccessful. The term Irreversible implies the inevitability of at least minor tissue loss irrespective of successful revascularization (e.g., necrosis of toes or forefoot) and neuropathy

Clinical/Physical Findings

- History

  ○ Same onset as other categories of ALLI
  ○ Pain is constant and severe unless sensation is absent
  ○ Pain is not relieved by dependency or walking

- Examination
  ○ Sensory function

    ■ Foot has profound sensory loss
    ■ Most clear-cut if anesthetic.
    ■ Proprioception gone

  ○ Motor function

    ■ Toe flexion is gone. Ankle movement is impaired or absent

  ○ Foot examination

    ■ COLD
    ■ Skin has fixed, marbled discoloration (purple and white)
    ■ Absent capillary refill
    ■ Calf muscle firmness with marked tenderness, unless limb is anesthetic

  ○ Muscle rigor (rock-hard dead muscle that cannot contract).

■ Revascularizing this tissue carries a significant risk of death due to the lethal systemic post-revascularization syndrome

○ The more proximal the leg involvement, the graver the prognosis
○ Purplish discoloration and coldness of thigh are associated with 50% mortality in surgical series.

Doppler Findings

• No audible Doppler signals in either arteries or veins in the feet
• Absence of venous flow despite foot compression is an ominous sign

○ Last Doppler finding to go
○ Indicates thrombosis of the veins as well as arteries of the foot

Angiographic Findings

• Usually extensive occlusions involving both proximal and distal vessels without reestablishment of flow into distal trifurcation and/or foot vessels.
• Profound/Irreversible = poorer results, higher risk; but lysis may be best therapeutic alternative.

○ 2 levels of occlusion and no trifurcation filling. Examples:

■ Femoropopliteal bypass graft + popliteal + (at least origins of) all trifurcation arteries.
■ Common femoral artery occlusion (usually embolus) without demonstrable filling of any distal vessels (rare).
■ Aortobifemoral + femoropopliteal bypass graft occlusions without demonstrable filling of distal vessels (usually due to associated stenosis of profunda femoris).
■ Popliteal artery occlusion + occlusion of all trifurcation arteries throughout the calf; usually popliteal embolus with secondary propogation throughout previously stenotic arteries (rare).

Action

• Systemic heparinization, including bolus.
• Do not lyse if calf muscles are not viable (rigid and non-functioning).
• These patients are considered poor candidates for lysis due to the long time required to lyse what is generally a large clot volume and ischemia that is rapidly advancing.
• If lysis attempted:

- ○ Mechanical clot removal associated with bolus of GIIb/IIIa
- ○ Follow with continuous lytic infusion if flow can be restored through at least one major trifurcation artery.
- ○ Consider a high dose of lytic for the first few hours after restoring flow
- ○ Systemically heparinize, but at low-end of therapeutic range if have given abciximab, but upper end if not.

- Restoration of flow will flush intracellular contents (potassium, myoglobin), lactic acid, fibrin–platelet aggregates, and pro-coagulants into systemic circulation leading to *Systemic Revascularization Syndrome.*

- ○ Hypotension, arrhythmias, hypoxemia, ARDS, ATN.
- ○ High likelihood of death, myocardial infarction.

- For those candidates deemed to be acceptable surgical candidates, operative removal of as much clot as possible, followed by intra-operative administration of lytic or amputation, if unsuccessful
- Blaisdell recommended administration of high-dose heparin followed by either delayed revascularization surgery or primary amputation depending upon the evolution of the ischemia.

- ○ The goal was to minimize the loss of life associated with thromboembolectomy of ALLI.
- ○ Improvements in anesthesia, cardiac care, and surgical management have reduced that risk. Nonetheless, the Blaisdell approach should not to be dismissed.

Key Points

- Combining angiographic, Doppler, and clinical findings enables one to quite accurately assess how rapidly one needs to restore blood flow.
- The combination also guides one in recommending interventional versus surgical treatments, as well as in deciding upon the intervention.
- For the most severely ischemic limbs there is the potential to rapidly restore flow by combining lytic agents and abciximab as well as with the enhancement provided by ultrasound (EKOS infusion catheter) and to effectively aspirate with the Angiojet or other mechanical devices.
- Viable category of ischemia

  - ○ Single segment of occlusion
  - ○ Normal sensorimotor exam
  - ○ ~10% of ALLI
  - ○ ~100% likelihood of success
  - ○ ~0% likelihood of major amputation
  - ○ ~0% likelihood of death

- Threatened category of ischemia

  ○ Two segments of occlusion (or equivalent) and >1 trifurcation patent
  ○ Impaired sensorimotor exam (minimal to marked)
  ○ ~80% of ALLI.
  ○ ~90% likelihood of success.
  ○ ~5% likelihood of major amputation
  ○ ~0% likelihood of death

- Irreversible/Profound category of ischemia.

  ○ Greater than two segments of occlusion and no trifurcation patent throughout.
  ○ Anesthesia +/– Paraysis
  ○ Low success rate and high morbidity.

Suggested Reading

1. Ansel GM, George BS, Botti CF, McNamara TO, Jenkins JS, Ramee, SR Rosenfield K, ANoethen, and Mehta T. Rheolytic thrombectomy in the management of limb ischemia: 30-day results from a multicenter registry. J Endovasc Ther 2002; 9(4): 395–402.
2. Bertele V, Roncaglioni MC, Pangrazzi J, Terzian E, Tognoni EG. Clinical outcome and its predictors in 1560 patients with critical leg ischaemia. Chronic Critical Leg Ischaemia Group. Eur J Vasc Endovasc Surg 1999;18: 401–410.
3. Callum K, Bradbury A. Clinical review ABC of arterial and venous disease. Br Med J 2000; 320: 764–767.
4. Davidian M, Powell A, Benenati J, Katzen B, Becker G, Zemel G. Initial results of reteplase in the treatment of acute lower extremity arterial occlusions. J Vasc Interventional Radiol 2000; 11(3): 289–294.
5. Earnshaw J, Whitman B, Foy C . National Audit of Thrombolysis for Acute Leg Ischemia (NATALI): clinical factors associated with early outcome. J Vasc Surg 2004; 39(5): 1018–1025.
6. Kasirajan K, Haskal Z, Ouriel K. The use of mechanical thrombectomy devices in the management of acute peripheral arterial occlusive disease. J Vasc Interventional Radiol 2001; 12(4): 405–411.
7. Kessel D, Berridge D, Roberston I. Infusion techniques for peripheral arterial thrombolysis. Cochrane Database Syst Rev 2004; 1: CD000985.
8. Kudo T, Chandra FA, Ahn SS. The effectiveness of percutaneous transluminal angioplasty for the treatment of critical limb ischemia: a 10-year experience. J Vasc Surg 2005; 41: 423–435.
9. McNamara TO, Dong P, Chen J, Quinn B, Gomes A, Goodwin S, Aban K. Bleeding complications associated with the use of rt-PA for peripheral arterial and venous thromboembolic occlusions. Techniques in Vasc Interventional Radiol 2001; 4(2): 92–98.
10. McNamara TO, Gardner KR, Bomberger RA, Greaser LE. Clinical and angiographic selection factors for thrombolysis as initial therapy for acute lower limb ischemia. J Vasc Interventional Radiol 1995; Nov–Dec 6: 36–47.
11. McNamara TO, Fischer JR. Thrombolysis of peripheral arterial and graft occlusions: improved results using high-dose urokinase. Am J Roentgenol 1985; 144(4): 769–775.

12. McNamara TO. Thrombolysis treatment for acute lower limb ischemia. In Vascular Diseases: Surgical and Interventional Therapy, edited by A. van Breda and D.E. Strandness 1994, Churchill Livingstone, New York, 355–377.

13. McNamara, TO. Thrombolysis as an alternative initial therapy for the acutely ischemic lower limb. Seminars Vasc Surg 1992; 5: 89–98.

14. Norgren L, Hiatt WR, Dormandy JA, Nehler MR, Harris KA, Fowkes FG. Inter-society consensus for the management of peripheral arterial disease (TASC II). J Vasc Surg 2007; 45(Suppl S): S5–S67.

15. Slovet DP, Sullivan TM. Critical limb ischemia: Medical and surgical management. Vasc Med 2008; 13(3): 281–291.

Endovascular Treatment of Acute Stroke

Ali R. Zomorodi and Tony P. Smith

Introduction

- Stroke is the clinical situation that follows neurological cell death due to decreased blood flow:

  - The area remaining where the cells are ischemic but not yet infarcted is called the ischemic penumbra.
  - Penumbra is of variable size dependent on numerous factors:

    - Collateral blood flow
    - Perfusion pressure
    - Patient's overall constitutional health

  - The restoration of blood flow to salvage this ischemic area is the goal in the treatment of acute stroke.

- Therapy for acute stroke consists of supportive care, intravenous tissue plasminogen-activating factor (tPA), endovascular measures, and some investigative approaches such as venous perfusion. Supportive care is involved regardless of the therapy undertaken and becomes the mainstay of treatment when intravenous (IV) or intraarterial (IA) measures cannot be undertaken.

  - Intravenous tPA has United States Food and Drug Administration (FDA) approval as a treatment for ischemic stoke in patients within 3 h of symptom onset.

- Endovascular treatment of stroke holds great promise for ameliorating one of the leading causes of morbidity and mortality in the United States.

  - Requires an established stroke program with a multidisciplinary stroke team:

    - Abides by written protocols that are continuously reviewed and modified in light of the ever changing clinical data
    - Scrupulous attention to institutional quality improvement and outcomes tracking.

R.A. Morgan, E. Walser (eds.), *Handbook of Angioplasty and Stenting Procedures*,
Techniques in Interventional Radiology, DOI 10.1007/978-1-84800-399-6_22,
© Springer-Verlag London Limited 2010

Clinical Features

- Estimated annual incidence of stroke is approximately 750,000 per year in the United States.
- Stroke is the third leading cause of death and the leading cause of long-term disability in the United States, with an estimated 60 deaths per 100,000 people.
- 83% of strokes are considered ischemic: due to large vessel thrombosis (31%), embolism (32%), and small vessel thrombosis (20%). The remaining 17% are hemorrhagic, of which approximately 10% are intracerebral hemorrhage and 7% are subarachnoid hemorrhage.
- Endovascular treatment shows promise in treating large vessel thrombotic and embolic ischemic stroke.

Diagnostic Evaluation

- The patient should be initially evaluated by the stroke team and the interventionist is notified if the patient has an ischemic stroke within the appropriate treatment window. Below is an outline of the key features of the diagnostic evaluation that will impact the endovascular treatment.

History

- Time of symptom onset is critical. If not obtainable exactly from the patient or family, the last time the patient was known to be normal is used.
- Recent history of trauma.
- Recent surgical procedures or lumbar puncture.
- Prior strokes.
- Seizures at time of stroke onset.
- Contrast allergy.

Physical Exam

- Determine vital signs and treat blood pressure to keep less than 180/100.
- Determine National Institute of Health Stroke Scale (NIHSS) presented at the end of this chapter.
- Determine likely vascular territory and cause of stroke based on physical exam findings (Table 1).

Table 1 Common stroke syndromes and likely location of occlusion

Artery	Syndrome	Pathophysiology
ACA	Motor and/or sensory deficit (foot >> face, arm)	Embolic >
	Grasp, sucking, rooting reflex	atherothrombotic
	Abulia, rigidity, gait apraxia	
MCA	Dominant: aphasia, motor and sensory deficit (face, arm > leg > foot), hemianopsia	Embolic > atherothrombotic
	Non-dominant: neglect, anosognosia, motor and sensory deficit, hemianopsia	
PCA	Hemianopsia, alexia, visual hallucination, spontaneous pain, motor deficit	Embolic > atherothrombotic
Perforators	Pure motor hemiparesis; Pure sensory deficit	Small artery
	Hemiparesis and ataxia; Dysarthria/clumsy hand	disease
VBA	CN palsies	Embolic =
	Crossed sensory deficit	atherothrombotic
	Diplopia, dizziness, nausea, vomiting, dysarthria, dysphagia	
	Coma	

ACA = anterior cerebral artery; MCA = middle cerebral artery; PCA = posterior cerebral artery; VBA = vertebrobasilar artery

Laboratory

- Determine blood glucose levels. Hypo- and hyperglycemia represent very common mimickers of stroke. Additionally, the incidence of intracranial hemorrhage following endovascular treatment increases if blood sugar is >200.
- Coagulation parameters: PT/INR, PTT, and platelet count. Hyper- and hypocoagulable states must be dealt with accordingly.

Imaging

- Non-contrast head CT (Fig. 1): Evaluate for the presence of intracerebral or subarachnoid hemorrhage. Quantify the extent of cerebral infarction, if present. Assess for the presence of intracranial tumors.
- CT angiogram if rapidly obtainable may be used to verify and localize large vessel occlusion; allows assessment of aortic arch, carotid and vertebral artery anatomy for planning endovascular treatment.
- CT perfusion if available, will allow detection of possibly salvageable ischemic penumbra. In the ischemic penumbra, mean transit time (MTT) is elevated and cerebral blood flow (CBF) is diminished, while cerebral blood volume (CBV) is preserved. In infarcted tissue, MTT is elevated, and both CBF and CBV are decreased.

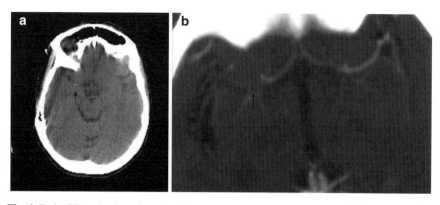

Fig. 1 Early CT evaluation of stroke. (**a**) Plain head CT demonstrates hyperdense right middle cerebral artery (*arrow*). The ipsilateral temporal lobe shows early loss of cortical differentiation.(**b**) Corresponding CTA demonstrates thrombus in the right middle cerebral artery

Indications

- NB: While there is widespread agreement on which patients are eligible for IV tPA, the indications for IA therapy vary from institution to institution. Some reserve IA therapy for patients not eligible for IV tPA; others routinely give eligible patients lower bridging doses of IV tPA to transition to IA therapy and still others proceed with IA therapy even after full dose IV tPA in clinically refractory patients. Below are the general indications for IA therapy of stroke.

  - Neurologic symptoms must be significant: Isolated aphasia or hemianopsia, or NIHSS >4.
  - Patient's symptoms must be concordant with the vascular territory of ischemia.
  - Currently, mechanical thrombolysis is possible only for proximal M2, M1, A1, P1, ICA, Basilar, and vertebral arteries. More distal occlusion can be treated with IA tPA.
  - Patients with anterior circulation occlusion are eligible for IA tPA if thrombolysis is possible within 6 h, and eligible for mechanical thrombolysis if revascularization is possible within 8 h of symptom onset.
  - Patients with basilar artery occlusion are eligible for treatment within 12–24 h of presentation.

Contraindications

- Any acute intracranial hemorrhage
- Parenchymal hypodensity in more than 1/3 of the affected vascular territory
- Mass effect with significant midline shift
- Intracranial tumor except small meningioma

Relative Contraindications

- Rapidly improving neurologic exam
- Seizures at the time of presentation
- Baseline NIHSS <10
- Head trauma within the past 90 days
- Stroke within the past 60 days
- Baseline INR >1.7, aPTT >1.5 ×, platelets <100 K
- Systolic blood pressure >180 and diastolic blood pressure >100

Relevant Anatomy

- The site of vessel occlusion can be ascertained by physical exam findings (Table 1) and by diagnostic angiography. The Qureshi system for grading the severity of intracranial vascular occlusion is presented below. Clinical outcome decreases significantly with each increase in grade on this scale.

Equipment

Catheters

- Five French diagnostic catheter for initial angiography
- Six French guiding catheter for thrombolysis, angioplasty, stenting, or Penumbra® mechanical thrombolysis (see mechanical thrombus disruption/removal below)
- Eight or nine French Concentric balloon occlusion catheter for Merci® thrombectomy (see mechanical thrombus disruption/removal below)
- Microcatheter for IA tPA, Penumbra®, or Merci® mechanical thrombolysis

Thrombolytic Agents

- Urokinase: typically given in 100,000 unit boluses over 10 min each for a maximum of 1 million units
- tPA: Given at 10 mg/h for a maximum of 20 mg
- Activase: 1.5 mg infused into clot, and 1.5 mg/h infused proximal to clot. Maximum duration of infusion is 3
- Retavase: 0.1 unit infused into clot and 0.1 unit/h infused proximally. Maximum duration of infusion is 3 h

  - NB: Doses vary somewhat among interventionists and institutions. Activase and retavase are third generation fibrinolytics. Their safety and efficacy remains unknown and their use should be limited to the Interventional Stroke Therapy Outcomes (INSTOR) registry or in the hands of those very familiar with these agents through use in other applications such as peripheral vascular thrombolytic therapy.

Angiography

Patient Preparation

- Dextrose containing solutions must not be used in stroke patients.
- Close attention is paid to blood pressure control and to ensure indications/contraindications are assessed.
- Sedation can have unpredictable effects on stroke patients who are often stuporous and altered at baseline. We prefer to perform stroke interventions under the more controlled conditions of general anesthesia.
- The use of heparin in stroke thrombolysis is controversial, as there is an increased risk of intracranial hemorrhage. Currently, a 2,000 unit bolus followed by a 500 U/h infusion as per the PROACTII trial is used in the registry protocols.

Access

- Micropuncture system should be used for gaining access to the femoral artery.
- A 6F sheath should be used initially.

Runs

- The goal of cerebral angiogram is to document the occlusive lesion and to assess the degree of cerebrovascular collateral, per the Qureshi grading system (Table 2).
- If time is limiting or the occlusion is fairly distal in the vessel, runs of the target vessel alone can be performed.
- The effectiveness of revascularization is measured using the thrombolysis in cerebral ischemia scale (Table 3).

Performing the Procedure

General Technique

- Intra-arterial thrombolysis: Placement of a microcatheter into the thrombus for administration of a thrombolytic agent
- Mechanical thrombus disruption and/or thrombectomy: placement of balloon catheters, stents, or clot extraction devices. The latter consists of two devices that currently have limited FDA approval in the United States

Table 2 Grading the severity of intracranial vascular occlusion

Grade		Type of Occlusion	
0	No occlusion		
1	MCA occlusion (M3 segment)	ACA occlusion (A2 or distal)	1 BA or VA branch
2	MCA occlusion (M2 segment)	ACA occlusion (A1 and A2)	≥ 2 BA or VA branch
3	MCA occlusion (M1 segment)		
3A	Lenticulostriate sparing or leptomeningeal collaterals reconstruct territory		
3B	No sparing of lenticulostriates and no leptomeningeal collaterals		
4	ICA occlusion with partial filling through collaterals	BA occlusion with partial filling through collaterals	
4A	Collaterals fill MCA	Collaterals allow anterograde filling	
4B	Collaterals fill ACA	Collaterals allow retrograde filling	
5	ICA occlusion no collaterals	BA occlusion no collaterals	

ICA=internal carotid artery; ACA=anterior cerebral artery; MCA= middle cerebral artery; BA=basilar artery; VA=vertebral artery

Table 3 Thrombolysis in cerebral ischemia (TICI)

Grade	TICI
0	No perfusion, no antegrade flow distal to occlusion
1	Penetration with minimal perfusion: contrast material passes beyond occlusion, but fails to opacify the entire cerebral bed distal to the obstruction for the duration of the run
2	Partial perfusion: Contrast material passes distal to the obstruction and opacifies the distal bed appreciably more slowly than normal vasculature
2a	Only partial filling (less than 2/3) of the distal vascular territory is visualized.
2b	Complete filling of the distal vascular territory is visualized, but occurs more slowly.
3	Normal flow is reestablished distal to the occlusion

Intra-arterial Thrombolysis

- A 6F guiding catheter is placed in the target vessel and connected to a continuous heparinized saline flush through a Y-connector.
- 0.014-inch microwire and catheter are advanced to the site of the occlusion.
- A microcatheter is passed through the lesion, and 5 cc of the thrombolytic agent is slowly injected into the thrombus as the catheter is withdrawn. Multiple passes can be performed until the thrombus is dissolved, a predetermined maximum dose of agent is administered, or the time allotted for revascularization expires.
- Proximal infusion is performed by placing the microcatheter just proximal to the clot. A syringe pump is then used to run a continuous infusion of thrombolytics into the occluded vessel. Progress is assessed with intermittent runs through the guiding catheter. The infusion continues until there is revascularization, a

predetermined maximum dose of thrombolytic is given, or the allotted time for revascularization expires (Fig. 2).
- Data regarding effectiveness is from a manufacturer sponsored randomized trial (see below and suggested reading)

Mechanical Thrombus Disruption/Removal

Balloon Angioplasty and Stenting

- Thought to be analogous to coronary intervention where thrombus is disrupted by ballooning and vessel patency restored by stent placement
- A 6F guiding catheter for coronary angioplasty balloons and coronary stent placement
- Wide variety of coronary devices, Gateway™ PTA dilation catheter/ Wingspan™ stent system (Boston Scientific Corp; Fremont CA)
- Most often follows failed or partially successful intra-arterial or intravenous thrombolysis, or when time from symptom onset precluded use of thrombolytics
- Only case reports and small series data to prove effectiveness

Merci® (Concentric Medical Inc; Mountain View CA) Mechanical Thrombolysis

- Requires 9F sheath in the common femoral artery in order to place the Merci® balloon occlusion catheter into the internal carotid artery or vertebral artery.
- One of a variety of corkscrew appearing Merci® devices is deployed through the provided microcatheter distal to the thrombus.
- The device and the microcatheter are withdrawn together through the balloon catheter to remove intact clot (Fig. 3).
- Only data regarding effectiveness is from manufacturer-sponsored trial (see suggested reading)

Penumbra Stroke System® (Penumbra, Inc; Alameda CA) Mechanical Thrombolysis

- A 6F guiding catheter is placed in the target vessel
- Specialized microcatheter is placed into the thrombus and the catheter tip separates revealing a suction lumen
- Thrombus can then be mechanically removed using controlled suction provided by a specialized pump
- Only data regarding effectiveness is from manufacturer-sponsored trial (abstract data only)

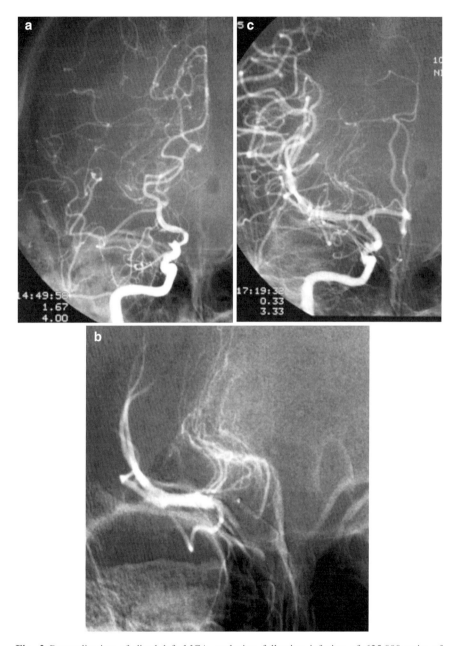

Fig. 2 Recanalization of distal left MCA occlusion following infusion of 625,000 units of Urokinase into the thrombus. (**a**) Initial angiogram demonstrating occlusion of right MCA just distal to its origin. (**b**). Microcatheter injection distal to thrombus delineates extent of clot. (**c**) Following infusion of urokinase, there is revascularization of the right MCA

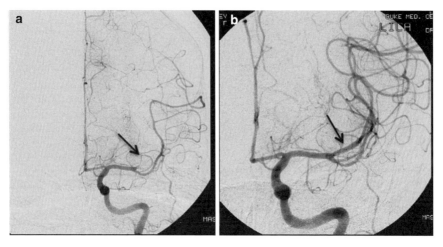

Fig. 3 Results of mechanical thrombolysis. (**a**) Pre-procedure runs demonstrate occlusion of the superior trunk left MCA. (**b**) Following mechanical thrombectomy with MERCI device, flow is restored to superior trunk of the right MCA

Aftercare

- The sheath is sutured in place if systemic thrombolytic therapy has been given.
- Otherwise a closure device should be used.
- Direct repair of the artery may be needed for 9F sheaths.
- Daily laboratory evaluation is necessary to detect clinically silent retroperitoneal hemorrhage and to detect and treat hyperglycemia.
- Close blood pressure control to keep systolic blood pressure between 120 and 160 mmHg.
- Fluid status should be controlled to prevent dehydration or fluid overload and cerebral edema.

Results

- Angiographic results are determined using the thrombolysis in cerebral ischemia (TICI) scale for reperfusion.
- Clinical results are determined using the modified Rankin Score (mRS) or the Barthel Index.

  - Best-published results to date are for intra-arterial thrombolysis and consists of the PROACT I and II trials. In these studies, patients with middle cerebral artery thrombus were randomized to receive prourokinase, a non-FDA approved agent similar to urokinase, versus heparin. The thrombolytic group had significantly better overall neurologic outcomes despite an early increased rate of intracranial hemorrhage.

Complications

- Intracranial hemorrhage:

  ○ Intraprocedure hemorrhage can be detected by sudden hemodynamic fluctuation due to increased intracranial pressure, and evidence of extravasation on angiogram.

  ○ Thrombolytic infusion should be discontinued immediately, and heparinization reversed with protamine at a dose of 1 mg per 100 units of heparin given, up to 50 mg total.

  ○ Stat head CT should be obtained. Medical management of ICP is initiated.

  ○ Ventriculostomy and ICP monitors should be used judiciously as there is increased risk of intracranial hemorrhage.

  ○ For clinically deteriorating patients who have significant mass effect and easily accessed hematomas, surgical evaluation should be considered.

Key Points

- Level 1 data is completely lacking to support the endovascular treatment of acute stroke. All of the results to date are based on small series, case reports, and manufacturer-sponsored studies but do show promising results.
- Time to treatment is critical. Must have a system in place to deliver appropriate patients to the interventional suite as quickly as possible.
- Techniques require considerable expertise in the neurointerventional arena and overall care of these patients is enhanced by a multidisciplinary stroke team.

Suggested Reading

1. Del Zoppo GJ, Higashida RT, Furlan AJ, et al. PROACT: a phase II randomized trail of recombinant pro-urokinase by direct arterial delivery in acute middle cerebral artery stroke. Stroke 1998; 29:1894–1900.
2. Ng PP, Higashida RT, Cullen SP, Malek R, Dowd CF, Halbach VV. Intraarterial thrombolysis trials in acute ischemic stroke. J Vasc Interv Radiol. 2004; 15:S77–S85.
3. Qureshi AI. New grading system for angiographic evaluation of arterial occlusions and recanalization response to intra-arterial thrombolysis in acute ischemic stroke. Neurosurgery 2002; 50: 1405–1415.
4. Smith WS, Sung G, Saver J, et al. Mechanical thrombectomy for acute ischemic stroke: final results of the Multi MERCI trial. Stroke 2008; 39: 1205–1212.

Venoplasty and Stenting

Haraldur Bjarnason

Introduction

- Venoplasty and venous stenting is commonly applied to chronically throm-bosed veins. Venous angioplasty by itself is usually not sufficient to keep a vein open, presumable because of the low intravascular blood pressure (compared to the arterial system). Therefore, metal stents are usually required for long-term patency in venous disease.

Clinical Feature

- Swelling or edema is the most common symptom of venous obstruction (occlu-sion or narrowing). The extremities, legs, and arms are most commonly affected, but the head can also be affected. Occasionally the trunk may be affected when the central veins (Inferior Vena Cava (IVC) or Superior Vena Cava (SVC)) are obstructed.
- SVC syndrome (SVCS) is typically caused by obstruction or occlusion of the SVC or both the Internal Jugular Vein's (IJV) and/or Innominate veins (INV). Symptoms typically only result from total obstruction to the venous outflow from the head and one open IJV down to the right atrium (RA) will avert symptoms.
- SVCS can be expressed by some or all of the following symptoms:

  - Neck and facial swelling (typically around the eyes)
  - Dyspnea, cough, and hoarseness or change in character of voice
  - Headaches
  - Tongue swelling, nasal congestion
  - Epistaxis, hemoptysis
  - Dysphagia
  - Dizziness, syncope
  - Lethargy

R.A. Morgan, E. Walser (eds.), *Handbook of Angioplasty and Stenting Procedures*,
Techniques in Interventional Radiology, DOI 10.1007/978-1-84800-399-6_23,
© Springer-Verlag London Limited 2010

- ○ Bending forward or lying down may aggravate the symptoms
- Characteristic physical findings of SVCS:

  - ○ Prominent neck veins and increased number of collateral veins on the anterior chest wall
  - ○ Edema of the face, arms, and chest
  - ○ Cyanosis

- Obstruction of the subclavian veins or axillary veins results in swelling of the affected arm, which usually improves without intervention. Similarly, unilateral and isolated innominate vein obstruction or occlusion commonly goes unnoticed as it is well-compensated by the jugular vein flow.
- Thoracic outlet syndrome (TOS), which is muscular or ligamentous compression of the vein as it leaves the chest, can cause persistent arm heaviness and swelling with chronic venous occlusion in typical locations on venography.
- Iliac vein obstruction and IVC occlusion will typically present with

  - ○ Lower extremity swelling, which can extend from the feet to the buttock area depending on the distribution of the thrombosis and can be bilateral in case of bilateral involvement or if the IVC is also occluded or obstructed
  - ○ Venous claudication – sensation of tightness and pain upon walking, typically in the thigh muscles
  - ○ Long-lasting obstruction will commonly result in post-thrombotic syndrome (PTS) which is characterized with, swelling, pain, skin changes, and even ulcers

Diagnostic Evaluation

Clinical

- Detailed history needs to be obtained:

  - ○ Previous malignant disease
  - ○ Previous surgical history including history of venous catheterization or trauma
  - ○ Previous history of radiation
  - ○ Family history of venous disease such as thrombosis history or hypercoagulable states
  - ○ Iodinated contrast allergy, history of renal dysfunction, history of cardiac valves or pacemaker, and history of claustrophobia in preparation for MRI, CT, or venography

- Careful physical examination is mandatory:

  - ○ Pulses in affected extremity

- ○ Diameter discrepancy between affected/unaffected extremity
- ○ Ulcerations or skin changes
- ○ Auscultation/palpation for bruits (rule out AV malformations, fistulae)
- ○ Palpation for adenopathy (rule out lymphedema)
- ○ Lung/cardiac exam to rule out congestive heart failure or valvular disease as cause of right heart dysfunction and lower extremity edema

Laboratory

- Patients with unprovoked chronic thrombotic obstruction require careful hematological evaluation for hyper-coagulable states:

  - ○ Factor V Leiden deficiency
  - ○ Antithrombin III deficiency
  - ○ Protein S or Protein C deficiency
  - ○ Anti-cardiolipin antibodies
  - ○ Heparin-induced thrombotic thrombocytopenia (HITT)
  - ○ Lupus anticoagulant

- Before any procedure is scheduled, check

  - ○ Creatinine
  - ○ Electrolytes
  - ○ Prothrombin time (PT) and activated partial thromboplastin time (APTT) if the patient is on anticoagulation
  - ○ Complete blood count with platelet assessment

- Non-invasive physiologic studies such as plethysmography can affect treatment decisions and monitor results of therapy for patients with lower extremity venous problems.

Imaging

- Ultrasound plays an important role in the evaluation and diagnosis of the venous system.

  - ○ Deep venous structures in the pelvis (iliac veins), abdomen (IVC), and chest (central veins) may not be accessible with ultrasound but occlusions in inaccessible segments can be inferred by dampened venous signals without cardiac pulsations or response to Valsalva maneuver in the upstream veins easily imaged by ultrasound (common femoral veins, subclavian veins)
  - ○ Pulse-wave Doppler and color Doppler analysis of veins provides substantial physiological information (flow volume, valvular incompetence) which other imaging studies do not offer.
  - ○ Acute venous occlusion:

- ■ Hypoechoic clot in distended, non-compressible vein with few collaterals and significant subcutaneous and fascial edema

  ○ Chronic venous occlusion:

  - ■ Linear, hyperechoic, occasionally calcified clot with partial flow and compressibility in venous segment surrounded by multiple collateral veins. Minimal subcutaneous edema evident.

- Venography (conventional) – gold standard imaging study for venous anatomic evaluation:

  ○ Injection of contrast through a peripheral vein in the affected foot or arm will in most cases give a very good image of anatomic structures and the location and degree of obstruction. Tourniquets or local compression allows visualization of deep venous structures or specific superficial venous pathways.
  ○ Venography will not give accurate hemodynamic information. The presence of collaterals bypassing an obstructed vein indicates a hemodynamically significant obstruction.
  ○ Image quality on venography diminishes in the more central veins near the heart due to contrast dilution.

- Catheter-based venography:

  ○ Negotiation of a catheter past an obstructed or stenotic venous segment with injection of contrast through and beyond it gives better images of the obstruction and integrity of the remaining venous outflow to the heart. Pressure measurements can also be obtained through the catheter on both sides of the obstruction (Fig. 1a) with a 3 mmHg pressure drop considered a significant gradient and indicative of venous flow impairment.

- Intravascular ultrasound (IVUS)
- Due to the inherent difficulties in visualizing the venous lumen with contrast due to contrast dilution, unopacified blood inflow, and the very thin and compliant nature of the venous wall, IVUS can obtain a more exact estimate of the degree of a venous stenosis as well as its nature (concentric or asymmetric stenoses, presence of clot, etc)
- Computer Tomographic Venography (CTV)

  ○ Essentially a delayed contrast-enhanced CT when venous opacification is optimal. Provides 3D and multiplanar venous imaging with excellent evaluation of endoluminal and perivenous pathology.

- Magnetic resonance venography (MRV) can be helpful under certain circumstances:

  ○ Serious iodinated contrast allergy and inability to have CTV
  ○ MRV with phase contrast imaging can provide flow speed, volume, and direction information not available by CT
  ○ MRV can perform real time cine venograpy in any specified plane

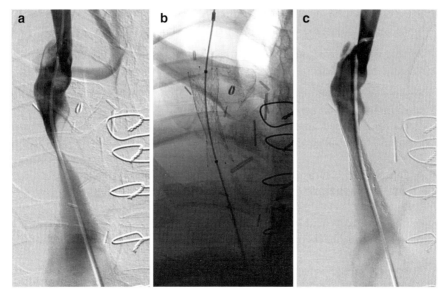

Fig. 1 A 29-year-old female patient with synovial cancer of the chest requiring right pneumonectomy in the past. She now has significant SVCS. (**a**) Access from the right CFV and venogram through the angiographic catheter depicts the obstruction just below the confluence area. Pressure measurement revealed a gradient of 14 mmHg across the obstruction. (**b**) A single 14-mm diameter by 40-mm long Protégé (EV3, Plymoth, MN) was placed across the obstruction. This was subsequently dilated with a 14-mm angioplasty balloon. (**c**) Follow-up venogram as in (a) reveals no collateral flow and the pressure gradient was 1 mmHg, down from 14 mmHg prior to stent placement

- ■ Requires respiratory and ECG gating

- ○ The experience with MRV is less than with CTV.

Indications

- Any symptomatic venous narrowing can be considered an indication for venoplasty and venous stenting.
- The accepted anatomic areas are the SVC, IVC, iliac veins, subclavian vein, and innominate vein.

Contraindications

- Stents are contraindicated in the subclavian vein across the first rib/clavicle junction in patients with Paget–Schroetter syndrome (venous thoracic outlet syndrome). After first rib resection for this condition, a stent is acceptable should restenosis occurs.

- Bacteremia is a relative contraindication for stent placement due to the potential for bacterial colonization of the stent causing a chronic infection:

  ○ This is a relative contraindication as there are exceptionally few reports of vascular stent infections, especially in the venous system.

- Impaired renal functional is a relative contraindication as for all other procedures based on use of contrast agents.
- Stents have limited applications below the common femoral vein (CFV) and peripheral to the subclavian vein due to poor long-term patency in these locations.

Patient Preparation

- During venoplasty and stent placement the patient receives full anticoagulation using unfractionated heparin. The Activated Clotting Time (ACT) should be 280–300 sec.
- The patient should be fasting according to guidelines established for each practice setting (typically 6–8 h).
- Patients need intravenous access for delivery of medications such as sedatives and fluids.
- Pre-procedure antibiotics are not routine but consider them in patients with

  ○ Prosthetic cardiac valves
  ○ Vascular grafts that may be accessed percutaneously (i.e., PTFE dialysis grafts)

Relevant Anatomy

Normal Anatomy

- The venous anatomy is more variable than that of the arterial system. Arteries and veins tend to travel side by side but venous aberrancy occurs in several important areas.

Aberrant Anatomy

- A duplicated SVC exist in 0.3% of cases where the left SVC drains into the right atrium, usually via an enlarged coronary sinus.
- A left only SVC is less common.
- A duplicated IVC is seen in 2% of patients in which case the left IVC drains into the left renal vein.
- Variation in anatomy is more common in the peripheral veins.

Equipment

- Stents: The stents used in the venous system should be self-expanding in most cases.
- Common stent diameters vary from 10 to 16 mm.
- There are many self-expandable stent types available including nitinol-based stents and stainless steel-based stents.
- The Gianturco Z-stent is unique for its large cell size and strong radial force:

    ○ Customizable in length – suture stents together
    ○ Customizable in diameter – create a "flared" end by cutting and re-tying encircling suture at either end of stent

- Balloon-expandable stents are only used when extra radial force is needed and should not be used in superficial areas.

    ○ Fibrotic SVC/IVC stenoses:

        ■ Cancer
        ■ Radiation
        ■ Fibrosing mediastinitis
        ■ Surgically ligated veins

- Catheters: 5F angled angiographic catheters, preferably with hydrophilic coating are optimal for navigating occluded or obstructed veins.
- Guidewire: To recanalize chronically occluded veins or torturous veins try hydrophilic guide wire such as the Glidewire (Terumo). Stiff wires can be very helpful. Once the occlusion is crossed, use braided guide wires as these give more stability. Stiffer wires give added support.
- Angioplasty balloons: We usually use high-pressure balloons to dilated chronically thrombosed veins. Frequently require >20 mmHg pressure to dilate chronic venous stenoses.

Pre-procedure Medications

- Antibiotics are not routinely given.
- Anti-anxiety medications (Ativan, Xanax) can be given pre-procedurally for very anxious patients.

Procedure

Venous Access

- Use ultrasound to guide venous access unless you are very confident in the ease of gaining access based on anatomic landmarks.

- Selection of venous access depends on the anatomic location of the obstruction to be treated:

  ○ For the SVC or IVC, the common femoral vein (CFV) provides ideal access (right if possible)
  ○ Right IJV access works well also and may be preferred for anatomic reasons – i.e., femoral veins occluded
  ○ The iliac veins are accessed from the ipsilateral CFV if it is not severely diseased or the right IJV otherwise.
  ○ The subclavian and innominate veins may be easiest accessed from the ipsilateral upper arm veins (basilic or brachial veins), but CFV access can also be used for these veins.
  ○ Use of both jugular and femoral venous access with "through and through" wire access (achieved by snaring a wire from one vein and out the other) can be a useful technique for advancing catheters and angioplasty balloons through very long or fibrotic venous occlusions/stenoses. This is because control of both ends of a guidewire allows maximum catheter pushability over the taut wire.

Intra-procedural Medications

- Heparin typically 4000 units–5000 units with a target activated clotting time (ACT) of 280–300 sec. If the procedure is prolonged, there may be need for additional doses based on periodic ACT determinations.
- Intravenous titration of midazolam hydrochloride and fentanyl citrate provides sedation and analgesia. Very rarely is more significant sedation or pain management needed.
- Administer narcotic doses (Fentanyl) as needed but especially preceding balloon angioplasty of venous strictures, which may cause significant pain.

Assessing the Narrowing or Occlusion

- Pre-existing studies such as ultrasounds, CT scans, and MRI will give important information with regards to location and severity. These imaging tools will also help to identify contributing factors such as tumors or aneurysms compressing the vein. The final evaluation occurs during the procedure using catheter-based venography and hemodynamics (venous pressure gradients):

  ○ **Morphology and location:** The length and severity can be determined at the time of the catheter-based venogram. It is helpful to use catheters with markers so more precise length and diameter measurements are obtained. The diameter of the chosen stent is based on the diameter of the normal vein adjacent to the lesion. As a reference the common iliac vein (CIV) is usually treated using a 14- or 16-mm diameter stent and the external iliac vein (EIV) by using a 14-mm diameter stent. The CFV is also 14-mm in diameter. For smaller people the diameter is decreased by about 2 mm.

- ■ The SVC and IVC measure about 20–25 mm in adults but can be over 30 mm in normal individuals. In practice, symptomatic SVC or IVC stenoses rarely require stents over 18 mm in diameter.

- ○ **Pressure Measurements:** Use of pressure measurements in the venous system is debated. A consensus has built around a pressure difference (gradient) of 2–3 mmHg as significant in the venous system. The pressure is measured with a angiographic catheter on each side of the obstruction. In practice, instrument inaccuracy, respiratory variation, and transducer positioning produce errors which exceed this 2–3 mmHg threshold and, therefore, the patient's symptoms and degree of stenosis should guide treatment rather than hemodynamics.

Choosing a Balloon or Stent

- • As a general rule, self-expanding stents work best in the venous system. Balloon-expandable stents are poor choices outside of the chest cavity or abdominal cavity.

  - ○ However, in the event that self-expanding stents are insufficient to overcome early elastic recoil in a peripheral vein, "nesting" a balloon-expandable stent within may provide adequate additional radial force for complete expansion.

- • Compression and deformation of balloon expandable stents does not spontaneously reverse as occurs with self-expanding stents. Placing balloon-expandable stents where they can undergo such external force can lead to severe consequences such as restenosis or re-occlusion which may be difficult to treat percutaneously.

Performing the Procedure

- • **Crossing the lesion:** Chronic thrombotic occlusion of the upper or lower extremity veins is frequently difficult to traverse. The combination of a glidewire and a 4 or 5F glide-coated angiographic catheter works best for this. A stiff-angled glidewire works better than a soft or regular glidewire. When the lesion is crossed, a stiff guidewire (braided) is placed, over which stents and balloons more easily travel.
- • **Deploying the balloon/Stent:** Endpoint: Free flow without residual pressure gradient. Collateral filling indicates persistent hemodynamically significant narrowing. Cover the entire if possible (Figs. 1 b, c and 2).

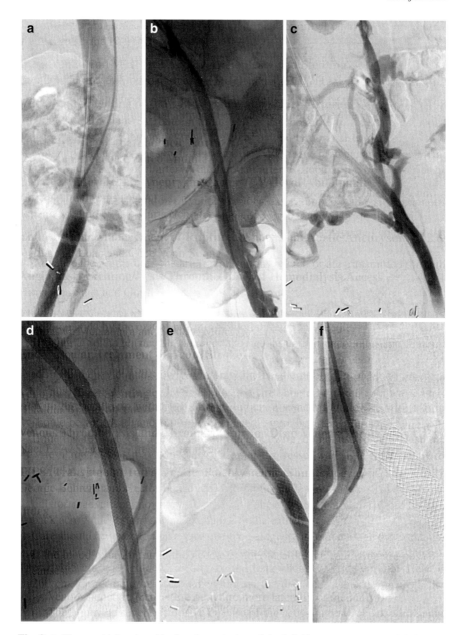

Fig. 2 A 60-year-old female with chronic occlusion of the left iliac venous system. (**a**) Access from the RIJV demonstrates normal right iliac veins and IVC. (**b, c**) A glide catheter has been passed through the chronically thrombosed left iliac venous system. Venograms at two levels reveal chronic thrombotic changes with collaterals. (**d–f**) 14-mm diameter Wallstents (Boston Scientific; Natick, MA) have been placed from the proximal CFV to the IVC ostium. Care is taken not to have the stents over-ride the contralateral CIV. The stents are dilated to their nominated diameter, 14 mm. Not that the collaterals have disappeared. There was no pressure gradient following stent placement compared to 7 mmHg before

- **Immediate post-procedure care:**

  ○ Observe the patient in post anesthesia unit until sedation has worn off (at least 1 h).
  ○ Observe for signs of bleeding or pericardial tamponade in superior vena cava stent cases.

Follow-Up and Post-procedure Medications

- Anticoagulation is usually not required after upper extremity stent placement unless patency is compromised by poor inflow.
- Iliac vein stents benefit from therapeutic anticoagulation for up to 2 months with a target INR of 2–3.5
- Clopidogrel is often given as 75 mg/day for 6 weeks following venous stent placement.
- For iliac vein and inferior vena cava recanalization, consider providing pain medication at discharge

  ○ Non-steroidal anti-inflammatory drugs suffice in most cases.
  ○ The pain wears off in 2–3 days in most cases.

Results

- Iliac vein stenting:

  ○ At 3 years, a study of over 400 limbs demonstrated a primary patency of 75%, primary-assisted patency of 92%, and secondary patency of 93%.

- IVC/SVC stenting:

  ○ Insertion of an SVC stent-relieved malignant SVC syndrome in 95%; 11% of those treated experienced reocclusion but recanalization was possible in the majority resulting in a long-term patency rate of 92%.

Alternative Therapies

- Conservative treatment with compression hosiery and limb elevation (and anticoagulation) is acceptable alternative therapy before more invasive procedures are attempted.
- Medical centers that possess the surgical expertise for venous bypass are few:

  ○ Iliac vein and IVC occlusions rarely undergo surgical bypass.
  ○ Surgical venous bypass is a viable option for SVCS, with a bypass from the innominate veins to the right atrium infrequently performed in the event of failed percutaneous procedures.

- Surgeons often create small arteriovenous fistulae in conjunction with large vein surgical bypasses in order to improve patency in these low flow vessels.

Complications

- Complications of venous angioplasty and stent placement are few:
- Bleeding complications are surprisingly rare. We have encountered procedure-related hemodynamically significant bleeding and venous perforation in the face of recent:
  - External beam radiation therapy
  - Surgery, such as regional lymph node dissection
- There are reported deaths from exsanguination or pericardial tamponade due to iatrogenic rupture of the SVC. Thus, the operator should be prepared to act quickly if patients deteriorate immediately or soon following SVC stent placement.

How to Treat

- Keep in mind that you can diagnose pericardial tamponade quickly with ultrasound and immediate placement of a pericardial drain is usually the treatment. A covered stent or surgery may be required if pericardial hemorrhage is persistent.
- Re-inflate the balloon in the SVC if extravasation occurs to halt active bleeding and prepare to place a covered stent or initiate surgical repair if extravasation persists after 15–30 min of balloon inflation.

How to Avoid

- Be careful in areas of previous radiation treatment or surgical intervention especially if recent dissection or radiation was directed toward the target vein. Consider a covered stent if treatment is absolutely necessary.
- Pericardial tamponade is hard to avoid. The length of the pericardial reflection varies much and can extend to the innominate vein confluence:
  - Be careful not to over dilate. We dilate rarely beyond 14 mm.
  - The primary use of covered stents may be an option.

Key Points

- Good inflow is a key requirement for successful venoplasty and stent placement. If the inflow is impaired, the treated segment will likely occlude (Fig. 2)

- Larger stents do better than smaller ones. Therefore, oversize by 10–20% compared to the normal-sized vessel.
- If the lesion exhibits significant recoil, consider placing stents with added support. Use balloon-expandable stents with their better radial force in deeply guarded locations as in the chest or pelvis.
- Be prepared to quickly respond to hemothorax or hemopericardium when dilating or stenting SVC stenoses, especially if the area has been radiated or surgically manipulated within the last 2–3 months.

Suggested Reading

1. Barshes NR, Annambhotla S, El Sayed HF, et al. Percutaneous stenting of superior vena cava syndrome: Treatment outcome in patients with benign and malignant etiology. Vascular 2007; 15(5): 314–321.
2. Ganesha A, Quen Hon L, Wrakaulle DR, et al. Superior vena caval stenting for SVC obstruction: Current status. Eur J of Radiol 2009; 71(2): 343–349.
3. Mussa FF, Peden EK, Zhou W, et al. Iliac vein stenting for chronic venous insufficiency. Tex Heart Inst J 2007; 34(1): 60–66.
4. Neglen P, Raju S. In-stent recurrent stenosis in stents placed in the lower extremity venous outflow tract. J Vasc Surg 2004; 39(1): 181–188.
5. Neglen P, Thrasher TL, Raju S. Venous outflow obstruction: An underestimated contributor to chronic venous disease. J Vasc Surg 2003; 38(5): 879–885.

Venous Thrombolysis and Thrombectomy for Deep Venous Thrombosis

Nael E. A. Saad and Suresh Vedantham

Clinical Features

- Venous thromboembolism (VTE) has an incidence of nearly 1 million cases per year in the United States alone. VTE encompasses deep vein thrombosis (DVT) and pulmonary embolism (PE) [1].
- Table 1 outlines the major risk factors for developing VTE.
- Although many DVT cases are clinically silent, DVT patients usually experience limb swelling, cramping, and/or pain:

  - With modern DVT care, commonly delivered in outpatient fashion, these presenting DVT symptoms may often be under managed from the affected patient's perspective.

- 85–90% of DVT cases involve lower extremity veins and 10–15% involve upper extremity veins.
- Lower extremity DVT is divided into several categories:

  - Isolated Calf DVT ("distal DVT") is associated with a low risk of causing PE. However, a minority of calf DVT cases will eventually propagate into the popliteal vein if untreated.
  - Proximal DVT, defined as DVT involving the popliteal vein and/or more cephalad deep veins, is associated with relatively high risk of PE.
  - Iliofemoral DVT refers to proximal DVT that involves the iliac vein and/or the common femoral vein. Iliofemoral DVT tends to cause more severe acute symptomatology, and is associated with a significantly higher risk of the Post-Thrombotic Syndrome (PTS) [2].

- Consequences of Venous Thromboembolism:

  - Early complications of acute DVT include

    - PE is the presenting manifestation in approximately one-third of VTE cases and is estimated to cause more than 100,000 deaths per year in the United States alone [1].

R.A. Morgan, E. Walser (eds.), *Handbook of Angioplasty and Stenting Procedures*,
Techniques in Interventional Radiology, DOI 10.1007/978-1-84800-399-6_24,
© Springer-Verlag London Limited 2010

Table 1 Major risk factors for developing DVT

Major risk factors for developing DVT

- Previous DVT or PE
- Orthopedic surgery of the lower extremity
- Major surgical procedure
- Increased patient age
- Malignancy
- Obesity
- Major trauma
- Congestive heart failure, myocardial infarction
- Estrogen therapy
- Immobilization
- Inherited thrombophilia

■ Paradoxical embolization, a rare condition in which a deep venous thrombus passes through an intracardiac shunt to enter the arterial circulation, may cause devastating complications, including stroke.
■ Phlegmasia cerulea dolens, a rare condition in which DVT causes massive swelling of the entire extremity, can lead to arterial insufficiency, compartment syndrome, venous gangrene, and/or limb amputation.

○ Despite use of anticoagulant therapy, complications of acute DVT include

■ Recurrent VTE episodes (5–10% per year for most subgroups) [3]
■ Chronic thromboembolic pulmonary hypertension.
■ Post-Thrombotic Syndrome (PTS) (Table 2)
■ As a result, acute DVT is actually a chronic disease!

Table 2 The post-thrombotic syndrome

The post-thrombotic syndrome

- PTS develops in 25–50% of patients with a first episode of proximal lower-extremity DVT
- PTS causes chronic lifestyle-limiting symptoms such as limb swelling, pain, limb heaviness/fatigue, venous claudication, and stasis dermatitis, and can progress to skin ulceration
- PTS causes significant quality of life (QOL) impairment in DVT patients. The severity of PTS parallels the degree of QOL impairment. The health impairment caused by established PTS is comparable to that of other chronic diseases such as chronic obstructive pulmonary disease
- Because established PTS and venous ulcers are difficult and expensive to treat and often result in work disability, the disease burden of PTS has major economic consequences to society as well
- The most consistent risk factor for PTS has been the development of recurrent ipsilateral DVT. Therefore, pending future studies, adequate anticoagulant therapy should be viewed as a key PTS prevention measure. However, many anticoagulated patients will still develop PTS
- Daily use of 30–40 mmHg, knee-high, elastic compression stockings (ECS) for 2 years after DVT decreases the incidence of PTS by about 50% (to around 25%)

Diagnostic Evaluation

Clinical

- A number of clinical decision tools assist the diagnostic evaluation of DVT. They incorporate:
  - Clinical suspicion level,
  - Results of imaging tests
  - Laboratory findings.

Laboratory

- A negative D-dimer has a high negative predictive value for DVT.

Imaging

- Duplex ultrasound almost always establishes the diagnosis of extremity DVT

  - High (>95%) accuracy for proximal DVT and moderate (70–80%) accuracy for isolated calf DVT.

- In patients with DVT isolated to the iliocaval veins, cross-sectional imaging using CT scan or MR venography may be used. In selected cases, one may resort to diagnostic venography.

Indications for Endovascular DVT Thrombolysis

- A highly individualized approach to selecting DVT patients for thrombolysis is recommended [4, 5].
- Urgent first-line endovascular thrombolysis is performed to treat phlegmasia cerulea dolens or progressive IVC thrombosis (to prevent fatal PE or renal failure from IVC/renal vein thrombosis).
- Non-urgent second-line endovascular thrombolysis is performed for patients with symptomatic proximal DVT who exhibit clinical and/or anatomic progression of DVT on anticoagulant therapy. This may include rapid iliocaval thrombus extension, exacerbation or persistence of major lower extremity symptoms, and/or failure to experience sufficient symptom relief to permit ambulation.
- Non-urgent first-line endovascular thrombolysis may be performed to enable faster symptom relief and/or long-term prevention of PTS in patients with symptomatic, acute extensive proximal DVT. Acute iliofemoral DVT patients are the best candidates for therapy. However, the risk–benefit ratio of this approach is uncertain due to a lack of supporting multicenter randomized controlled trials.

- Rationale for undertaking endovascular thrombolysis for the prevention of PTS:

  - PTS is caused by the development of ambulatory venous hypertension, which is thought to be caused by two main factors after an episode of DVT: Valvular reflux and venous obstruction.
  - Venous thrombosis causes progressive valvular reflux in both involved venous segments (by direct valvular damage due to the inflammation accompanying thrombosis) and in uninvolved segments (by increasing venous pressures below the obstruction). Veins in which rapid endogenous clot lysis is observed tend to develop valvular reflux much less frequently [6].
  - In iliofemoral DVT, complete venous recanalization rarely occurs with anticoagulation alone.
  - Small randomized trials of systemic thrombolysis and surgical thrombectomy have observed reduced rates of reflux, late venous obstruction, and PTS in proximal DVT patients [7–10].

- Table 3 reviews the contraindications and other factors that impact the decision process.

Patient Preparation

- If the patient is on warfarin, ensure that the INR is below 2.0 (preferably 1.5) before starting.
- If the patient has mild-moderate contrast allergy, pre-medicate with steroids and histamine antagonists.
- In selected patients, placement of a retrievable IVC filter prior to starting therapy is reasonable:

  - IVC filter is probably unnecessary when infusion-first catheter-directed thrombolysis (CDT – see below) is used since PE occurs rarely with this method.
  - The need for IVC filter placement prior to single-session pharmacomechanical CDT (PCDT) therapy is unclear and may be indicated, especially in patients with a large thrombus burden.

Anatomical Considerations

- Know the anatomy and proper names of the lower extremity and pelvic veins. The term "superficial femoral vein" is no longer used – the correct term for this important deep vein is "femoral vein".
- Remember that the femoral vein is duplicated in 5–20% of patients

Table 3 Major factors that impact the decision process for thrombectomy/thrombolysis of DVT

Factor	Good candidate	Poor candidate
Life-expectancy	Long	Short
Activity level	Ambulatory before DVT episode	Non-ambulatory, poor performance status before DVT
Bleeding risk profile	Low-risk	High-risk: • Intracranial disease (history of stroke, central nervous system tumor, aneurysm, arteriovenous malformation, or other intracranial lesion) • Very recent surgery or trauma • Ongoing pregnancy or very recent delivery • Recent gastrointestinal bleeding or other internal bleeding • Thrombocytopenia or hepatic dysfunction • Severe hypertension
Anatomical extent of DVT	• IVC Thrombosis • Iliofemoral DVT	• Isolated calf vein DVT, because the rate of PTS may be lower in these patients and the risk–benefit ratio of endovascular therapy is therefore questionable
Symptom duration and severity	• Acute DVT (less than 2 weeks) • Rapidly progressive DVT despite initial anticoagulant therapy • Debilitating symptoms	• Asymptomatic DVT, because they rarely develop PTS • Chronic femoropopliteal DVT – lytic therapy ineffective
Signs of circulatory compromise	• Emergency thrombolysis unless a strong contraindication is present; if so, consider the use of surgical venous thrombectomy	

Percutaneous Options for Acute DVT

Catheter-Directed Pharmacological Thrombolysis ("Infusion-First CDT")

- Mechanism of action:

  ○ Direct intra-thrombus drug delivery increases local concentration
  ○ Drug enhances conversion of plasminogen to plasmin, which cleaves fibrin

- Technique:

  ○ The basic method [12] of initiating CDT involves several steps:
  ○ Perform the procedure with conscious sedation with local anesthesia.
  ○ Access a lower-extremity vein (ideally below the lowest extent of thrombus) under real-time ultrasound guidance – the popliteal vein and posterior tibial vein are two commonly used veins, although other veins are also available. An internal jugular vein can also be used.
  ○ Use a diagnostic catheter to perform venography and define the clot extent.
  ○ A multisidehole catheter bridges the thrombosed venous segment and distributes the infusion of a thrombolytic drug.
  ○ A new infusion catheter (EKOS, Bothell, WA) emits low power ultrasound energy during infusion to loosen fibrin strands and speed lysis [13].

- Drug dosing, monitoring, and adjunctive procedures:

  ○ Urokinase (120,000–180,000 units/h), recombinant tissue plasminogen activator (0.5–1.0 mg/h), reteplase (0.50–0.75 units/h), or tenecteplase (0.25–0.50 mg/h) are used for infusion-CDT [4].
  ○ The drug is infused continuously through the catheter, and concomitant unfractionated heparin is given at subtherapeutic levels (300–600 units/h)
  ○ Hematocrit, PTT, and platelet count evaluated every 6 h. You can monitor the Fibrinogen level, although there is no data establishing its value.
  ○ Patients transfer to an ICU or step-down unit. If active bleeding occurs or if the PTT is subtherapeutic, discontinue the infusion.
  ○ Re-assess lytic progress venographically at 8- to 16-h intervals.
  ○ If only partial thrombolysis occurs, an angioplasty balloon can be used to macerate the softened residual thrombus to increase its surface area and speed the thrombolytic process. Thrombolytic infusion is then continued.
  ○ After thrombolysis is completed, repeat venography and venoplasty any visualized stenoses or consider venous stent placement. Repeat venography confirms patency of the venous system.
  ○ Full-dose anticoagulant therapy is re-started and patients' transition to long-term oral vitamin K-antagonist therapy (warfarin) and are asked to wear 30–40 mmHg graduated compression stockings for PTS prevention [14].

- Results:

  ○ 80–90% of patients with acute DVT (symptom duration <2 weeks) achieve significant clot lysis and marked relief of symptoms [11].
  ○ Three comparative studies suggest that successful CDT results in prevention of valvular reflux, late venous obstruction, and PTS. However, none of these studies were multicenter randomized controlled trials [15–17].
  ○ In a large multicenter venous registry, infusion CDT was associated with major bleeding in 11% of patients, and with intracranial bleeding in 0.4% [11]. Successful thrombolysis required an average of 48 h infusion with 1–3 days ICU monitoring.

Stand-Alone Percutaneous Mechanical Thrombectomy(PMT)

- Mechanism of action:

  ○ "Aspirating" devices aspirate and remove thrombus from the venous lumen
  ○ "Non-Aspirating" devices macerate thrombus into tiny fragments, which are spontaneously lysed by the body

- Advantage:

  ○ Can perform in patients with contraindications to the use of fibrinolytic drugs

- Disadvantages:

  ○ Increased on-table procedure time
  ○ Potential for displacing thrombus with mechanical manipulation:

    ■ Increased risk for PE, paradoxical embolus

  ○ Theoretical potential for causing venous valve injury

- Technique:

  ○ Varies among available devices. The AngioJet (Possis Medical, Minneapolis, MN) is an FDA-approved device for removal of iliac and femoral vein thrombus. It features a mainframe unit attached to a 5–6 French rheolytic catheter. The catheter advances to-and-fro over a guidewire within the clot while depressing a foot pedal. If it is necessary to direct the device to various positions within a clotted vein, a guiding catheter may be used.

- Results:

  ○ In general, the available aspirating-type devices do not remove sufficient thrombus to be therapeutically useful in DVT.
  ○ The non-aspirating devices (without placement of an inferior vena cava (IVC) filter) can result in symptomatic PE.

- For these reasons, the use of stand-alone PMT is generally restricted to patients with clinically severe DVT in whom fibrinolytic drugs are contraindicated:

  - Consider the use of retrievable IVC filters when treatment is undertaken under these circumstances.

Pharmacomechanical Catheter-Directed Thrombolysis (PCDT)

- Mechanism of action:

  - Combine both mechanisms of action for CDT and PMT
  - All available devices macerate thrombus and thereby increase the surface area of residual thrombus and improve thrombolytic drug dispersion within the thrombus

- Advantages:

  - Accelerates thrombolysis, reducing drug dose and infusion time by 40–50%
  - Reduces ICU utilization, which may reduce hospital costs
  - Newer techniques may enable complete DVT treatment in a single procedure session, which eliminates the need for prolonged drug infusions or ICU monitoring

- Disadvantages:

  - Thrombolytic drugs contraindicated in patients with a high-risk bleeding profile.
  - The disadvantages of PMT are also present with PCDT

- Technique:

  - Older "first-generation" PCDT techniques involve a sequential use of infusion CDT with PMT:

    - For example, after a short (6–18 h) CDT infusion, PMT can be used to clean up residual thrombus, shorten treatment time, and reduce drug dose.
    - Or, initiate therapy with PMT to debulk the thrombus, followed by infusion CDT to clean up.

  - With "Powerpulse PCDT", the Angiojet [18] is used to forcefully pulse-spray a bolus dose of thrombolytic drug into the thrombus. The drug dwells in the clot for 20–30 min, then the Angiojet is used to aspirate the residual softened thrombus.
  - With "Isolated Thrombolysis", the Trellis Peripheral Infusion System (Bacchus Vascular, Santa Clara, CA) is used [19]. This device features two catheter-mounted balloons that "isolate" a segment of vein for treatment after the balloons are inflated.

- ■ With the balloons inflated, a bolus dose of a thrombolytic drug is injected directly into the thrombus. Activation of an oscillating wire for 10 min is then used to disperse the drug within the thrombus, then the drug is aspirated through a port on the device.

- Results:
  - ○ Retrospective comparisons show that first-generation PCDT provides at least equal clot removal efficacy as infusion CDT, but reduces drug dose and infusion time.
  - ○ Very limited observational data on the single-session PCDT methods suggest that they allow therapy completion in a single procedure over 50% of the time.
  - ○ There are no published prospective studies demonstrating long-term results of any PCDT technique in terms of PTS prevention or venous valvular function.

Conclusion

- Endovascular DVT thrombolysis offers the potential to provide faster relief of presenting DVT symptoms and to prevent PTS and its associated major disability.
- To confirm that existing percutaneous methods of treating acute DVT indeed produce favorable outcomes, we urgently need supporting randomized clinical trials. Until they are completed, a highly individualized approach to patient selection optimizes clinical benefit.

Key Points

- Urgent thrombolysis is required to treat phlegmasia cerula dolens or progressive IVC thrombosis.
- Thrombolysis may also be useful to prevent post thrombotic syndrome, which occurs in 25–50% of patients after first DVT.
- Can use thrombolysis alone, mechanical devices alone, or a combination.
- Optional filter placement may be necessary for pharmacomechanical therapy.

Suggested Reading

1. Heit JA, Cohen AT, Anderson FA, for the VTE Impact Assessment Group. Estimated annual number of incident and recurrent, non-fatal and fatal venous thromboembolism (VTE) events in the USA (abstract). Blood 2005; 106:267a.

2. Kahn SR, Shrier I, Julian JA, et al. Determinants and time course of the postthrombotic syndrome after acute deep venous thrombosis. Ann Intern Med 2008; 149:698–707.

3. Kearon C, Kahn SR, Agnelli G, Goldhaber SZ, Raskob GE, Comerota AJ. Antithrombotic therapy for venous thromboembolic disease. American College of Chest Physicians Evidence-Based Clinical Practice Guidelines (8th Ed). Chest 2008; 133:454S–545S.

4. Vedantham S, Thorpe PE, Cardella JF, et al for the CIRSE and SIR Standards of Practice Committees. Quality improvement guidelines for the treatment of lower extremity deep vein thrombosis with use of endovascular thrombus removal. J Vasc Interv Radiol 2006; 17: 435–448.

5. Vedantham S. Interventions for deep vein thrombosis: re-emergence of a promising therapy. Am J Med 2008; 121:S28–S39.

6. Meissner MH, Manzo RA, Bergelin RO, Markel A, Strandness DE. Deep venous insufficiency: the relationship between lysis and subsequent reflux. J Vasc Surg 1993; 18:596–608.

7. Plate G, Akesson H, Einarsson E, Ohlin P, Eklor B. Long-term results of venous thrombectomy combined with a temporary arterio-venous fistula. Eur J Vasc Surg 1990; 4:483–489.

8. Elliot MS, Immelman EJ, Jeffery P, Benatar SR, Funston MR, Smith JA, Shepstone BJ, Ferguson D, Jacobs P, Walker W, Louw JH. A comparative randomized trial of heparin versus streptokinase in the treatment of acute proximal venous thrombosis: an interim report of a prospective trial. Br J Surg 1979; 66:838–843.

9. Arnesen H, Hoiseth A, Ly B. Streptokinase or heparin in the treatment of deep vein thrombosis. Acta Med Scand 1982; 211:65–68.

10. Turpie AGG, Levine MN, Hirsh J, Ginsberg JS, Cruickshank M, Jay R, Gent M. Tissue plasminogen activator (rt-PA) vs. heparin in deep vein thrombosis: results of a randomized trial. Chest Suppl 1990; 97(4):172S–175S.

11. Mewissen WM, Seabrook GR, Meissner MH, et al. Catheter-directed thrombolysis for lower extremity deep vein thrombosis: report of a national multicenter registry. Radiology 1999; 211:39–49.

12. Semba CP, Dake MD. Iliofemoral deep venous thrombosis: aggressive therapy with catheter-directed thrombolysis. Radiology 1994; 191:487–494.

13. Parikh SR, Motarjeme A, McNamara TO, et al. Ultrasound-accelerated thrombolysis for the treatment of deep vein thrombosis: initial clinical experience. J Vasc Interv Radiol 2008; 19(4):521–528.

14. Prandoni P, Lensing AW, Prins MH, et al. Below-knee elastic compression stockings to prevent the post-thrombotic syndrome. Ann Intern Med 2004; 141:249–256.

15. Comerota AJ, Throm RC, Mathias SD, et al. Catheter-directed thrombolysis for iliofemoral deep vein thrombosis improves health-related quality of life. J Vasc Surg; 32:130–137.

16. AbuRahma AF, Perkins SE, Wulu JT, et al. Iliofemoral deep vein thrombosis: conventional therapy versus lysis and percutaneous transluminal angioplasty and stenting. Ann Surg 2001; 233:752–760.

17. Elsharawy M, Elzayat E. Early results of thrombolysis vs anticoagulation in iliofemoral venous thrombosis. Eur J Vasc Endovasc Surg 2002; 24:209–214.

18. Cynamon J, Stein EG, Dym J, et al. A new method for aggressive management of DVT: retrospective study of the power pulse technique. J Vasc Interv Radiol 2006; 17:1043–1049.

19. O'Sullivan GJ, Lohan DG, Gough N, et al. Pharmacomechanical thrombectomy of acute deep vein thrombosis with the Trellis-8 isolated thrombolysis catheter. J Vasc Interv Radiol 2007, 18:715–724.

20. Kim HS, Patra A, Paxton BE, et al. Adjunctive percutaneous mechanical thrombectomy for lower-extremity deep vein thrombosis: clinical and economic outcomes. J Vasc Interv Radiol 2006; 17:1099–1104.

TIPS (Transjugular Intrahepatic Portosystemic Shunts)

George Behrens and Hector Ferral

General Concept and Definition

- The Transjugular Intrahepatic Portosystemic Shunt (TIPS) is a non-selective portosystemic shunt that is created using percutaneous endovascular techniques.
- The procedure consists of creating a transhepatic communication between one of the hepatic veins and a portal vein branch by using a needle system.
- The transhepatic tract is kept open with the use of metallic stents.
- The purpose of creating a TIPS is to decompress a hypertensive portal system.
- The TIPS procedure should be performed in state-of-the-art angiography suites with digital subtraction capabilities.
- The procedure can be completed with the use of conscious sedation, avoiding the risks of general anesthesia, although some operators prefer the use of general anesthesia to avoid patient discomfort.
- The procedure is usually well tolerated. If performed electively, the patient is hospitalized a mean of 1–3 days.
- Close follow-up is recommended for clinical assessment as well as assessment of shunt patency.

Pre-procedure Evaluation

Clinical Evaluation

- Careful patient evaluation before TIPS is critical:

  - Focused clinical history and physical exam.
  - Physical exam should include evaluation of degree of encephalopathy, ascites, and hemodynamic status.
  - The indication for TIPS should be clearly established.

- Etiology of liver disease needs to be documented, ideally with biopsy results.

R.A. Morgan, E. Walser (eds.), *Handbook of Angioplasty and Stenting Procedures*,
Techniques in Interventional Radiology, DOI 10.1007/978-1-84800-399-6_25,
© Springer-Verlag London Limited 2010

Imaging and Endoscopy

- Evaluation of imaging studies:

  ○ Three-phase CT scan of the liver
  ○ Doppler ultrasound

- Evaluation of endoscopic studies. In case of bleeding: Confirm presence and localization of varices (esophageal versus gastric varices or hypertensive gastropathy)

Laboratory

- Liver function tests
- Kidney function
- Coagulation status
- Hemoglobin and hematocrit

Prognostic Models

- Useful to predict patient outcomes
- Elective TIPS: Child-Pugh score and MELD score
- Emergency TIPS: Prognostic Index and APACHE II score

Child-Pugh Score

- Designed to predict mortality of patients with chronic liver disease during surgery.
- Based on five variables: Serum bilirubin level, serum albumin, INR, clinical evaluation of encephalopathy, and clinical evaluation of ascites.
- Score range: 5–15 points (Table 1)
- Employed by interventionalist to assess the prognosis of cirrhotic patient for elective TIPS procedure.

Table 1 Child-Pugh classification for liver disease

Child class	Points	Perioperative mortality
A	5–6 points	0–10%
B	7–9 points	15–30%
C	10–15 points	30–50%

Meld Score

- Pronostic model created as predictor of 3-month mortality in patients undergoing elective TIPS procedures
- Based on three variables: Serum creatinine, serum bilirubin, and INR.
- Formula: MELD Score $= 10\{0.957 \times Ln \text{ (serum creatinine)} + 0.378 \times Ln \text{ (total bilirubin)} + 1.12 \times Ln \text{ (INR)} + 0.643\}$
- Web calculator: www.thedrugmonitor.com/meld.html
- Prognosis according to MELD score:

    ○ MELD < 17: 3 month mortality: 16%
    ○ MELD > 18: 3 month mortality: 35%
    ○ MELD > 24: 3 month mortality: 65%
                        30-day mortality: 50%

APACHE II

- Designed to measure the severity of disease for adult patients admitted to intensive care units.
- Used basically in emergency settings (non-elective cases).
- The score is calculated from 12 variables, routine physiological measurements (such as blood pressure, body temperature, heart rate) during the first 24 h after admission. However, interventionalist measures the variables before the shunt creation.
- Weakness of the score is related to subjective variables such as encephalopathy (mild, moderate, severe), ascites (medically treated versus not treated), and lack of definition of etiology of liver disease.
- An APACHE II Score <18 is associated with an improved survival rate after emergency TIPS (70–80%).
- APACHE II Score >18 combined with a Child-Pugh Class C is associated with 98–100% 30-day mortality rate:

    ○ The most common cause of early death is multiorgan failure.

Prognostic Index

- Is the only model specifically designed for patients undergoing emergency TIPS
- Five factors were associated with a poor prognosis: ascites (moderate or severe), need for ventilation, white blood cell count, creatinine, and aPTT (activated partial thromboplastin time)
- Formula: PI = 1.54 (ascites) + 1.27 (ventilation) + 1.38 log e (white blood cell count) + 2.48 log e (aPTT) + 1.55 log e (creatinine) – 1.05 log e (platelet count)
- A PI greater than 18.52 is associated with a 6-week mortality of 100%

Indications for Tips

- Recurrent variceal bleeding not controlled by endoscopic or medical therapy
- Acute Variceal Bleeding refractory to endoscopic and medical therapy
- Refractory ascites
- Refractory hepatic hydrothorax
- Budd–Chiari syndrome
- Hepato-renal syndrome
- Hepato-pulmonary syndrome

Contraindications

- **Absolute**

  - Right heart failure
  - Elevated central venous pressures and severe pulmonary hypertension
  - Polycystic liver disease
  - Uncontrolled sepsis or systemic infection
  - Biliary obstruction
  - Severe liver failure

- **Relative**

  - Severe encephalopathy
  - Severe coagulopathy
  - Portal vein thrombosis
  - Liver tumors

Procedure Preparation

- **General**

  - Obtain informed consent
  - Decide if the procedure should be performed under conscious sedation or general anesthesia
  - Complete patient resuscitation
  - Correction of coagulopathy
  - Standard monitoring: ECG, O_2 saturation, and blood pressure
  - Intravenous antibiotic prophylaxis should be provided. (1 h before the procedure)

    - Cephalosporins
    - Vancomycin 1gr. IV

Material Selection

Materials

- TIPS access set which is selected based on operator experience:
  - Colapinto transjugular and biopsy set (Cook, Bloomington, IN)
  - Ring TIPS set (Cook, Bloomington, IN)
  - Haskal TIPS Access Set (Cook, Bloomington, IN)
  - Rosch-Uchida (Cook, Bloomington, IN)
  - Angiodynamics TIPS set (Angiodynamics, Queensbury, NY)
- Guidewires:
  - Bentson wire
  - Amplatz super-stiff
  - Angled stiff glidewire (Terumo Medical Corporation, Somerset, NJ)
- CO_2 delivery system (Angiodynamics, Queensbury, NY)
- A 5-French multipurpose catheter
- A 5-French straight marker catheter
- A 6–10-mm angioplasty balloons
- Metallic stents
- Metallic coils
- Pressure transducer for recording portal and central venous pressures

Stents

- Stent-graft:
  - Viatorr (W. L. Gore & Associates, Inc., Newark, DE). FDA approved for TIPS application
- Non-covered stents:
  - Wallstent (Boston Scientific Medi-Tech, Natick, MA) FDA approved for TIPS application
  - Memotherm (C.R. Bard, Inc., Covington, GA)
  - Intrastent (IntraTherapeutics, St. Paul, MN)
  - SMART Stent (Cordis Corp.)
  - Zilver stent (Cook Inc, Bloomington, IN)

Procedure

General considerations:

- Technical success: 95–100%
- Procedural time: 2 (1–3) h

- Early Mortality: 3–15%
- Procedural Mortality: 1–4%

Steps:

- The right internal jugular vein is the preferred access.
- Left internal jugular vein and external jugular vessels may also be used.
- Isolated reported cases of femoral, transhepatic, and transcaval approaches.
- 10F × 40-cm vascular sheath is then advanced into the right atrium
- Multipurpose catheter is used to catheterize the hepatic veins and hepatic venogram is performed.
- Wedge hepatic vein, free hepatic vein, inferior vena cava, and right atrial pressures should be obtained
- The right hepatic vein is again catheterized and wedged into the hepatic parenchyma in order to perform CO_2 portogram. An occlusion balloon can be used:

    - The use of CO_2 delivery system is recommended.
    - Gentle injection of 30–40 cc of CO_2 is recommended.
    - Hand injection is the simplest method for delivery.
    - Approximately 50 mL can be injected manually at one time injected in 1–2 sec.
    - Enables excellent visualization of the intra- and extrahepatic portal veins.

- The catheter system is then exchanged for the trocar of the corresponding TIPS access set.
- The transhepatic puncture system is advanced.
- Transhepatic puncture is performed. The needle is withdrawn and the catheter system is carefully withdrawn while gentle aspiration is performed until venous blood is obtained. Then, small amount of contrast is injected.
- If entry into the portal system is confirmed, a guidewire is carefully advanced into the portal system.
- A catheter is then advanced into the portal vein and a direct portogram is performed.
- The portal vein pressure is measured.
- A guidewire is advanced and next, tract dilation is performed using 8–10 mm angioplasty balloons
- A 5-French marking catheter is advanced and contrast injection is performed.
- The length of the tract is measured to calculate the size of the stent.
- Stent selection is then conducted. In general 8–12-mm diameter metal self-expanding stents are used.
- The most commonly used stent is the 10-mm diameter stent.
- Once the stent has been deployed, stent dilation is performed using 8–10 mm angioplasty balloons.

- Portogram and pressure measurement is again performed. If portogram shows a patent stent and the portosystemic gradient has been reduced to the target level (usually less than 12 mmHg), the procedure is complete
- Variceal or gastro-splenic shunt embolization is optional but recommended in patients with continued variceal opacification, despite adequate portal decompression:

    ○ Primarily to prevent rebleeding
    ○ Also may decrease competitive shunting and prolong TIPS patency

Post-procedure Management

- Hemodynamic changes after TIPS are expected. The patient may experience an increase in the central venous pressure:

    ○ Diuretic administration after TIPS is recommended (40 mg of Furosemide intravenously)

- The risk of encephalopathy ranges between 5 and 35%; it is usually well managed with medications:

    ○ Lactulose, e.g., 30 mL q day
    ○ Rifaximin (Xifaxan, Salix Pharmaceuticals, Inc, Morrisville, NC) PO, 400 mg q 8 h

- Prophylactic antibiotics are recommended (however, a benefit has not been documented by prospective, randomized trials)
- Doppler ultrasound should be performed 10–14 days after shunt creation if the tract was created with a covered stent:

    ○ Covered stents contain air initially and block ultrasound transmission – mimicking findings for shunt occlusion.
    ○ The Doppler study may be performed immediately after the TIPS if a bare stent has been employed.
    ○ Serve as a baseline for follow-up and to detect early complications.

Complications

- **Fatal complications :** Fatal complications during TIPS are rare and include

    ○ Hepatic arterial injury
    ○ Capsular perforation
    ○ Access into the bare segment of the portal vein or main portal vein

        ■ Peritoneal hemorrhage may result

    ○ Right atrial perforation caused by a misplaced stent

- **Procedural complications**

    - Biliary duct injury
    - Hemobilia
    - Intraparenchymal hematoma
    - Stent migration

        - Right atrium
        - Pulmonary artery

- **Shunt-related complications**

    - Hemodynamic changes causing right heart failure
    - Liver failure
    - Encephalopathy

- **Late complications**

    - TIPS to biliary fistula leading to shunt occlusion or sepsis
    - Shunt occlusion
    - Shunt infections
    - Liver failure

Results

- Comparison of TIPS to endoscopic treatment for esophageal variceal bleeding:

    - TIPS does not increase the survival rate in cirrhotic patients (57 versus 56%) but significantly reduces the incidence of variceal rebleeding 18% versus 66% ($P < 0.001$) without increasing the rate of encephalopathy (47 versus 44%).

- Recurrent bleeding is usually associated with recurrent portal hypertension due to shunt stenosis or thrombosis:

    - This finding has dramatically decreased after the use of stent grafts
    - Can be corrected in 95% with the use of angioplasty, bare stent, or a stent-graft

- Comparison of TIPS to surgical treatment:

    - A prospective randomized controlled clinical trial at five centers comparing distal splenorenal shunt versus TIPS in Child-Pugh class A and B cirrhosis and refractory variceal bleeding showed no significant difference in rebleeding rates (DSRS, 5.5%; TIPS, 10.5%; $P = .29$)
    - No difference on first encephalopathy event (DSRS, 50%; TIPS, 50%).
    - Survival rates at 2 and 5 years (DSRS, 81 and 62%; TIPS, 88 and 61%, respectively) ($P = .87$).
    - TIPS patients had a significantly higher shunt thrombosis, stenosis, and reintervention rates (DSRS, 11%; TIPS, 82%) ($P < 0.001$)
    - No differences were seen in rates of ascites, need for transplant, or quality of life.

- Randomized clinical trials comparing TIPS and paracentesis with or without volume expanders for cirrhotic patients with refractory ascites demonstrated:

  - No significant difference in mortality at 30 days
  - TIPS significantly reduced the re-accumulation of ascites at 3-months ($P < 0.01$) and 12 months ($P < 0.01$).

Key Points

- TIPS is a validated therapeutic alternative for the management of patients with complications related to portal hypertension.
- Careful patient evaluation before the procedure is critical. A valid indication for the creation of TIPS should always be established before embarking on this complex procedure.
- Ideally, the decision to proceed with a TIPS should be a multidisciplinary decision, involving a gastroenterologist or hepatologist, a transplant surgeon, and an interventional radiologist.
- Prognostic models help the interventional radiologist establish an anticipated outcome to both referring physician and patient's family members.
- Use a covered stent for longer patency (Viatorr).
- Target for pressure gradient is less than 12 mmHg.
- Most prospective randomized trials have documented that TIPS is effective in controlling variceal bleeding and reaccumulation of ascites; however, a benefit on patient survival has not been established.

Suggested Reading

1. Boyer TD, Haskal ZJ. American Association for the Study of Liver Diseases Practice Guidelines: The role of Transjugular Intrahepatic Portosystemic Shunt Creation in the Management of Portal Hypertension. J Vasc Intervent Radiol 2005; 16: 615–629.
2. Ferral H, Gamboa P, Postoak DW, Albernaz VS, Young CR, Speeg KV, McMahan CA. Survival after elective transjugular intrahepatic portosystemic shunt creation: prediction with model for end-stage liver disease score. Radiology 2004; 231: 231–236.
3. Pomier-Layrargues G, Villeneuve J-P, Deschênes M, Bui B, Perreault P, Fenyves D, Willems B, Marleau D, Bilodeau M, Lafortune M, Dufresne M-P. Transjugular intrahepatic portosystemic shunt (TIPS) versus endoscopic variceal ligation in the prevention of variceal rebleeding in patients with cirrhosis: a randomised trial Gut 2001; 48: 390–396.
4. Henderson JM, Boyer TD, Kutner MH, Galloway JR, Rikkers LF, Jeffers LJ, Abu-Elmagd K, Connor J. DIVERT Study Group. Distal splenorenal shunt versus transjugular intrahepatic portal systematic shunt for variceal bleeding: a randomized trial. Gastroenterology 2006; 130: 1643–1651.

5. Khan S, Tudur Smith C, Williamson P, Sutton R. Portosystemic shunts versus endoscopic therapy for variceal rebleeding in patients with cirrhosis. Cochrane Database Syst Rev 2006; 18(4):CD000553.
6. Saab S, Nieto JM, Lewis SK, Runyon BA. TIPS versus paracentesis for cirrhotic patients with refractory ascites. Cochrane Database Syst Rev 2006; 18(4).

Index

Note: Locators followed by 'f' and 't' refer to figures and tables respectively.